Multiple Sclerosis: Diagnosis and Treatment II

Multiple Sclerosis: Diagnosis and Treatment II

Editor

Víctor M. Rivera

MDPI • Basel • Beijing • Wuhan • Barcelona • Belgrade • Manchester • Tokyo • Cluj • Tianjin

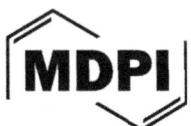

Editor
Víctor M. Rivera
Department of Neurology,
Baylor College of Medicine
USA

Editorial Office
MDPI
St. Alban-Anlage 66
4052 Basel, Switzerland

This is a reprint of articles from the Special Issue published online in the open access journal *Biomedicines* (ISSN 2227-9059) (available at: https://www.mdpi.com/journal/biomedicines/special_issues/multiple_sclerosis_2).

For citation purposes, cite each article independently as indicated on the article page online and as indicated below:

LastName, A.A.; LastName, B.B.; LastName, C.C. Article Title. *Journal Name* **Year**, *Volume Number*, Page Range.

ISBN 978-3-0365-2916-5 (Hbk)
ISBN 978-3-0365-2917-2 (PDF)

© 2021 by the authors. Articles in this book are Open Access and distributed under the Creative Commons Attribution (CC BY) license, which allows users to download, copy and build upon published articles, as long as the author and publisher are properly credited, which ensures maximum dissemination and a wider impact of our publications.

The book as a whole is distributed by MDPI under the terms and conditions of the Creative Commons license CC BY-NC-ND.

Contents

About the Editor vii

Victor M. Rivera
Editorial of Special Issue "Multiple Sclerosis: Diagnosis and Treatment II"
Reprinted from: *Biomedicines* **2021**, *9*, 1605, doi:10.3390/biomedicines9111605 1

Valentina Gatta, Guadalupe Mengod, Marcella Reale and Ada Maria Tata
Possible Correlation between Cholinergic System Alterations and Neuro/Inflammation in Multiple Sclerosis
Reprinted from: *Biomedicines* **2020**, *8*, 153, doi:10.3390/biomedicines8060153 7

Domenico De Rasmo, Anna Ferretta, Silvia Russo, Maddalena Ruggieri, Piergiorgio Lasorella, Damiano Paolicelli, Maria Trojano and Anna Signorile
PBMC of Multiple Sclerosis Patients Show Deregulation of OPA1 Processing Associated with Increased ROS and PHB2 Protein Levels
Reprinted from: *Biomedicines* **2020**, *8*, 85, doi:10.3390/biomedicines8040085 23

Vicki Mercado, Deepa Dongarwar, Kristen Fisher, Hamisu M. Salihu, George J. Hutton and Fernando X. Cuascut
Multiple Sclerosis in a Multi-Ethnic Population in Houston, Texas: A Retrospective Analysis
Reprinted from: *Biomedicines* **2020**, *8*, 534, doi:10.3390/biomedicines8120534 35

Simon Thebault, Ronald A. Booth and Mark S. Freedman
Blood Neurofilament Light Chain: The Neurologist's Troponin?
Reprinted from: *Biomedicines* **2020**, *8*, 523, doi:10.3390/biomedicines8110523 47

Mariano Marrodan, María I. Gaitán and Jorge Correale
Spinal Cord Involvement in MS and Other Demyelinating Diseases
Reprinted from: *Biomedicines* **2020**, *8*, 130, doi:10.3390/biomedicines8050130 59

Stanley Cohan, Elisabeth Lucassen, Kyle Smoot, Justine Brink and Chiayi Chen
Sphingosine-1-Phosphate: Its Pharmacological Regulation and the Treatment of Multiple Sclerosis: A Review Article
Reprinted from: *Biomedicines* **2020**, *8*, 227, doi:10.3390/biomedicines8070227 85

André Huss, Makbule Senel, Ahmed Abdelhak, Benjamin Mayer, Jan Kassubek, Albert C. Ludolph, Markus Otto and Hayrettin Tumani
Longitudinal Serum Neurofilament Levels of Multiple Sclerosis Patients Before and After Treatment with First-Line Immunomodulatory Therapies
Reprinted from: *Biomedicines* **2020**, *8*, 312, doi:10.3390/biomedicines8090312 109

Leire Iparraguirre, Danel Olaverri, Telmo Blasco, Lucía Sepúlveda, Tamara Castillo-Triviño, Mercedes Espiño, Lucienne Costa-Frossard, Álvaro Prada, Luisa María Villar, David Otaegui and Maider Muñoz-Culla
Whole-Transcriptome Analysis in Peripheral Blood Mononuclear Cells from Patients with Lipid-Specific Oligoclonal IgM Band Characterization Reveals Two Circular RNAs and Two Linear RNAs as Biomarkers of Highly Active Disease
Reprinted from: *Biomedicines* **2020**, *8*, 540, doi:10.3390/biomedicines8120540 121

Kristen S. Fisher, Fernando X. Cuascut, Victor M. Rivera and George J. Hutton
Current Advances in Pediatric Onset Multiple Sclerosis
Reprinted from: *Biomedicines* **2020**, *8*, 71, doi:10.3390/biomedicines8040071 137

About the Editor

Víctor M. Rivera is a Distinguished Emeritus Professor at Baylor College of Medicine in Houston, Texas, US, and Honorary Neurologist at Houston Methodist Hospital. Prof. Rivera is the founder and inaugural director of the Maxine Mesinger MS Comprehensive Care Center in Houston. He has trained and mentored numerous international MS and neuroimmunology specialists. He serves as an advisor on MS issues, including socioeconomic aspects affecting Latin American populations and access to care, and contributed to planning initiatives to support people with MS in the United Arab Emirates, for the Abu Dhabi Crown Prince Court. Prof. Rivera received the Life Achievement Awards from the National MS Society (US) and the Consortium of MS Centers

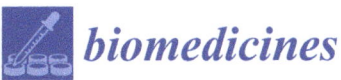

Editorial

Editorial of Special Issue "Multiple Sclerosis: Diagnosis and Treatment II"

Victor M. Rivera

Department of Neurology, Baylor College of Medicine, One Baylor Plaza, Houston, TX 77030, USA; vrivera@bcm.edu; Tel.: +1-832-407-0668

Abstract: The special issue on Multiple Sclerosis: Diagnosis and Treatment II, reflects advances and discoveries in the molecular and cellular mechanisms of disease, and novel laboratory techniques providing more sensitivity to diagnostic techinques and the understanding of neuroinflammation. Mitochondrial-mediated apoptosis in isolated peripheral blood mononuclear cells and the role of reactive oxygen species are studied as indicators of activity of MS. In these cells, downregulation of circular and linera RNAs are reported as markers of highly active disease in MS. Progress and importance of Neurofilaments determinations in early diagnosis and as a marker of disease activity, and the analysis of the complex mechanisms and therapeutic potential of Sphingosine-1-phosphate receptor modulator are discussed. Epidemiologic observations from a highly diversified area of the world provide more insights into this important aspect of MS; discussions on the clinical challenges posed by spinal cord involvement in demyelinatind disorders and the latest aspects of pediatric onset MS, complement this fine collection of scientific papers.

Keywords: multiple sclerosis; acetylcholine; PBMCs; minority populations; spinal cord; sphingosine-1-phosphate modulators; neurofilaments light chain; biomarkers; microRNAs; child neurology

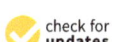

Citation: Rivera, V.M. Editorial of Special Issue "Multiple Sclerosis: Diagnosis and Treatment II". *Biomedicines* **2021**, *9*, 1605. https://doi.org/10.3390/biomedicines9111605

Received: 29 October 2021
Accepted: 30 October 2021
Published: 3 November 2021

Publisher's Note: MDPI stays neutral with regard to jurisdictional claims in published maps and institutional affiliations.

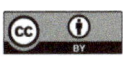

Copyright: © 2021 by the author. Licensee MDPI, Basel, Switzerland. This article is an open access article distributed under the terms and conditions of the Creative Commons Attribution (CC BY) license (https://creativecommons.org/licenses/by/4.0/).

Evolution in the knowledge of previously obscure molecular mechanisms underlying clinical manifestations of multiple sclerosis (MS) has been truly remarkable and has added to the progress of diverse branches of neurosciences. Understanding new molecular (beyond some of the known immunologic mechanisms) and biochemical aspects contributing to the intimate mechanism of the disease, while definitely adding to the complexity of MS, concomitantly provides the potential to translate alterations of these paths into therapeutic interventions for this multifaceted neurological disorder.

Epidemiologically, MS is the most common inflammatory, demyelinating, and degenerative disease of the central nervous system (CNS). In the US, Canada, the British Isles, Scandinavia, Northern Europe, and other areas of the world where MS has a considerable prevalence, this condition constitutes the most common cause of neurological disability in young adults after head injury. In addition, current data indicate the presence of MS in practically every ethnic group in the world.

Etiologically, MS represents a multifactorial complex whereby numerous environmental elements with epigenetic effects contribute to triggering the disease in a genetically susceptible individual.

Mechanistically, MS is an autoimmune disease, with its typical erroneous immune cascade initiating by activation of peripheral T-cell lymphocytes by antigen-presenting cells. Under influences from B-cell lymphocytes and other molecular stimulations, cell division increases, and the permeability of the blood–brain barrier is favored by the release of pro-inflammatory cytokines by T-cells. This setting facilitates the trafficking of immune cells into the CNS with the consequent attack of myelin and eventually axonal injury. A gamut of clinical neurological manifestations will result from damage to these CNS structures.

Many of the molecular mechanisms involved in this process are unknown. Acetylcholine (Ach) participates in the modulation of central and peripheral inflammation irrespective of the causation, ergo in neuroinflammation in MS. T and B cells, macrophages, dendritic cells, microglia, astrocytes, and oligodendrocytes all play a consequential role in the immunology involved in the disease, and all express cholinergic markers and receptors of muscarinic and nicotinic type. The Ach hydrolyzing enzymes acetylcholinesterase and butyrylcholinesterase are reportedly reduced in MS while (not necessarily in a homeostatic response) pro-inflammatory cytokines (IL-6, Tumor Necrosis Factor, and interferon-gamma among others) are released in excess by activated T-cells. Genetic influences are shown by the influence of polymorphisms in the enzymatic activity, and the expression of cholinergic markers in serum and cerebrospinal fluid (CSF) during clinical exacerbation in patients with relapsing disease, and in the chronic phases of the animal model with experimental autoimmune encephalomyelitis (EAE), demonstrate the possible correlation between cholinergic system alterations and neuroinflammation in MS [1].

Since MS pathophysiology largely depends on cellular behavior, the proliferation and increased division of activated lymphocytes are confounded when mitochondria-mediated apoptosis is impaired. Several mechanisms and proteins—including optic atrophy 1 (OPA1) protein, PHB2 protein, and increased reactive oxygen species (ROS)—regulate mitochondrial dynamics and release pro-apoptotic factors. These phenomena were studied utilizing sophisticated techniques in isolated peripheral blood mononuclear cells (PBMCs), demonstrating deregulation of OPA1 processing and increased PHB2 and ROS. As postulated by the investigators, these molecular parameters could also be useful to evaluate MS activity [2]. In addition, increased ROS and its role in the senescence of the immune system are being studied at present.

Epidemiological observations have shown that in addition to global differences in MS prevalence among ethnic and racial groups, disease severity and clinical features appear to differ among populations. A retrospective analysis performed on multi-ethnic cohorts in Houston, Texas, US, disclosed substantial disparities in epidemiological distributions, risk factors, neurological disability, and magnetic resonance imaging (MRI) findings among the groups [3]. Houston is reportedly the most ethnically diverse city in the US. In this study, African Americans (AA) and Hispanics (people of Latin American extraction) had a lower incidence than White patients but had greater disease encumbrance and disability in earlier stages of the disease. At the onset, however, mean age and degree of brain atrophy were similar, as was the degree of volume loss progression over time and the burden of T1, T2, and gadolinium-enhancing lesions. The study showed that active smokers had significantly increased odds of greater disability both at diagnosis and at last clinical encounter compared to nonsmokers (OR: 2.44, 95% CI: 1.10–7.10, OR = 2.44, 95% CI: 1.35–6.12, $p = 0.01$, respectively).

This study also disclosed the importance of access to care. Patients who were evaluated by a neurologist at symptom onset had significantly decreased disability (defined by the investigators as Expanded Disability Status Scare (EDSS) > 4.5) at last presentation compared to patients who were not evaluated by a neurologist (OR: 0.04, 95% CI: 0.16–0.9).

The accurate diagnosis of clinically definite MS continues to be a challenging task, involving a great responsibility for the practitioner since the current paradigm of *"early diagnosis, early treatment"* will reflect an improved prognosis. The internationally used McDonald Criteria 2017 version [4] is an essential diagnostic tool designed to amalgamate the clinical presentation (first event) along with specific MR imaging criteria and CSF analysis demonstrating the presence of Oligoclonal Bands. The conjunction of all these elements provides the cardinal principles of lesions *disseminated in space* and *disseminated in time*, and that is not a *better explanation* for the clinical picture. The proper utilization of the McDonald Criteria considerably reduces the possibilities of misdiagnosis as well.

Despite the progress accomplished in MS diagnostic identification, disease biomarkers have been notably lacking. Blood neurofilament light chain (NfL), neuronal-specific heteropolymers, have been established as a marker of neuronal and axonal injury in diverse neurodegenerative and inflammatory disorders. NfLs are light (low-molecular-weight) chains with a specific carboxy-terminal domain. Following synthesis and assembly in the neuron cell body, tetramers of NfL proteins are transported bidirectionally along axons by the microtubular apparatus, forming an overlapping array that runs parallel to axons. Once formed, however, in a healthy state, they remain stable for months to years. In the presence of neuronal–axonal disease, NfL is released into the CSF and blood compartments, becoming specific indicators of CNS structural damage. NfL is reported to be significantly elevated in amyotrophic lateral sclerosis, Alzheimer's disease, frontotemporal dementia, and other CNS-degenerative conditions, and even in some peripheral neuropathies. NfL was initially studied in CSF, but the invasive nature of the lumbar puncture procedure limited its utilization. More recently, the advent of ultrasensitive digital immunoassay technologies has enabled reliable detection and measurement in serum/plasma. A comprehensive review of the diagnostic potential of NfL in MS, and the association with clinical outcomes, emphasizes the next steps to overcome before this test is adopted on a routine clinical basis [5].

The presence of numerous clinical phenotypes and the development of a monophasic course (the majority of cases exhibit a relapsing/remitting course) are special challenges to consider in the differential diagnosis of MS, particularly in cases where the spinal cord is involved.

An actualized review of clinical aspects, MRI spinal cord lesion patterns, CSF profiles, and autoantibodies in conditions such as neuromyelitis optica (anti-Aquaporin-4 IgG), anti-Myelin oligodendrocyte glycoprotein (MOG), and anti-glial fibrillary acidic protein IgG-associated diseases underlines the understanding of individual case etiology to make adequate therapeutic decisions, crucial for the prognosis and long-term outcomes in patients with MS or its mimickers [6].

Treatment of MS has experienced remarkable progress since the advent of disease-modifying therapies (DMT) as injectable interferons and glatiramer acetate in the decade of 1990, considered at present as first-line or platform treatments. Pharmacological agents of more recent approval include some monoclonal antibodies (MABs) with specific molecular targets; three of these agents are administered by periodic intravenous infusion, and one is injected subcutaneously. An important addition to the therapeutic armamentarium constituted the emergence of oral medications: sphingosine-1-phosphate receptor (S1PR) modulators, fumarates, and cladribine. MABs and oral medications are rated in general in the range of moderate-to-high efficacy agents. The US Food and Drug Administration approved the first S1PR modulator, fingolimod, in 2010, and the European Medicine Agency approved in the following year.

The molecule sphingosine-1-phosphate, via its G-protein-coupled receptors, signals lymphocytes to egress from peripheral lymphoid organs. S1PR-antagonist agents promote sequestration of lymphocytes in the lymph glands and hence reducing lymphocyte-driven inflammatory damage of the CNS. Five S1P receptors have been identified (S1PR1-5). In 2020–2021, other S1PR-modulator drugs became available: Siponimod, Ozanimod, and Posenimod.

These agents reduce relapse risk, sustained disability progression, MRI markers of disease activity, and whole-brain atrophy. A review [7] of the molecular characteristics of this family of therapeutic modulators addresses the possibility of the development of more selective and intracellular S1PR-driven downstream pathway modulators for MS.

While the role of NfL as a diagnostic marker for MS is being considered (see above), an exploratory observational study assessed serum levels behaviors measured longitudinally before and after 24 months of treatment with first-line immunotherapy, carried out in patients with relapsing–remitting MS [8]. The medications utilized were the traditional platform therapies: interferon-beta and glatiramer acetate. Overall serum NfL was higher at time points concurrent with relapse than during remission periods (12.8 pg/mL vs. 9.7 pg/mL, $p = 0.011$). At follow-up, relapse-free patients showed significantly reduced serum NfL starting from 9 months compared to baseline ($p = 0.05$) and reduced levels after 12 months compared to baseline ($p = 0.013$) in patients without EDSS progression for 12 months. These data suggest that longitudinal measurements of serum NfL to monitor disease activity and therapy response in MS are one more potential aspect to explore for this biomarker.

Observations in MS patients with highly active disease (defined as a clinical course with frequent and repeated relapses and new T2 or gadolinium-enhancing lesions by MRI) show the presence of anti-myelin lipid-specific oligoclonal IgM bands (LS-OCMBs) in CSF to be an accurate predictor of an aggressive evolution of the disease. A disadvantage of this assessment is the need for an invasive spinal tap procedure. Investigators have studied the expression profile of circular RNA and linear RNA arrays in PBMCs from patients with LS-OCMBs. Two circular (hsa_circ_0000478 and hsa_circ_0116639) and two linear RNAs (*IRF5* and *MTRNR2L8*) were downregulated in PBMCs from patients with positive CSF bands (70% accuracy). The investigators propose that RNAs' expression in peripheral blood cells might serve as minimally invasive biomarkers of highly active MS [9].

The clinical, laboratory, and experimental studies in this Special Issue address novel immunologic and molecular findings and their impact and influence on clinical manifestations in adult patients with MS. It is estimated that between 3 and 5% of all patients have an onset of disease under de age of 18 (considered as the pediatric age), and although MS is rare in children, it carries a significant physical and cognitive disability in these groups. Progress in the understanding of MS in children and the availability of pediatric MS diagnostic criteria is essential in differentiating this disorder from a myriad of complex neurological diseases affecting children. The incidence between males and females diagnosed before puberty is relatively equivalent. In adolescents, the ratio of females to males with MS increases to 2 to 3:1, similar to the gender distribution in adults. A review study [10] emphasizes the development of the International Pediatric MS Study Group in 2005 as a milestone in the progress of the knowledge base surrounding pediatric MS, including clinical manifestations and possibilities of treatment.

Knowledge of MS over recent decades has flourished substantially, resulting in notable scientific findings, the development of sensitive laboratory technologies, and enrichment of the understanding of the clinical aspects of this complex neurological disorder.

Funding: This research received no external funding.

Institutional Review Board: Not applicable.

Informed Consent Statement: Not applicable.

Data Availability Statement: Exclude.

Conflicts of Interest: The author declares no conflict of interest.

References

1. Gatta, V.; Mengog, G.; Reale, M.; Tata, A.M. Possible Correlation between Cholinergic System Alterations and Neuro/Inflammation. *Biomedicines* **2020**, *8*, 153. [CrossRef] [PubMed]
2. De Rasmo, D.; Ferretta, A.; Russo, S.; Ruggieri, M.; Lasorella, P.; Paolicelli, D.; Trojano, M.; Signorile, A. PBMC of Multiple Sclerosis Patients Show Deregulation of OPA1 Processing Associated with Increased ROS and PHB2 Protein Levels. *Biomedicines* **2020**, *8*, 85. [CrossRef] [PubMed]
3. Mercado, V.; Dongarwar, D.; Fisher, K.; Salihu, H.M.; Hutton, G.J.; Cuascut, F.X. Multiple Sclerosis in a Multi-Ethnic Population in Houston, Texas: A Retrospective Analysis. *Biomedicines* **2020**, *8*, 534. [CrossRef] [PubMed]
4. Thompson, A.; Banwell, B.L.; Barkhof, F.; Carroll, W.M.; Coetzee, T.; Comi, G.; Correale, J.; Fazekas, F.; Filippi, M.; Freedman, M.S.; et al. Diagnosis of multiple sclerosis: 2017 revisions of the McDonald criteria. *Lancet Neurol.* **2017**, *17*, 162–173. [CrossRef]
5. Thebault, S.; Booth, R.A.; Freedman, M.S. Blood Neurofilament Light Chain: The Neurologist's Troponin? *Biomedicines* **2020**, *8*, 523. [CrossRef] [PubMed]
6. Marrodan, M.; Gaitán, M.I.; Correale, J. Spinal Cord Involvement in MS and Other Demyelinating Diseases. *Biomedicines* **2020**, *8*, 130. [CrossRef] [PubMed]
7. Cohan, S.; Lucassen, E.; Smoot, K.; Brink, J.; Chen, C. Sphingosine-1-Phosphate: Its Pharmacological Regulation and the Treatment of Multiple Sclerosis: A Review Article. *Biomedicines* **2020**, *8*, 227. [CrossRef] [PubMed]

8. Huss, A.; Senel, M.; Abdelhak, A.; Mayer, B.; Kassubek, J.; Ludolph, A.C.; Otto, M.; Hayrettin, T. Longitudinal Serum Neurofilament Levels of Multiple Sclerosis Patients Before and After Treatment with First-Line Immnunomodulatory Therapies. *Biomedicines* **2020**, *8*, 312. [CrossRef] [PubMed]
9. Iparraguirre, L.; Olaverri, D.; Blasco, T.; Sepúlveda, L.; Castillo-Triviño, T.; Espiño, M.; Costa-Frossard, L.; Prada, A.; Villar, L.M.; Otaegui, D.; et al. Whole-Transcriptome Analysis in Peripheral Blood Mononuclear Cells from Patients with Lipid-Specific Oligoclonal IgM Band Characterization Reveals Two Circular RNAs and Two Linear RNAs as Biomarkers of Highly Active Disease. *Biomedicines* **2020**, *8*, 540. [CrossRef] [PubMed]
10. Fisher, K.S.; Cuascut, F.X.; Rivera, V.M.; Hutton, G.J. Current Advances in Pediatric Onset Multiple Sclerosis. *Biomedicines* **2020**, *8*, 71. [CrossRef] [PubMed]

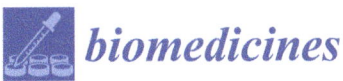

Review

Possible Correlation between Cholinergic System Alterations and Neuro/Inflammation in Multiple Sclerosis

Valentina Gatta [1], Guadalupe Mengod [2], Marcella Reale [3] and Ada Maria Tata [4,5,*]

[1] Department of Psychological, Health and Territorial Sciences, School of Medicine and Health Sciences, "G. d'Annunzio" University, 66100 Chieti, Italy; valentina.gatta@unich.it
[2] IIBB-CSIC, IDIBAPS, CIBERNED, 08036 Barcelona, Spain; guadalupe.mengod@iibb.csic.es
[3] Department of Medical, Oral and Biotechnological Science, University "G. d'Annunzio" Chieti-Pescara, 66100 Chieti, Italy; m.reale@unich.it
[4] Department of Biology and Biotechnologies C. Darwin, "Sapienza" University of Rome, 00185 Rome, Italy
[5] Research Center of Neurobiology Daniel Bovet, "Sapienza" University of Rome, 00185 Rome, Italy
* Correspondence: adamaria.tata@uniroma1.it; Tel.: +39-06-4991-2822

Received: 12 May 2020; Accepted: 6 June 2020; Published: 8 June 2020

Abstract: Multiple sclerosis (MS) is an autoimmune and demyelinating disease of the central nervous system. Although the etiology of MS is still unknown, both genetic and environmental factors contribute to the pathogenesis of the disease. Acetylcholine participates in the modulation of central and peripheral inflammation. The cells of the immune system, as well as microglia, astrocytes and oligodendrocytes express cholinergic markers and receptors of muscarinic and nicotinic type. The role played by acetylcholine in MS has been recently investigated. In the present review, we summarize the evidence indicating the cholinergic dysfunction in serum and cerebrospinal fluid of relapsing–remitting (RR)-MS patients and in the brains of the MS animal model experimental autoimmune encephalomyelitis (EAE). The correlation between the increased activity of the cholinergic hydrolyzing enzymes acetylcholinesterase and butyrylcholinesterase, the reduced levels of acetylcholine and the increase of pro-inflammatory cytokines production were recently described in immune cells of MS patients. Moreover, the genetic polymorphisms for both hydrolyzing enzymes and the possible correlation with the altered levels of their enzymatic activity have been also reported. Finally, the changes in cholinergic markers expression in the central nervous system of EAE mice in peak and chronic phases suggest the involvement of the acetylcholine also in neuro-inflammatory processes.

Keywords: cholinergic system; acetylcholine; multiple sclerosis; inflammation; cytokines; EAE

1. Acetylcholine and Immune System

Acetylcholine (ACh) is known as one of the main neurotransmitters in the central (CNS) and the peripheral nervous system (PNS) [1]. It plays relevant roles in several organisms: in multicellular organisms and in particular in mammalian species, it mediates the communication between the nervous system and several peripheral organs such as muscle cells, heart, glands, gut, etc.....[2,3]. Interestingly, ACh can be produced also by non-neuronal cells, such as keratinocytes and endothelial cells, contributing to local regulation of the cell physiology [4–6].

Evidence has been accumulated over the past 20 years on the ability of immune cells to respond to cholinergic stimuli, focusing on the cholinergic modulation of the immune response and inflammatory processes both in the immune system and in the brain [7,8].

The first evidence suggested that the vagus nerve was responsible of the control of immune cells responses by inflammatory reflex mediated by the cholinergic stimulation [9]. Albeit the vagus nerve stimulation can modulate the peripheral inflammation, it has been proposed that it may control ACh production directly by the immune cells in the spleen or in other lymphoid organs through adrenergic stimulation [10,11]. This hypothesis appears more realistic considering that the ACh has an extremely short half-life in vivo as a consequence of the ubiquitous distribution of its hydrolytic enzymes acetylcholinesterase (AChE) and butirylcholinesterase (BChE) [12], which rapidly degrade it. Therefore, the cholinergic source of ACh must be very close to the site of action (paracrine function). It has been shown that several immune cells are able to produce ACh and to respond to cholinergic stimuli. T and B cells, macrophages and dendritic cells (DCs) express most of the components of the cholinergic system [13,14]. The presence of choline acetyltransferase (ChAT) and AChE in immune cells has been demonstrated by different techniques [8,15,16]. Immunological activation of T cells up-regulates cholinergic activity, as well as the toll-like receptor activation by selective agonists, induces ChAT expression in DCs and macrophages [7]. These data support a clear cholinergic involvement in the regulation of the immune functions.

The acetylcholine signaling in the immune system is mediated by two types of cholinergic receptors: the muscarinic and nicotinic receptors.

The muscarinic receptors (mAChRs) are metabotropic receptors able to activate different signal transduction pathways [17]. The immune cells express muscarinic receptors whose selective activation modulates the synthesis and production of pro-inflammatory cytokines contributing to modulating the inflammatory processes and, albeit they are not involved in the regulation of the antibodies' synthesis, they favor the antibody class switching from IgM to IgG1 [18,19].

Nicotinic receptors (nAChRs) are classical ionotropic receptors. The immune cells express different nicotinic receptor subunits ($\alpha 2$, $\alpha 4$, $\alpha 5$, $\alpha 9$, $\alpha 7$ and $\beta 1$, $\beta 2$) whose combination contributes to the hetero- or homopentameric receptor subtype formation. The expression of these receptors is differently distributed in the immune cells and in some cases correlates with their differentiation state [20]. The homopentameric $\alpha 7$ nAChR is the best characterized nicotinic receptor subtype in the immune system. This receptor appears mainly involved in the inhibition of inflammatory processes modulating the production of the anti-inflammatory cytokine, suppressing dendritic cells and macrophage activity and leading to the suppression of T cell differentiation [21,22].

Considering the relevant role of the ACh and its receptors in immune cells functions and in the modulation of the inflammatory processes, it is not difficult to hypothesize that a better understanding of the roles played by ACh and its receptors in inflammatory-related diseases such as neurodegenerative diseases, is of great clinical relevance.

In the present review, we summarize the data indicating the possible involvement of ACh also in demyelinating disease such as multiple sclerosis (MS), reporting recent data demonstrating how the alteration of the cholinergic system activity is present in MS patients and in experimental autoimmune encephalomyelitis (EAE) mice, may be correlated with the immune system dysfunction and alterations of the neuro-inflammatory processes characterizing the MS pathology.

2. Cholinergic Dysfunction in Multiple Sclerosis

MS is an autoimmune disease characterized by demyelination and chronic inflammation. The progressive phases of the disease are associated with myelin sheets alteration and degradation and decreased oligodendrocyte differentiation. The involvement of the cholinergic system in MS is poorly known. However, several studies on EAE mice have suggested how the treatment with cholinesterase inhibitors may improve motor and cognitive impairment and reduce the neuro-inflammation [23]. These effects were significantly abolished by $\alpha 7$ nAChR antagonists [24]. Moreover, as reviewed by Nizri and Brenner [25], the $\alpha 7$ nAChRs also play a relevant role in the immune system where they control the number of dendritic cells and the proliferation of the autoreactive T cells [26].

According to this evidence, the ACh production and cholinergic marker expression and activity in serum and cerebrospinal fluid (CSF) of MS patients were reported [27]. The first data have demonstrated that ACh levels were significantly lower in MS patients with a relapsing–remitting course of the disease

(RR-MS) compared with healthy subjects (HS), both in sera and CSF [27,28]. However, no relationship was found between ACh levels and patient gender or demographic and clinical aspects [27].

Interestingly the enzymatic activity of the ACh hydrolyzing enzymes AChE and BChE resulted significantly increased in sera of MS patients [29]. The studies of the expression of AChE and BChE transcripts in peripheral blood mononuclear cells (PBMC) of MS patients have demonstrated an increase in the transcript levels of both hydrolyzing enzymes, in particular for BChE [28,29]. Moreover, the levels of ACh biosynthetic enzyme ChAT were higher in MS patients compared with HS. Finally, the expression of transcript for OCTN-1 and mediatophore, the two proteins typically expressed in immune cells and responsible for the non-vesicular ACh release were also upregulated in MS patients [29].

These results suggest that the decreased levels of ACh observed in MS patients, may mainly be dependent on the increased expression and activity of cholinergic hydrolyzing enzyme BChE and AChE (Figure 1).

The dysregulated homeostasis of ACh has already been described in other neurological and neurodegenerative diseases (i.e., schizophrenia, Alzheimer's, Parkinson diseases) [30]. For these pathologies, as well as for MS, it is difficult to understand whether the cholinergic dysregulation is the cause or the effect of the pathology.

Interestingly, also some autoimmune diseases present alterations of cholinergic receptors expression or activity (i.e., Sjogren's disease, sepsis, myasthenia gravis) [31–33], confirming a relevant role of cholinergic receptors also in immune system activity. Thus, the MS may be a new pathology possibly correlated with cholinergic dysfunction.

3. The Interface between Cholinergic System and Inflammatory Cytokines in MS

Cytokines orchestrate all phases of immune responses, act in highly complex and dynamic networks in a paracrine and/or autocrine manner and often perform overlapping and partly redundant functions through multicomponent molecules that can be shared by different cell types. For the homeostatic balance, a dynamic equilibrium between pro and anti-inflammatory cytokines is required. Cytokines play a key role in the pathogenesis of MS through the activation of the immune system in the periphery and in the central nervous system. Aberrant immune responses occur in MS and it is likely that the spectrum of the cytokines produced decisively influences the outcome of the disease, as evidenced by the cytokine profiles altered in the central nervous system [34] and in the biological fluid of MS patients. As reported above, the serum levels of ACh were found to be lower in MS patients with respect to levels detected in HS. Considering that ACh plays a central role in the crosstalk between the immune and nervous system and that may act as a suppressor of inflammatory responses, the relationship between the ACh synthesizing and degrading enzymes and pro-inflammatory cytokines was evaluated. Interestingly, AChE and BChE are present at high levels in MS patients, contributing to alter the steady-state equilibrium of the ACh [29]. The balance between the levels of pro- and anti-inflammatory cytokines and their sequential release can be decisive for the severity of inflammatory responses. Alteration of this balance can convert a beneficial effect into a pathological inflammatory reaction. The well-known contribution of the inflammatory component to the progression of multiple sclerosis has led to new attempts to discover ways to attenuate inflammation. The cholinergic system has been suggested as a mediator of the crosstalk between the immune and nervous systems playing an important role as a modulator of immune responses. The effect of dysregulated balance between ACh, AChE and BChE on cytokines levels was studied in order to understand the role of the cholinergic system on inflammatory environment present in MS patients. In the CSF and sera of RR-MS patients and control subjects, the levels of IL-10 and IL-4 were evaluated and no statistical differences were detected [27]. Conversely in both CSF and serum from RR-MS patients, the levels of IL-1β were significantly higher than those detected in CSF and serum of control subjects. Interesting, in both MS and control groups, also the mean level of IL-17 was higher in the CSF than in serum, and serum levels of IL-1β were about four times higher than in CSF of MS subjects. These data confirmed the active pro-inflammatory state characterizing the MS patients [27,28,35]. Moreover, significant differences in TNFα, IL-12/IL-23p40 and IL-18 levels were observed between MS patients and controls. However, a not significant association between ACh hydrolyzing enzymes and the levels of these cytokines was found [27,29].

However, in the serum of MS patients undergoing IFN-β treatment substantially lower levels of IL-1β, IL-12/23p40, IL-18, TNF-α, and HMGB-1 and higher levels of IL-18BP and ACh were detected. These results, other than reinforce the previous observation that a reduction in ACh levels is involved in RR-MS and that ACh and circulating cytokines are mutually influenced [29], have suggested the ability of IFN-β to modulate inflammatory cytokines also by restoring of the ACh levels [36].

ACh was present in inflammatory sites, probably synthesized from immune cells, and cytokines produced to represent an inflammatory input signal to activate afferent vagus nerve fibers that transmit information to the brain. Therefore, the cytokines produced by blood peripheral cells might affect the function of the CNS by crossing the blood–brain barrier (BBB) for direct interaction with CNS tissue. On the other hand, the cells of the immune systems may respond to neurotransmitters released by autonomic nerves and communicate through neurotransmitters [11].

The higher gene expression level of several cytokines, such as IL-1β, IL-12/IL-23p40, IL-17, IL-18 and TNFα was detected in RR-MS compared to HS, according to with the levels measured in the serum; this confirms the relationship between expression and production of pro-inflammatory cytokines in MS patients [35].

These results led to evaluating which components of the cholinergic system could be relevant in terms of the therapeutic tool in controlling the inflammatory state in MS patients. It is known that α7 nicotinic receptors stimulate the cholinergic anti-inflammatory pathway [37]. The expression of α7 and α4 nicotinic receptor subunits, in RR-MS patients and HS, was documented [35]. The expression of the α7 receptor protein by western blot analysis, confirmed the gene expression data, showing higher protein levels in MS patients. The stimulation with phytohaemagglutinin (PHA) was also able to differently modulate the α7 nicotinic receptor expression in RR-MS patients and HS. In fact, PHA stimulation significantly decreased mRNA levels for the α7 receptor subunit only in RR-MS patients. Instead, the increased α7 nAChR expression after nicotine stimulation in PBMC of RR-MS patients correlated with a reduction of the pro-inflammatory cytokines [35]. In fact, the ability of nicotine to modulate the inflammatory cytokines in RR-MS patients was also evaluated. The effects of nicotine on the production of IL-1β and IL-17 from PHA-stimulated PBMC of RR-MS and HS were described. In both groups, nicotine decreased the levels of IL-1β and IL-17 released, but a more significant decrease was observed in RR-MS patients. The expression of the cytokine transcript levels after nicotine treatment was also evaluated [35]. In particular, the treatment of PBMC with PHA plus nicotine significantly reduced the expression of IL-1β, especially in MS patients. Interestingly the co-treatment of PBMC with PHA and 10 μM nicotine did not modify the expression of α7 subunit mRNA in HS, while inducing a significant increase of α7 transcript levels in RR-MS patients [35]. Globally, these data suggest that the locally expressed and released components of the non-neuronal cholinergic system may play paracrine or autocrine effects and contribute to modulate inflammatory cytokines (Figure 1). This may suggest strategies involving the use of selective agonists of α7 nAChRs in the modulation of the inflammatory responses also in demyelinating disease.

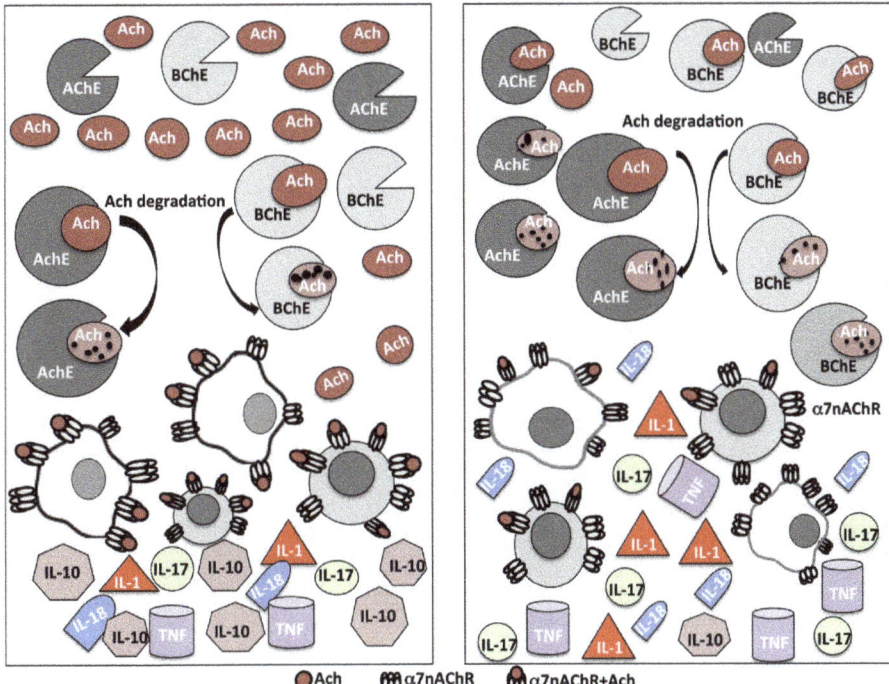

Figure 1. Schematic representation of the mechanism associated with Acetylcholine (Ach) degradation by acetylcholinesterase (AChE) and butirylcholinesterase (BChE) (see arrows), in healthy (left) and multiple sclerosis patients' immune cells (right). The decreased ACh levels may contribute to a reduced α-7 nicotinic receptor activation and a consequent increase of pro-inflammatory cytokines.

4. Genetic Polymorphisms for BChE and AChE and MS

The etiology of MS can be considered multifactorial, based on the interaction between genetic and several environmental factors (Figure 2). A hereditary basis of MS is suggested by epidemiological studies. This can be supported by the recurrence risk of MS in twins, siblings, conjugal MS individuals, and lower recurrence risk in adoptees [38–40]. In the general population, the risk of developing MS is about 0.00125%, including the variability for geographic areas. Overall, about 15% of the patients with MS have an affected relative. Studies in twins reveal a concordance of 25% in monozygotic twins and only 2.4% in dizygotic twins [41]. Recently, the following meta-analysis estimate was reported: 0.50 (95% CI: 0.39–0.61) for heritability, 0.21 (95% CI: 0.11–0.30) for shared environmental component and 0.29 (95% CI: 0.26–0.33) for unique environmental component [42]. The authors conclude that these results support the efforts to fill the gap of 'missing heritability' by genome-wide association studies (GWAS) on large populations as well as massive sequencing analysis by next-generation sequencing (NGS). The risk of developing the disease is 15-fold higher when MS is present in a first-degree relative. Siblings of patients with MS have a risk of ~2.6%, parents have a risk of 1.8% and sons have a risk of ~1.5%. Accordingly, considering the distinction between monogenic and complex traits, no single gene or environmental factor causes MS and it does not follow the Mendelian model.

MS is believed to be dependent on multiple independent or interacting polymorphism genes with small or moderate effects, as well as their interaction with behavioral and environmental factors (Figure 2) [43]. Several studies also aim to disclose the genetic basis of MS. For decades, only several variants of the *HLA* antigen were known to have the strongest effect on the risk of MS [44,45]. Carrying *HLA-DRB1*1501* is associated with about three-fold greater odds of developing MS, while carrying

HLA-A*02 is associated with meaningfully reduced odds. So far, genome-wide association studies, carried out in populations worldwide, provided strong evidence for the association of approximately >230 genetic variants. All these variants only account for 20% to 30% of MS heritability, suggesting that its remaining part is likely related to epigenetic factors and gene-gene or gene-environment interactions. Considerable attention has been focused on studies evaluating disease-modifying effects in MS that identified genes such as the *APOE, CXCR5, IL2RA, IL7R, IL7, IL12RB1, IL22RA2, IL12A, IL12B, IRF8, TNFRSF1A, TNFRSF14, TNFSF14, CBLB, GPR65, MALT1, RGS1, RIC3, STAT3, TAGAP, TYK2, CYP27B1* and *CYP24A1* [44,45].

Recently, it was reported in genome-wide association studies, that the implication of RIC3, a chaperone of nAChRs, in multiple sclerosis (MS) and neuroinflammatory disease. RIC3 promotes the functional expression of α7 nAChR, and it was shown a dynamic regulation of RIC3 in macrophages and in lymphocytes, following an immune activation in human and murine cells.

Moreover, increased average expression of *RIC3* and *CHRNA7* in lymphocytes from MS patients but not in healthy donors was observed. These data are consistent with a role for RIC3 and in its regulated expression in inflammatory processes and in neuroinflammatory diseases [45].

The variation in some genes of the cholinergic system, such as those encoding BChE (gene *BChE*, chrom. 3q26.1–q26.2) and AChE (gene *AChE*, chrom. 7q22.1) [http://www.genatlas.org] has also been studied in MS patients in relation to altered levels of their enzymatic activity.

Variants in these genes have been largely investigated in relation to the onset of Alzheimer's disease [46,47], since the levels of these enzymes were found increased in the brains of patients, as well as a number of low-grade systemic inflammation pathologies [48,49].

In particular, two specific polymorphisms within these genes have been studied, namely rs1803274 for *BChE* and rs2571598 for *AChE*. It is reported that rs1803274 for *BChE* is able to reduce the enzymes' activity by about 30%–50% [50]. The *BChE* rs1803274 is characterized by a G/A substitution inducing the Ala/Tr change at the codon 539 and it produces the so-called K-allele. This variation causes the reduction of 30%–60% of ACh's hydrolyzing activity and 30% of the capacity to hydrolyze butyryl-thiocholine. BChE K-carriers, showing lowered hydrolytic activity of BChE K-allele, could potentially improve cholinergic activity.

There are 19 single nucleotide polymorphisms (SNPs) for *AChE* [51]. The only rs1799806 on exon 6, a functional intronic C/T substitution, was associated with activity changes. The AChE activity of homozygote Pro/Pro genotype was significantly lower than Arg/Arg genotypes. The presence of these variants is controversially considered a risk factor for Alzheimer's disease, as well as other conditions such as stroke, Parkinson's disease and related dementia [52,53]. Even if cholinergic neurotransmission regulates the immune response and inhibits cytokine release after stroke, only the variant alleles of *BChE* have been identified as risk factors for ischemic stroke [54] and associated with reduced BChE activity in patients with post-stroke dementia (PSD) [49], while *AChE* rs1799806 do not influence the AChE activity.

As above-described the ACh levels in serum of RR-MS patients were inversely correlated with the increased activity of the hydrolyzing enzymes AChE and BChE [29]. The observed lower circulating ACh levels in sera of MS patients are probably dependent on the higher activity of cholinergic hydrolyzing enzymes [29].

In this context, it was recently investigated whether lower ACh concentration observed in RR-MS compared to HS may be related to the ability to regulate the extracellular ACh levels, when needed, or to the variation of AChE or BChE activity related to the association with rs1803274 for *BChE* and rs2571598 for *AChE* genetic variations [55]. An association between the *BChE* K-allele and *AChE* rs2571598 in 102 relapsing remitting-MS patients compared to 117 healthy controls was reported. These data underlined that in RR-MS patients carrying the K-allele, higher BChE activity was observed [55]. Although this is in contrast with the reported role of this SNP in *BChE* gene, this excess of circulating BChE removes ACh, negatively influencing the levels of all investigated pro-inflammatory cytokines (Figure 1). Conceivably, other pathways, such as increased transduction of BChE, microRNAs or other gene modulators acting in combination with BChE-K, could be involved in the balance of the BChE as well as a higher BChE enzymatic activity induced by the presence of the polymorphic allele may reduce the amounts of circulating ACh.

These evidences may suggest that specific genetic endo-phenotypes are able to modulate the pro-inflammatory immune responses in MS patients, altering the activity of AChE through ACh hydrolysis. These data highlight the potential role of the non-neuronal cholinergic system in immune cell function, even if studies on larger populations are needed in order to better discover MS etiology and progression and to develop new disease-modifying therapies for MS with AChE and ACh as targets.

The reported literature about genetic biomarkers in MS is not always consistent in the worldwide population. The detection of a single nucleotide polymorphism related to MS pathogenesis is very hard given that several genetic polymorphisms are implicated, each with a small contribution to the susceptibility or resistance to MS. Although numerous causal genes have been detected by genome-wide association studies (GWAS), these susceptibility genes are linked to relatively low disease risk, indicating the important role of environmental factors in the pathogenesis of the disease. Next-generation sequencing (NGS) technology, with high-throughput capacity and accuracy, could be a powerful tool to discover the genetic basis of MS. NGS can be applied to sequence analysis in any part of the genome and the resulting transcriptome, including the whole genome, exons, and other interesting regions, and accordingly can be roughly classified as whole-genome sequencing (WGS), whole-exome sequencing (WES), RNA sequencing (RNA-seq), and DNA methylation sequencing. So far, only rare variants of modest effect on MS risk affecting a subset of patients have been detected by NGS including *CYP27B1* and *TYK2* genes [56,57]. Epigenetic mechanisms that have been detected for MS pathogenesis are DNA methylation, histone modification and some microRNAs' alternations. Several cellular processes including apoptosis, differentiation and evolution can be modulated along with epigenetic changes [58]. All these data support the idea of a complex basis of MS with clear gene–environment interactions and epigenetic alterations triggered by environmental exposures in individuals with a particular genetic profile (Figure 2) [59].

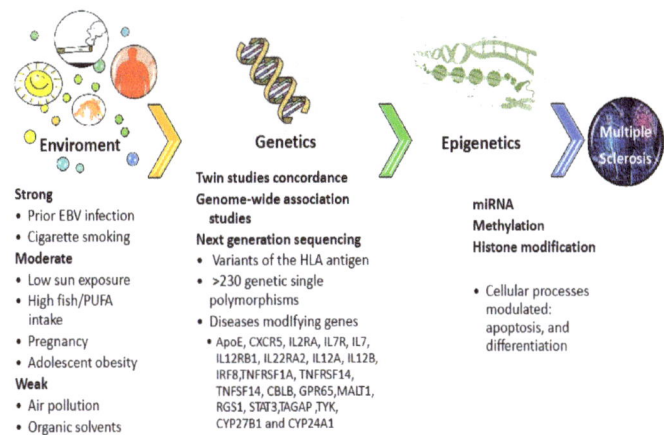

Figure 2. Risk factors for multiple sclerosis (MS). A hereditary basis of MS is suggested by epidemiological studies and recurrence risk of MS in twins, siblings, conjugal MS individuals. MS is believed to result from multiple independent or interacting polymorphism genes as well as their interaction with behavioral and environmental factors with strong, moderate, or weak effects. Epigenetic mechanisms that have been detected for MS pathogenesis are DNA methylation, histone modification and some microRNAs alternations.

5. Cholinergic Markers Alteration in the Brain of EAE Mice

One of the animal models of MS, EAE can be obtained after active immunization with myelin oligodendrocyte glycoprotein (MOG) 35–55 peptide as antigen in C57BL6 mice, and reproduces many pathological features observed in MS [60]. Several days after immunization, it is possible to observe immune cells infiltrating the CNS and activation of microglia. These events take place predominantly in the spinal cord but also in other brain structures such as the cerebellum and the optic tract [61], which lead to axonal damage and demyelination [62]. The MOG$_{35-55}$-induced model of EAE is characterized by the peak inflammatory phase, followed by a chronic phase of neurological deficit.

ACh may play a role in the development or in the remission of MS. Recent analyses of cholinergic markers in the brain and spinal cord of EAE mice revealed specific alterations in their expression in different brain areas and cellular populations associated to the different phases of the disease [63]. The mRNA coding for ChAT, the enzyme responsible for the synthesis of ACh from choline and acetyl-CoA that serves as a marker of cholinergic cells, presents alterations in the expression levels in different brain regions and spinal cord and in different disease phases of EAE mice [63]. Several cholinergic nuclei of EAE mice in the chronic phase present an increment in ChAT expression levels and an increase of the AChE activity and mRNA expression at peak of disease, suggesting that the balance of ACh levels may contribute to the chronicity of the disease.

The BChE activity, a non-selective cholinesterase enzyme that catalyzes the ACh hydrolysis, is altered in the habenula and solitary nucleus in both disease phases of EAE mice and in higher proportion in astroglia and microglia/macrophage cells in the chronic group [63]. BChE activity is detected in both glial cell populations and presents a significant increment in EAE animals in the chronic phase compared to the peak phase or control brains. The high ratio of BChE to AChE found in astrocytes of EAE mice in peak phase [63] may suggest this ratio as a potential marker for brain areas selectively vulnerable to this neuropathology as it was described for Alzheimer's disease brains [64]. However, the treatment of EAE mice with a BChE/AChE inhibitor (rivastigmine) resulted in an amelioration of the clinical symptoms associated also with a reduction in the demyelination [24], supporting the role of BChE in neuroinflammation and demyelination (Figure 3).

As reported above, several studies show that α7 nAChR is the key subtype involved in nAChR-mediated immune regulation [20,26,65]. α7 nAChR mRNA expression in the EAE chronic group is increased in habenula and decreased in the dorsal tegmental nucleus. Conversely, the mRNA levels of this receptor are increased in the dorsal tegmental nucleus of animals in the peak phase [63]. The altered expression of this receptor subunit in EAE mice during the chronic phase compared to the peak phase of the disease may sustain its role in the neuro-inflammation regulation also in the brain (Figure 3).

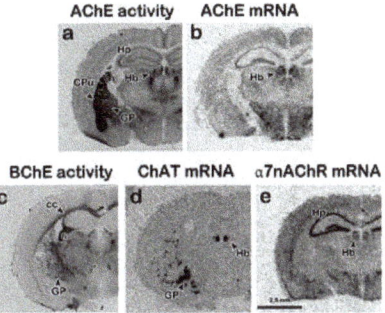

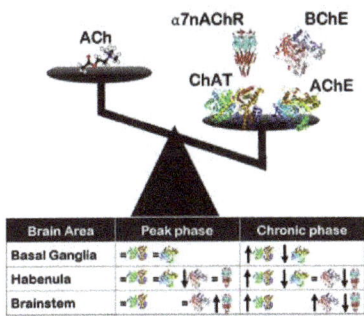

Figure 3. Cholinergic system changes in some brain areas (basal ganglia, habenula, and nuclei of the brainstem) of experimental autoimmune encephalomyelitis (EAE) mice at peak and chronic phases of the disease. (**A**) Photomicrographs showing AChE (**a**) and BChE (**c**) enzymatic activities stained histological brain sections and photomicrographs from autoradiograms of control mouse brain tissue sections visualizing brain areas expressing mRNAs coding for *AChE* (**b**), *ChAT* (**d**) and *α7nAChR* (**e**). (**B**) Representation of the homeostatic balance of cholinergic markers expression in brain areas of EAE mice. The table summarizes the quantification of enzymatic activities and mRNAs expression of cholinergic markers at peak and chronic phases of the disease. Abbreviations and symbols: CPu, caudate-putamen; CC, cerebral cortex; fi, fimbria; GP, globus pallidus; Hb, habenula; Hp, hippocampus;

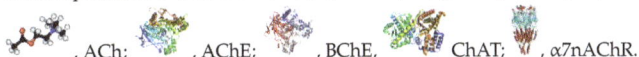

, ACh; , AChE; , BChE; ChAT; , α7nAChR.

6. Cholinergic Receptors in the Glial Cells

New ideas have emerged during the past several years on how the neurotransmitters, including Ach, can actively participate in neuron–glia cross talk. This interaction is relevant both during nervous system development to improve and address neuron and glial cell survival, proliferation and differentiation, and in adulthood, to maintain axonal function and myelin integrity [66]. It is now known that glial cells express receptors for different neurotransmitters, suggesting that these molecules, most probably when released in extra-synaptic regions [67–69], may modulate glial cell survival, proliferation, and myelination [67,70].

The expression of ACh receptors has been reported in several glial cells indicating these cells as potential targets for ACh action [70,71]. Oligodendrocyte (OLs), the main target in MS, express muscarinic receptors whose activation triggers different signal transduction pathways [67,70,72–74]. The presence of nicotinic receptor subunits (α3, α4, α5, α7, β2, and β4) was also revealed by RT-PCR and immunocytochemistry in oligodendrocytes precursor cells (OPC), but not in mature cells [75]. Oligodendrocytes express also acetylcholine muscarinic receptors. M1, M3, and M4 ACh receptors were the muscarinic subtypes expressed in OPCs, whereas all five muscarinic receptor subtypes were found to be expressed at low levels in mature OLs; thus muscarinic receptors favor the maintenance of immature proliferating progenitor cells and counteract progression toward a mature state [75]. Accordingly, with this evidence, more recent research demonstrated that antagonists of muscarinic receptors promote oligodendrocyte differentiation and rescue of the lesions in white matter in EAE mice [76]. In fact benztropine, a typical muscarinic antagonist used as a drug for Parkinson's disease treatment has been proposed for MS treatment considering that MS symptoms in the EAE mouse model were reverted [76,77]. Moreover, the benztropine appears to favor oligodendrocyte differentiation and myelination by a specific antagonism of M1 and M3 receptors on oligodendrocyte precursor cells (OPCs) [76]. Another important aspect to consider is that muscarinic receptors are able to modulate pro-inflammatory cytokine production [18,28], so it may be possible to hypothesize that the antagonism of muscarinic receptors can support not only oligodendrocyte differentiation but also the neuro-inflammation decrease.

The presence of muscarinic receptors was demonstrated in cultured astrocytes [78] as well as the expression of functional nAChRs subunits ($a4$, $a7$, $β2$, $β3$) has been reported in rat astrocytes [39,79]. In particular, the expression of $a7$ nAChR in astrocytes plays a relevant role in neuroprotection in several neurodegenerative diseases (i.e., Alzheimer and Parkinson) [80,81].

Finally, microglia also express both muscarinic and nicotinic receptors. Zhang and collaborators [82] described for the first time the expression of functional muscarinic receptors in human microglia. Interestingly the upregulated expression of M3 receptor subtype in these cells causes an increase of MHC-I and MHC-II expression, suggesting the pro-inflammatory microglia phenotype [83]. Microglia also display nicotinic receptors, with a prevalence of $a7$ subunit [84–87]. For these reasons, this nicotinic receptor subtype may be considered an interesting therapeutic target for several neurological disorders considering its ability to modulate the cholinergic anti-inflammatory pathway and the synaptic plasticity.

Taking all these into account, it cannot be excluded that cholinergic stimulation in the brain may influence a complex network controlling both neuronal and glial functions and play a relevant role in the control of the neuro-inflammation.

7. Conclusions

Understanding the mechanisms leading to aberrant immune response and the severe neuro-inflammation in MS plays a relevant role in the development of new treatments directed to decrease pro-inflammatory cytokine production and to ameliorate the clinical symptoms, slowing the disease outcome and delaying or arresting the onset of the disabilities. In this review we have presented recent data in EAE mice and in MS patients, supporting the role of ACh in MS. The dysregulated ACh homeostasis in MS, suggest how its altered functions might represent an additional pathogenetic mechanism negatively influencing the cytokines production with consequent disease outcome.

Interestingly, using the EAE mice model, it has also been described as the alteration of ACh synthesis or degradation may impact on neuron function, contributing to the motor and cognitive disabilities characteristics of MS patients, also influencing the glia network, the differentiation and survival of the oligodendrocytes, and triggering the neuro-inflammation.

The relevant role played by ACh in this context, is supported by the evidence that modulating the cholinergic system activity or cholinergic receptor functions, the clinical disabilities, at least in mice, are significantly reduced. In fact, the altered balance of ACh also in cholinergic area of the brain or spinal cord of EAE mice (i.e., basal ganglia or spinal motoneuros), suggested that the decreased ACh levels may influence the MS motor disabilities both reducing the levels of the neurotransmitter in the cholinergic neurons and increasing the neuro-inflammation with consequent impact on myelin disruption and axonal conduction [63,76,77].

This aspect appears supported by additional studies performed with conventional drugs used in the treatment of MS, as INFβ or dimethyl fumarate [36,88], that demonstrate a significant amelioration of the cholinergic activity with a possible consequent reduction of the clinical symptoms-MS associated. Therefore, further studies will be necessary to evaluate the impact of different immune modulators on the cholinergic system activity both in the immune system and in the brain.

In conclusion, the data described in this review highlight as ACh and its receptors may be implicated in MS pathogenesis. However, further investigation on the genetic aspects and epigenetic modulation of cholinergic markers gene expression could significantly improve the knowledge about MS onset and progression as well as to contribute to identifying new possible therapeutic strategies.

Author Contributions: Conceptualization A.M.T., Original draft preparation, writing—review and editing V.G., G.M., M.R., A.M.T. All authors have read and agreed to the published version of the manuscript.

Funding: Supported by FISM—Fondazione Italiana Sclerosi Multipla (Project number 2009-R-29; 2013-R-25).

Conflicts of Interest: The authors declare there are no conflicts of interest.

References

1. Mesulam, M.M. Central cholinergic pathways: Neuroanatomy and some behavioral implications. In *Neurotransmitters and Cortical Function*; Avoli, M., Reader, T.A., Dikes, R.W., Gloor, P., Eds.; Plenum Publishing: New York, NY, USA, 1988; pp. 237–260.
2. Wessler, I.; Kilbinger, H.; Bittinger, F.; Unger, R.; Kirkpatrick, C.J. The biological role of non-neuronal acetylcholine in plants and humans. *Jpn. J. Pharmacol.* **2001**, *85*, 2–10. [CrossRef] [PubMed]
3. Picciotto, M.R.; Higley, M.J.; Mineur, Y.S. Acetylcholine as a neuromodulator: Cholinergic signaling shapes nervous system function and behavior. *Neuron* **2012**, *76*, 116–129. [CrossRef] [PubMed]
4. Kawashima, K.; Fujii, T. Basic and clinical aspects of non-neuronal acetylcholine: Overview of non-neuronal cholinergic systems and their biological significance. *J. Pharmacol. Sci.* **2008**, *106*, 167–173. [CrossRef] [PubMed]
5. Furchgott, R.F.; Carvalho, M.H.; Khan, M.T.; Matsunaga, K. Evidence for endothelium-dependent vasodilation of resistance vessels by acetylcholine. *Blood Vessel.* **1987**, *24*, 145–149. [CrossRef]
6. Grando, S.A.; Pittelkow, M.R.; Schellreunter, K.U. Adrenergic and cholinergic control in the biology of epidermis: Physiological and clinical Significance. *J. Invest. Dermatol.* **2006**, *126*, 1948–1965. [CrossRef]
7. Cox, M.A.; Bassi, C.; Saunders, M.E.; Nechanitzky, R.; Morgado-Palacin, I.; Zheng1, C.; Mak, T.W. Beyond neurotransmission: Acetylcholine in immunity and inflammation. *J. Int. Med.* **2020**, *287*, 120–133. [CrossRef]
8. Fujii, T.; Mashimo, M.; Moriwaki, Y.; Misawa, H.; Ono, S.; Horiguchi, K.; Kawashima, K. Physiological functions of the cholinergic system in immune cells. *J. Pharmacol. Sci.* **2017**, *134*, 1–21. [CrossRef]
9. Borovikova, L.V.; Ivanova, S.; Zhang, M.; Yang, H.; Botchkina, G.I.; Watkins, L.R.; Wang, H.; Abumrad, N.; Eaton, J.W.; Tracey, K.J. Vagus nerve stimulation attenuates the systemic inflammatory response to endotoxin. *Nature* **2000**, *405*, 458–462. [CrossRef]
10. Carnevale, D.; Perrotta, M.; Pallante, F.; Fardella, V.; Iacobucci, R.; Fardella, S.; Carnevale, L.; Carnevale, R.; de Lucia, M.; Cifelli, G.; et al. A cholinergic sympathetic pathway primes immunity in hypertension and mediates brain-to-spleen communication. *Nat. Commun.* **2016**, *7*, 13035. [CrossRef]
11. Rosas-Ballina, M.; Olofsson, P.S.; Ochani, M.; Valdés-Ferrer, S.I.; Levine, Y.A.; Reardon, C.; Tusche, M.W.; Pavlov, V.A.; Andersson, U.; Chavan, S.; et al. Acetylcholine-synthesizing T cells relay neural signals in a vagus nerve circuit. *Science* **2011**, *334*, 98–101. [CrossRef]
12. Soreq, H.; Seidman, S. Acetylcholinesterase–new roles for an old actor. *Nat. Rev. Neurosci.* **2001**, *2*, 294–302. [CrossRef] [PubMed]
13. Kawashima, K.; Fujii, T. The lymphocytic cholinergic system and its contribution to the regulation of immune activity. *Life Sci.* **2003**, *74*, 675–696. [CrossRef] [PubMed]
14. Fujii, T.; Mashimo, M.; Moriwaki, Y.; Misawa, H.; Ono, S.; Horiguchi, K.; Kawashima, K. Expression and Function of the Cholinergic System in Immune Cells. *Front. Immunol.* **2017**, *8*, 1085. [CrossRef] [PubMed]

15. Ogawa, H.; Fujii, T.; Watanabe, Y.; Kawashima, K. Expression of multiple mRNA species for choline acetyltransferase in human T-lymphocytes. *Life Sci.* **2003**, *72*, 2127–2130. [CrossRef]
16. Kawashima, K.; Fujii, T. Extraneuronal cholinergic system in lymphocytes. *Pharmacol. Ther.* **2000**, *86*, 29–48. [CrossRef]
17. Tata, A.M. Muscarinic acetylcholine receptors: New potential therapeutic targets in antinociception and in cancer therapy. *Rec Pat. CNS Drug Discov.* **2008**, *3*, 94–103. [CrossRef]
18. Kawashima, K.; Fujii, T.; Watanabe, Y.; Misawa, H. Acetylcholine synthesis and muscarinic receptor subtype mRNA expression in T-lymphocytes. *Life Sci.* **1998**, *62*, 1701–1705. [CrossRef]
19. Fujii, T.; Watanabe, Y.; Inoue, T.; Kawashima, K. Upregulation of mRNA encoding the M5 muscarinic acetylcholine receptor in human T- and B-lymphocytes during immunological responses. *Neurochem. Res.* **2003**, *28*, 423–429. [CrossRef]
20. Wang, H.; Yu, M.; Ochani, M.; Amella, C.A.; Tanovic, M.; Susarla, S.; Li, J.H.; Wang, H.; Yang, H.; Ulloa, L.; et al. Nicotinic acetylcholine receptor [alpha] 7 subunit is an essential regulator of inflammation. *Nature* **2003**, *421*, 384–388. [CrossRef]
21. Skok, M.V.; Grathe, K.; Agenes, F.; Changeux, P.J. The role of nicotinic receptorsi in B-lymphocites development and activation. *Life Sci.* **2007**, *80*, 2324–2336. [CrossRef]
22. Kawashima, K.; Fuji, T.; Moriwaki, Y.; Misawa, H.; Horiguchi, K. Non-neuronal cholinergic system in regulation of immune function with a focus on α7 nAChRs. *Int. Immunopharmacol.* **2015**, *29*, 127–134. [CrossRef] [PubMed]
23. Nizri, E.; Hamra-Amitay, Y.; Sicsic, C.; Lavon, I.; Brenner, T. Anti-inflammatory properties of cholinergic up-regulation: A new role for acetylcholinesterase inhibitors. *Neuropharmacology* **2006**, *50*, 540–547. [CrossRef] [PubMed]
24. Nirzi, E.; Jromy-Tir-Sinai, M.; Faranesh, N.; Layon, I.; Lavi, E.; Weinstock, M.; Brenner, T. Supprssion of neuroinflammationby the acetylcholinesterase inhibitor rivastigamine. *J. Neuroimmunol.* **2008**, *203*, 12–22.
25. Nirzi, E.; Brenner, T. Modulation of inflammatory pathways by the immune-cholinergic system. *Amino Acids* **2013**, *45*, 75–85.
26. Nizri, E.; Irony-Tur-Sinai, M.; Lory, O.; Orr-Urtreger, A.; Lavi, E.; Brenner, T. Activation of the cholinergic anti-inflammatory system by nicotine attenuates neuroinflammation via suppression of Th1 and Th17 responses. *J. Immunol.* **2010**, *183*, 6681–6688. [CrossRef] [PubMed]
27. Reale, M.; De Angelis, F.; Di Nicola, M.; Capello, E.; Di Ioia, M.; De Luca, G.; Lugaresi, A.; Tata, A.M. Relation Between Pro-Inflammatory Cytokines and Acetylcholine Levels in Relapsing-Remitting Multiple Sclerosis Patients. *Int. J. Mol. Sci.* **2012**, *13*, 12656–12664. [CrossRef]
28. Di Bari, M.; Di Pinto, G.; Reale, M.; Mengod, G.; Tata, A.M. Cholinergic system and neuroinflammation: Implication in multiple sclerosis. *CNS Agents Med. Chem.* **2017**, *17*, 109–115. [CrossRef]
29. Di Bari, M.; Reale, M.; Di Nicola, M.; Orlando, V.; Galizia, S.; Porfilio, I.; Costantini, E.; D'Angelo, C.; Ruggieri, S.; Biagioni, S.; et al. Dysregulated homeostasis of acetylcholine levels in immune cells of RR-multiple sclerosis patients. *Int. J. Mol. Sci.* **2016**, *17*, E2009. [CrossRef]
30. Tata, A.M.; Velluto, L.; D'Angelo, C.; Reale, M. Cholinergic system dysfunctions and neurodegenerative diseases: Cause or effect? *CNS Neurol. Disord. Drug Targets* **2014**, *13*, 1294–1303. [CrossRef]
31. Yilmaz, V.; Oflazer, P.; Aysal, F.; Durmus, H.; Poulas, K.; Yentur, S.P.; Gulsen-Parman, Y.; Tzartos, S.; Marx, A.; Tuzun, E.; et al. Differential Cytokine Changes in Patients with Myasthenia Gravis with Antibodies against AChR and MuSK. *PLoS ONE* **2015**, *10*, e0123546. [CrossRef]
32. Baggi, F.; Antozzi, C.; Toscani, C.; Cordiglieri, C. Acetylcholine receptor-induced experimental myasthenia gravis: What have we learned from animal models after three decades? *Arch. Immunol. Ther. Exp.* **2012**, *60*, 19–30. [CrossRef] [PubMed]
33. Peña, G.; Cai, B.; Ramos, L.; Vida, G.; Deitch, E.A.; Ulloa, L. Cholinergic regulatory lymphocytes re-establish neuromodulation of innate immune responses in sepsis. *J. Immunol.* **2011**, *187*, 718–725. [CrossRef] [PubMed]
34. Wang, K.; Song, F. The Properties of Cytokines in Multiple Sclerosis: Pros and Cons. *Am. J. Med. Sci.* **2018**, *356*, 552–560. [CrossRef] [PubMed]
35. Reale, M.; Di Bari, M.; Di Nicola, M.; D'Angelo, C.; De Angelis, F.; Velluto, L.; Tata, A.M. Nicotinic receptor activation negatively modulates pro-inflammatory cytokine production in multiple sclerosis patients. *Int. Immunopharmacol.* **2015**, *29*, 152–157. [CrossRef] [PubMed]

36. D'Angelo, C.; Reale, M. IFN-β-Treatment and Canonical and Non-Traditional Cytokine Levels. *Front. Immunol.* **2018**, *9*, 1240. [CrossRef] [PubMed]
37. Báez-Pagán, C.A.; Delgado-Vélez, M. Activation of the Macrophage α7 Nicotinic Acetylcholine Receptor and Control of Inflammation. *J. Neuroimmune Pharmacol.* **2015**, *10*, 468–476. [CrossRef]
38. Marrosu, M.G.; Lai, M.; Cocco, E.; Loi, V.; Spinicci, G.; Pischedda, M.P.; Massole, S.; Marrosu, G.; Contu, P. Genetic factors and the founder effect explain familial MS in Sardinia. *Neurology* **2002**, *58*, 283–288. [CrossRef]
39. Kahana, E. Epidemiologic studies of multiple sclerosis: A review. *Biomed. Pharmacother.* **2000**, *54*, 100–112. [CrossRef]
40. Carton, H.; Vlietinck, R.; Debruyne, J.; De, K.J.; D'Hooghe, M.B.; Loos, R.; Medaer, R.; Truyen, L.; Yee, I.M.; Sadovnick, A.D. Risks of multiple sclerosis in relatives of patients in Flanders, Belgium. *J. Neurol. Neuros. Psych.* **1997**, *62*, 329–333. [CrossRef]
41. Miller, J.R. Esclerose múltipla. In *Tratado de Neurologia*, 10th ed.; Sociedad de Neurología: Santiago, Chile, 2002; pp. 670–686.
42. Buscarinu, M.C.; Fornasiero, A.; Ferraldeschi, M.; Romano, S.; Reniè, R.; Morena, E.; Romano, C.; Pellicciari, G.; Landi, A.C.; Fagnani, C.; et al. Disentangling the molecular mechanisms of multiple sclerosis: The contribution of twin studies. *Neurosci. Biobehav. Rev.* **2020**, *111*, 194–198. [CrossRef]
43. Hollenbach, J.A.; Oksenberg, J.R. The immunogenetics of multiple sclerosis: A comprehensive review. *J. Autoimmun.* **2015**, *64*, 13–25. [CrossRef] [PubMed]
44. Kallaur, A.P.; Kaimen-Maciel, D.R.; Morimoto, H.K.; Watanabe, M.A.; Georgeto, S.M.; Reiche, E.M. Genetic polymorphisms associated with the development and clinical course of multiple sclerosis. *Int. J. Mol. Med.* **2011**, *28*, 467–479. [PubMed]
45. Ben-David, Y.; Kagan, S.; Cohen Ben-Ami, H.; Rostami, J.; Mizrahi, T.; Kulkarni, A.R.; Thakur, G.A.; Vaknin-Dembinsky, A.; Healy, L.M.; Brenner, T.; et al. RIC3, the cholinergic anti-inflammatory pathway, and neuroinflammation. *Int. Immunopharmacol.* **2020**, *83*, 106381. [CrossRef] [PubMed]
46. Jasiecki, J.; Wasag, B. Butyrylcholinesterase Protein Ends in the Pathogenesis of Alzheimer's Disease-Could BCHE Genotyping Be Helpful in Alzheimer's Therapy. *Biomolecules* **2019**, *9*, 592. [CrossRef]
47. Jasiecki, J.; Limon-Sztencel, A.; Żuk, M.; Chmara, M.; Cysewski, D.; Limon, J.; Wasag, B. Synergy between the alteration in the N-terminal region of butyrylcholinesterase K variant and apolipoprotein E4 in late-onset Alzheimer's disease. *Sci. Rep.* **2019**, *9*, 5223. [CrossRef]
48. Scacchi, R.; Ruggeri, M.; Corbo, R.M. Variation of the butyrylcholinesterase (BChE) and acetylcholinesterase (AChE) genes in coronary artery disease. *Clin. Chim. Acta* **2011**, *412*, 1341–1344. [CrossRef]
49. Chen, Y.C.; Chou, W.H.; Fang, C.P.; Liu, T.H.; Tsou, H.H.; Wang, Y.; Liu, Y.L. Serum Level and Activity of Butylcholinesterase: A Biomarker for Post-Stroke Dementia. *J. Clin. Med.* **2019**, *8*, 1778. [CrossRef]
50. Lockridge, O.; Norgren, R.B., Jr.; Johnson, R.C.; Blake, T.A. Naturally Occurring Genetic Variants of Human Acetylcholinesterase and Butyrylcholinesterase and Their Potential Impact on the Risk of Toxicity from Cholinesterase Inhibitors. *Chem. Res. Toxicol.* **2016**, *29*, 1381–1392. [CrossRef]
51. Valle, A.M.; Radic, Z.; Rana, B.K.; Mahboubi, V.; Wessel, J.; Shih, P.A.; Rao, F.; O'Connor, D.T.; Taylor, P. Naturally occurring variations in the human cholinesterase genes: Heritability and association with cardiovascular and metabolic traits. *J. Pharmacol. Exp. Ther.* **2011**, *338*, 125–133. [CrossRef]
52. Santarpia, L.; Grandone, I.; Contaldo, F.; Pasanisi, F. Butyrylcholinesterase as a prognostic marker: A review of the literature. *J. Cachexia Sarcopenia Muscle* **2013**, *4*, 31–39. [CrossRef]
53. Dong, M.X.; Xu, X.M.; Hu, L.; Liu, Y.; Huang, Y.J.; Wei, Y.D. Serum Butyrylcholinesterase Activity: A Biomarker for Parkinson's Disease and Related Dementia. *BioMed. Res. Int.* **2017**, *2017*, 1524107. [CrossRef] [PubMed]
54. Oguri, M.; Kato, K.; Yokoi, K.; Yoshida, T.; Watanabe, S.; Metoki, N.; Yoshida, H.; Satoh, K.; Aoyagi, Y.; Tanaka, M.; et al. Association of a polymorphism of BCHE with ischemic stroke in Japanese individuals with chronic kidney disease. *Mol. Med. Rep.* **2009**, *2*, 779–785. [PubMed]
55. Reale, M.; Costantini, E.; Di Nicola, M.; D'Angelo, C.; Franchi, S.; D'Aurora, M.; Di Bari, M.; Orlando, V.; Galizia, S.; Ruggieri, S.; et al. Butyrylcholinesterase and Acetylcholinesterase polymorphisms in Multiple Sclerosis patients: Implication in peripheral inflammation. *Sci. Rep.* **2018**, *8*, 1319. [CrossRef] [PubMed]
56. Dyment, D.A.; Cader, M.Z.; Chao, M.J.; Lincoln, M.R.; Morrison, K.M.; Disanto, G.; Morahan, J.M.; De Luca, G.C.; Sadovnick, A.D.; Lepage, P.; et al. Exome sequencing identifies a novel multiple sclerosis susceptibility variant in the TYK2 gene. *Neurology* **2012**, *79*, 406–411. [CrossRef]

57. Ramagopalan, S.V.; Dyment, D.A.; Cader, M.Z.; Morrison, K.M.; Disanto, G.; Morahan, J.M.; Berlanga-Taylor, A.J.; Handel, A.; de Luca, G.C.; Sadovnick, D.P.A.D.; et al. Rare variants in the CYP27B1 gene are associated with multiple sclerosis. *Ann. Neurol.* **2011**, *70*, 881–886. [CrossRef]
58. Jamebozorgi, K.; Rostami, D.; Pormasoumi, H.; Taghizadeh, E.; Barreto, G.E.; Sahebkar, A. Epigenetic aspects of multiple sclerosis and future therapeutic options. *Int. J. Neurosci.* **2020**, 1–15. [CrossRef]
59. Waubant, E.; Lucas, R.; Mowry, E.; Graves, J.; Olsson, T.; Alfredsson, L.; Langer-Gould, A. Environmental and genetic risk factors for MS: An integrated review. *Ann. Clin. Transl. Neurol.* **2019**, *9*, 1905–1922. [CrossRef]
60. Swanborg, R.H. Experimental autoimmune encephalomyelitis in rodents as a model for human demyelinating disease. *Clin. Immunol. Immunopathol.* **1995**, *77*, 4–13. [CrossRef]
61. Brown, D.A.; Sawchenko, P.E. Time course and distribution of inflammatory and neurodegenerative events suggest structural bases for the pathogenesis of experimental autoimmune encephalomyelitis. *J. Comp. Neurol.* **2007**, *502*, 236–260. [CrossRef]
62. Soulika, A.M.; Lee, E.; McCauley, E.; Miers, L.; Bannerman, P.; Pleasure, D. Initiation and progression of axonopathy in experimental autoimmune encephalomyelitis. *J. Neurosci.* **2009**, *29*, 14965–14979. [CrossRef]
63. Di Pinto, G.; Di Bari, M.; Martin-Alvarez, R.; Sperduti, S.; Serrano-Acedo, S.; Gatta, V.; Tata, A.M.; Mengod, G. Comparative study of the expression of cholinergic system components in the CNS of experimental autoimmune encephalomyelitis mice: Acute vs. remitting phase. *Eur. J. Neurosci.* **2018**, *48*, 2165–2181. [CrossRef] [PubMed]
64. Wright, C.I.; Geula, C.; Mesulam, M.M. Neuroglial cholinesterases in the normal brain and in Alzheimer's disease: Relationship to plaques, tangles, and patterns of selective vulnerability. *Ann. Neurol.* **1993**, *34*, 373–384. [CrossRef] [PubMed]
65. Jiang, W.; St Pierre, S.; Roy, P.; Morley, B.J.; Hao, J.; Simard, A.R. Infiltration of CCR2+Ly6Chigh Proinflammatory Monocytes and Neutrophils into the Central Nervous System Is Modulated by Nicotinic Acetylcholine Receptors in a Model of Multiple Sclerosis. *J. Immunol.* **2016**, *196*, 2095–2108. [CrossRef] [PubMed]
66. Taveggia, C.; Feltri, M.L.; Wrabetz, L. Signals to promote myelin formation and repair. *Nat. Rev. Neurol.* **2010**, *6*, 276–287. [CrossRef] [PubMed]
67. Karadottir, R.; Attwell, D. Neurotrasmitter receptors in the life and death of oligodendrocytes. *Neuroscience* **2007**, *145*, 1426–1438. [CrossRef] [PubMed]
68. Corsetti, V.; Mozzetta, C.; Biagioni, S.; Augusti Tocco, G.; Tata, A.M. Acetylcholine release: The mechanisms and the site of release during chick dorsal root ganglia ontogenesis. *Life Sci.* **2012**, *91*, 783–788. [CrossRef]
69. Bernardini, N.; Srubek Tomassy, G.; Tata, A.M.; Augusti Tocco, G.; Biagioni, S. Detection of basal and potassium-evoked acetylcholine release from embryonic DRG explants. *J. Neurochem.* **2004**, *88*, 1533–1539. [CrossRef]
70. Jamebozorgi, K.; Rostami, D.; Pormasoumi, H.; Taghizadeh, E.; Barreto, G.E.; Sahebkar, A. Cholinergic signaling in myelination. *Glia* **2017**, *65*, 687–698.
71. Magnaghi, V.; Procacci, P.; Tata, A.M. Novel pharmacological approaches to Schwann cells as neuroprotective agents for peripheral nerve regeneration. *Int. Rev. Neurobiol.* **2009**, *87*, 295–315.
72. Larocca, J.N.; Almazan, G. Acetylcholine Agonists Stimulate Mitogen-Activated Protein Kinase in Oligodendrocyte Progenitors by Muscarinic Receptors. *J. Neurosci. Res.* **1997**, *50*, 743–754. [CrossRef]
73. Ragheb, F.; Molina-Holgado, E.; Cui, Q.L.; Khorchid, A.; Liu, H.N.; Larocca, J.N.; Almazan, G. Pharmacological and functional characterization of muscarinic receptor subtypes in developing oligodendrocytes. *J. Neurochem.* **2001**, *77*, 1396–1406. [CrossRef] [PubMed]
74. Molina-Holgado, E.; Khorchid, A.; Liu, H.; Almazan, G. Regulation of muscarinic receptor function in developing oligodendrocytes by agonist exposure. *Br. J. Pharmacol.* **2003**, *138*, 47–56. [CrossRef] [PubMed]
75. De Angelis, F.; Bernardo, A.; Magnaghi, V.; Minghetti, L.; Tata, A.M. Muscarinic receptor subtypes as potential targets to modulate oligodendrocyte progenitor survival, proliferation and differentiation. *Dev. Neurobiol.* **2012**, *72*, 713–728. [CrossRef] [PubMed]
76. Deshmukh, V.A.; Tardif, V.; Lyssiotis, C.A.; Green, C.C.; Kerman, B.; Kim, H.J.; Padmanabhan, K.; Swoboda, J.G.; Ahmad, I.; Kondo, T.; et al. The regenerative approaches for the treatment of multiple sclerosis. *Nature* **2013**, *502*, 327–332. [CrossRef] [PubMed]

77. Thompson, K.K.; Nissen, J.C.; Pretory, A.; Tsirka, S.E. Tuftis combines with remyelinating therapy and improves outcomes in models of CNS demyelinating disease. *Front. Immunol.* **2018**, *9*, 2784. [CrossRef] [PubMed]
78. Hertz, L.; Schousboe, I.; Hertz, L.; Schousboe, A. Receptor expression in primary cultures of neurons or astrocytes. *Prog Neuropsychopharmacol. Biol. Psych.* **1984**, *8*, 521–527. [CrossRef]
79. Lykhmus, O.; Voytenko, L.P.; Lips, K.S.; Bergen, I.; Krasteva-Christ, G.; Vetter, D.E.; Kummer, W.; Skok, M. Nicotinic acetylcholine receptor α9 and α10 subunits are express in the brain of mice. *Front. Cell Neurosci.* **2017**, *11*, 282. [CrossRef]
80. Zhang, X.; Lao, K.; Qiu, Z.; Rahman, M.S.; Zhang, Y.; Gou, X. Potential Astrocytic receptors and transporters in the pathogenesis of Alzheimer's disease. *J. Alzheimers Dis.* **2019**, *67*, 1109–1122. [CrossRef]
81. Kume, T.; Takada-Takatori, Y. Nicotinic acetylcholine receptor signaling: Roles in neuroprotection. In *Nicotinic Acetylcholine Receptor Signaling in Neuroprotection*; Akaike, A., Shimohama, S., Misu, Y., Eds.; Springer: Singapore, 2018.
82. Zhang, L.; McLarnon, J.G.; Goghari, V.; Lee, Y.B.; Kim, S.U.; Krieger, C. Cholinergic agonists increase intracellular Ca2+ in cultured human microglia. *Neurosci. Lett.* **1998**, *255*, 33–36. [CrossRef]
83. Pannell, M.; Meier, M.A.; Szulzewsky, F.; Matyash, V.; Endres, M.; Kronenberg, G.; Prinz, V.; Waiczies, S.; Wolf, S.A.; Kettenmann, H. The subpopulation of microglia expressing functional muscarinic acetylcholine receptors expands in stroke and Alzheimer's disease. *Brain Struct. Funct.* **2016**, *221*, 1157–1172. [CrossRef]
84. Shytle, R.D.; Mori, T.; Townsend, K.; Vendrame, M.; Sun, N.; Zeng, J.; Ehrhart, J.; Silver, A.A.; Sanberg, P.R.; Tan, J. Cholinergic modulation of microglial activation by a7 nicotinic receptors. *J. Neurochem.* **2004**, *89*, 337–343. [CrossRef] [PubMed]
85. Ke, P.; Shao, B.Z.; Xu, Z.Q.; Chen, X.W.; Wei, W.; Liu, C. Activation of α7 nicotinic acetylcholine receptor inhibits NLRP3 inflammasome through reulation of β-arrestin. *Neurosci. Ther.* **2017**, *23*, 875–884. [CrossRef] [PubMed]
86. De Simone, R.; Ajimone-Cat, M.A.; Carnevale, D.; Minghetti, L. Activation of α7 nicotinic acetylcholine receptor by nicotine selectively upregulates ciclooxygenase 2 and prostaglandin E2 in rat microglial cultures. *J. Neuroinflamm.* **2005**, *2*, 1–10. [CrossRef] [PubMed]
87. Egea, J.; Buendia, I.; Parada, E.; Navarro, E.; Leon, R.; Lopea, M.G. Anty inflammatory role of microglia α7 nAChRs and its role in neuroprotection. *Biochem. Pharmacol.* **2015**, *97*, 463–472. [CrossRef]
88. Nicoletti, C.G.; Landi, D.; Monteleone, F.; Mataluni, G.; Albanese, M.; Lauretti, B.; Rocchi, C.; Simonelli, I.; Boffa, L.; Buttari, F.; et al. Treatment with Dimethyl Fumarate Enhances Cholinergic Transmission in Multiple Sclerosis. *CNS Drugs* **2019**, *33*, 1133–1139. [CrossRef]

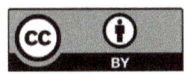

© 2020 by the authors. Licensee MDPI, Basel, Switzerland. This article is an open access article distributed under the terms and conditions of the Creative Commons Attribution (CC BY) license (http://creativecommons.org/licenses/by/4.0/).

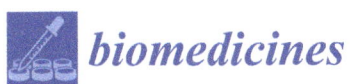

Article

PBMC of Multiple Sclerosis Patients Show Deregulation of OPA1 Processing Associated with Increased ROS and PHB2 Protein Levels

Domenico De Rasmo [1,*], Anna Ferretta [2], Silvia Russo [2], Maddalena Ruggieri [2], Piergiorgio Lasorella [2], Damiano Paolicelli [2], Maria Trojano [2] and Anna Signorile [2,*]

1 CNR-Institute of Biomembranes, Bioenergetics and Molecular Biotechnologies, 70126 Bari, Italy
2 Department of Basic Medical Sciences, Neurosciences and Sense Organs, University of Bari "Aldo Moro", 70124 Bari, Italy; anna.ferretta@uniba.it (A.F.); silvia.russo92@gmail.com (S.R.); maddalena.ruggieri@uniba.it (M.R.); p.lasorella@studenti.uniba.it (P.L.); damiano.paolicelli@uniba.it (D.P.); maria.trojano@uniba.it (M.T.)
* Correspondence: d.derasmo@ibiom.cnr.it (D.D.R.); anna.signorile@uniba.it (A.S.); Tel.: +39-080-547-8529 (D.D.R. & A.S.)

Received: 23 March 2020; Accepted: 10 April 2020; Published: 11 April 2020

Abstract: Multiple sclerosis (MS) is an autoimmune disease in which activated lymphocytes affect the central nervous system. Increase of reactive oxygen species (ROS), impairment of mitochondria-mediated apoptosis and mitochondrial alterations have been reported in peripheral lymphocytes of MS patients. Mitochondria-mediated apoptosis is regulated by several mechanisms and proteins. Among others, optic atrophy 1 (OPA1) protein plays a key role in the regulating mitochondrial dynamics, cristae architecture and release of pro-apoptotic factors. Very interesting, mutations in OPA1 gene, have been associated with multiple sclerosis-like disorder. We have analyzed OPA1 and some factors involved in its regulation. Fifteen patients with MS and fifteen healthy control subjects (HC) were enrolled into the study and peripheral blood mononuclear cells (PBMCs) were isolated. H_2O_2 level was measured spectrofluorimetrically, OPA1, PHB2, SIRT3, and OMA1 were analyzed by western blotting. Statistical analysis was performed using Student's t-test. The results showed that PBMC of MS patients were characterized by a deregulation of OPA1 processing associated with increased H_2O_2 production, inactivation of OMA1 and increase of PHB2 protein level. The presented data suggest that the alteration of PHB2, OMA1, and OPA1 processing could be involved in resistance towards apoptosis. These molecular parameters could also be useful to assess disease activity.

Keywords: multiple sclerosis; PBMCs; mitochondria; ROS; OPA1; PHB2; OMA1

1. Introduction

Multiple sclerosis (MS) is a complex neurodegenerative disease that involves immune and central nervous system (CNS) [1,2]. MS is expressed in different clinical forms including primary progressive (PP), secondary progressive (SP), progressive relapsing (RP) and relapsing-remitting (RR), which is the most prevalent form [3]. The pathogenesis of MS involves the loss of blood–brain barrier integrity with the consequent invasion of lymphocytes into the CNS resulting in tissue damage [4].

Despite the knowledge of genetics, cell biology and immunology, obtained in the last years, the ultimate etiology or specific elements that trigger MS remain unknown. The etiopathogenesis and pathophysiology of MS involves different factors, among others mitochondrial dysfunction and oxidative stress (OS) play a key role and have a further modulatory effect on many aspects of the disease. OS plays an important role in activation of immune cells, especially T cells [5–7], and recently it has been reported that peripheral blood mononuclear cells (PBMCs) of MS patients show impaired redox status associated with mitochondrial alterations [5]. A number of mechanisms participate in the maintenance of the immune homeostasis avoiding the development of autoimmune diseases. The apoptosis is an important anti-autoimmune process that deletes potentially pathogenic autoreactive lymphocytes, limiting the immune response-dependent tissue damage [8,9]. It has been shown that deletion of autoreactive lymphocytes by apoptosis is defective in patients with MS, thereby permitting these cells to perpetuate a continuous cycle of inflammation within the CNS [10,11]. In particular, the impairment of mitochondria-mediated apoptosis in Cd4+ T lymphocytes [12], as well as, a reduction of mitochondrial respiration are reported in MS patients [13]. Mitochondria have a main role in both cell death and life and they are a major source of reactive oxygen species (ROS) production. At the same time, mitochondria are responsive to OS and are critical in modulating apoptosis in response themselves to a variety of stress signals.

Several mitochondria parameters such as mitochondrial respiratory chain activity, ROS production, dynamics (fusion and fission), and mitochondria cristae architecture are involved in mitochondria-mediated apoptosis [14–16]. Among mitochondrial proteins involved in apoptosis mechanism, optic atrophy 1 (OPA1) is a mitochondrial dynamin like GTPase that has attracted great attention for its role in the regulating mitochondrial fusion and fission, the stability of the mitochondrial respiratory chain complexes, pro-apoptotic cytochrome c release and the maintenance of mitochondrial cristae architecture [17]. Very interesting, it is reported that mutations in OPA1 gene, resulting in autosomal dominant optic atrophy (ADOA), are associated with multiple sclerosis-like disorder in patients [18].

OPA1 undergoes constitutive processing leading to the conversion of the un-cleaved long OPA1 (L-OPA1) in a cleaved short OPA1 (S-OPA1) forms. Various stress conditions, including apoptotic stimulation are associated with the conversion of L-OPA1 into S-OPA1. The processing and activity of OPA1 is regulated by mitochondrial proteases, such as OMA1, cellular energetic condition [19], post-translational modification, such as acetylation status [20,21], and oxidative stress [20,22]. OMA1-mediated processing of OPA1 is a cellular stress response, in fact, although OMA1 is constitutively active, it display strongly enhanced activity in response to OS [23]. Furthermore, OPA1 stability is controlled by prohibitin 2 (PHB2) [24] a chaperon like protein, localizes in nucleus, plasma membrane, and mitochondria. Evidences indicate that mitochondrial PHB2 is over expressed under conditions of oxidative stress [25]. Interesting, PHB2 has been found up-regulated in lymphocytes of MS patients [26]. OPA1 processing is also modulated by its acetylation status mediated by SIRT3 enzyme, a mitochondrial deacetylase that also plays an important role in apoptosis [20]. In this work we have analyzed the protein level, and proteolytic processing of OPA1 and its stress-associated regulators, OMA1, SIRT3, and PHB2 in PBMCs of MS patients.

2. Experimental Section

2.1. Patients

Fifteen patients with MS according to McDonald criteria [27] and fifteen healthy volunteers control subjects (HC) were enrolled into the study. The patients and HC subjects were selected by the Centre of Multiple Sclerosis at Department of Basic Medical Sciences Neurosciences and Sense Organs, University of Bari. All patients had to be without any immunomodulatory treatment at least 6 months prior to study entry. All subjects gave their informed consent for inclusion before they participated in the study. The study was conducted in accordance with the Declaration of Helsinki and the protocol was approved by the Ethics Committee of Azienda Policlinico di Bari (Project identification code 5275). Table 1 reports demographic and clinical characteristics of MS patients and healthy subjects. For all data, no significant difference was observed between males and females as well as between RR and SP forms of MS.

Table 1. Demographic and clinical characteristics of patients with multiple sclerosis (MS) and healthy control subjects (HC) enrolled into the study. (SP: secondary progressive, RR: relapsing-remitting, EDSS: Expanded Disability Status Scale, SEM: standard error of mean.

	MS	HC
Subject (number)	15	15
Age (year)	45 ± 2.46 SEM	44.92 ± 3.92 SEM
Gender	12 Females 3 Males	6 Females 9 Males
MS form	11 RR 4 SP	
Disease duration(year)	14.4 ± 1.70 SEM	
EDSS	4.2 ± 0.34 SEM	

2.2. Sample Preparation

Peripheral blood mononuclear cells (PBMCs) were isolated from K3-EDTA blood by centrifugation on a Ficoll-Hypaque density gradient (density: 1.077 g/mL; Amersham Pharmacia Biotech, Buckinghamshire, UK), washed twice and resuspended in PBS. Total protein concentration was determined by Bio Rad protein assay.

2.3. Electrophoretic Procedures and Western Blotting

Protein of PBMCs were resuspended in RIPA lysis buffer, separated by 7.5% SDS-polyacrylamide gel electrophoresis (PAGE) and transferred into a nitrocellulose membrane. The membrane was blocked with 5% fatty acid free dry milk in 500 mM NaCl, 0.05% Tween 20, 20 mM Tris, pH 7.4 (TTBS) for 3 h at 4 °C and probed over night with antibodies against OPA1 (whole molecule of OPA1 protein was used as the immunogen) (Thermo scientific, Pierce Antibodies, Lausanne, Switzerland), PHB2 (Invitrogen, Paisley, UK), OMA1, SIRT3 (Cell Signalling, Danvers, MA, USA) and β-actin (Sigma-Aldrich, St. Louis, MO, USA). After being washed in TTBS, the membranes were incubated for 60 min with anti-rabbit or anti-mouse IgG peroxidase-conjugated. Immunodetection was then performed, after further TTBS washes, with the enhanced chemiluminescence (ECL) (Euroclone, Paignton, UK). Densitometric analysis, expressed as arbitrary densitometric units (ADU), electrophoretic profile and relative front (Rf) determinations were performed by Image Lab Touch 2.4 software (BioRad, Milan, Italy). Rf indicates the relative movement of the band from the top.

2.4. H_2O_2 Assay

H_2O_2 level was determined by the cell permeant probe 2′-7′-dichlorodihydrofluorescin diacetate (DCFDA). PBMCs were incubated with 10 µM DCFDA in the dark at 37 °C for 20 min, pelleted at 600× g for 5 min, washed and resuspended in the assay buffer (100 mM potassium phosphate, pH 7.4, 2 mM $MgCl_2$). An aliquot was used for protein determination. The H_2O_2 dependent oxidation of the fluorescent probe (507 nm excitation and 530 nm emission wavelengths) was measured by a Jasco FP6200 spectrofluorimeter (Jasco SRL, Cremella, Italy).

2.5. Data Analysis

All presented data are means ± standard error of mean (SEM). Statistical difference was determined by Student' t-test. p-value of 0.05 was considered as statistically significant (*** $p < 0.001$; ** $p < 0.01$; * $p < 0.05$).

Correlation plots for controls and MS have been performing with Excel Microsoft software using Pearson's correlation analysis. P-values less than 0.05 were considered statistically significant.

3. Results

Fifteen HC and fifteen MS subjects (see Table 1) were enrolled in the study. The patients group included 12 females and 3 males and 11 RR forms and 4 SP forms of MS (see Table 1). The PBMC cellular lysate was used to investigate on the OPA1 protein level and processing by Western blotting analysis using a specific antibody (Figure 1).

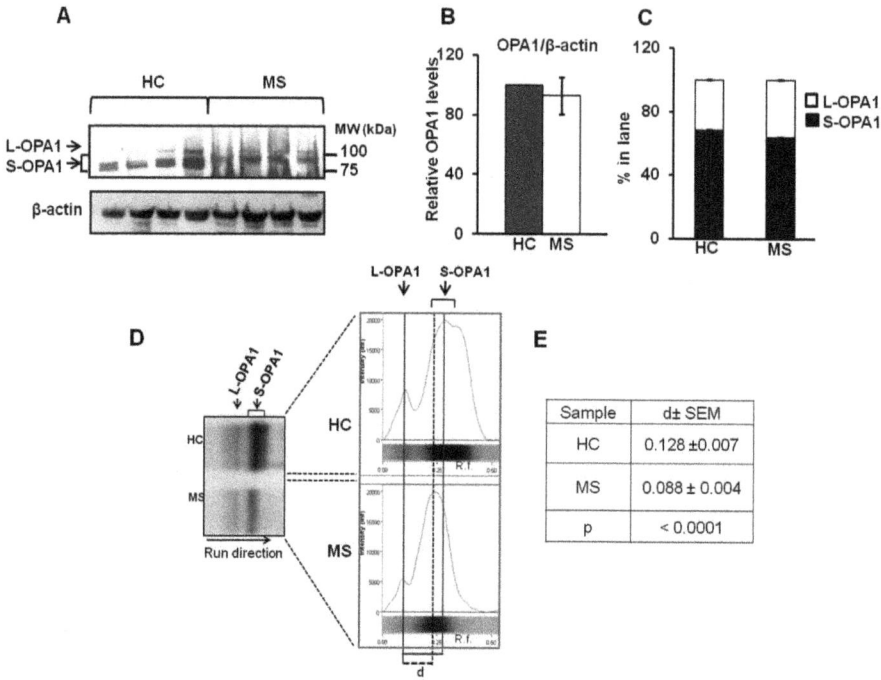

Figure 1. Optic atrophy 1 (OPA1) protein level and processing in peripheral blood mononuclear cells (PBMCs) from HC and MS patients. (**A**) Representative images of western blotting analysis. The PBMC proteins from HC and MS were loaded on 7.5% SDS-PAGE. After separation, the proteins were transferred on nitrocellulose membranes and immunoblotted with the antibody against OPA1. Protein loading was assessed with β-actin antibody. (**B**) The total protein level of OPA1 (L+S forms) was evaluated by densitometric analysis. The arbitrary densitometric units (ADU) of OPA1 were normalized to ADU of β-actin and the mean of HC set to 100%. The histograms represent the percentage values MS patients with respect to HC. The values are means ± SEM of different samples. (**C**) The histograms represent the percentage of ADU of long (L) and short (S), forms of OPA1 in each lane. The values are means ± SEM of samples. (**D**) Left panel, representative image of electrophoretic mobility of immune-revealed bands of OPA1 in PBMCs from HC and MS. Right panel, the images of the western blotting were analyzed by Image Lab Touch 2.4 software (BioRAD) for determination of electrophoretic profile of each lane and calculation of relative front (Rf) of L-OPA1 and S-OPA1 bands (see Table S1). Rf indicates the relative movement of the band from the top of the gel. "d" represents the difference between Rf of S-OPA1 and Rf of L-OPA1 in each lane. (**E**) The table reports the means values of "d" ± SEM of different samples. ($p < 0.001$, Student's t-test).

The antibody against OPA1 protein, immuno-revealed in both HC and MS groups a long form (L) and short forms (S) of OPA1 (Figure 1A). Densitometric analysis of immuno-revealed bands of OPA1 (L+S) showed the same level of total OPA1protein in MS group with respect to HC (Figure 1B). No difference was observed in percentage of L and S form of OPA1 between HC and SM samples

(Figure 1C). Interestingly, the image analysis of western blotting revealed two bands of S-OPA1 in HC and one band of S-OPA1with a different electrophoretic mobility with respect to HC samples in MS (Figure 1A,D). Analysis by Image Lab Touch 2.4 software confirmed the presence of two S-OPA1 bands in HC and one S-OPA1 band in MS as shown by curve peaks (Figure 1D). Moreover, the determination of Rf of L-OPA1 and S-OPA1 bands revealed a significant decrease in Rf of S-OPA1 in MS sample with respect to HC (see Table S1). No differences were observed in Rf of L-OPA1 between HC and MS samples (Table S1). Calculation of difference between Rf of S-OPA1 band and L-OPA1 band in each lane ("d"), revealed a significant decrease of "d" in MS samples with respect to HC (Figure 1D,E). This suggested that processing of OPA1, in MS samples, generated a S-OPA1 form at a higher molecular weight with respect to HC.

Processing of OPA1 is regulated by different proteins and cellular conditions such as oxidative stress. Measurement of H_2O_2 level, detected by the redox-sensitive fluorescent probe DCFDA, showed increased ROS production in the PBMCs of MS patients compared to HC (Figure 2).

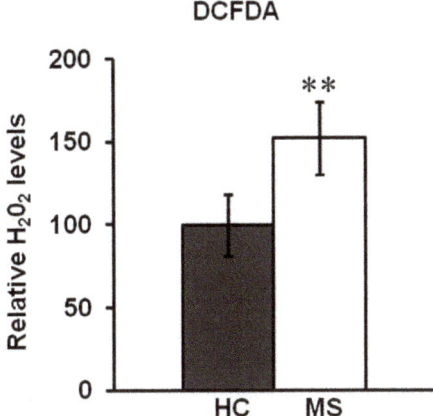

Figure 2. H_2O_2 production in PBMC of HC and MS patients. H_2O_2 level was detected spectrofluorimetrically by dichlorodihydrofluorescin (DCFDA) probe. The mean of HC was set to 100% and the mean value of MS expressed as percentage of intensity of fluorescence respect to HC. The histograms represent the means of values ± SEM. (** $p < 0.01$; Student's t-test).

This result prompted to investigate on stress regulated protein OMA1, PHB2 and SIRT3 that are involved in OPA1 processing and stabilization [20,22,25]. Activation of OMA1 protease is accompanied by its autocatalytic degradation that results in the complete turnover of protein [22]. Western blotting analysis of OMA1 did not show the activation of this protease in PBMCs from MS samples as revealed by the increased ratio between inactive and active forms (Figure 3A,B). We next examined PHB2 level by western blot analysis with specific antibody. An increased PHB2 protein level was observed in MS patients (Figure 3C,D) compared to HC samples, while no difference was observed for SIRT3 protein level (Figure 3C,D).

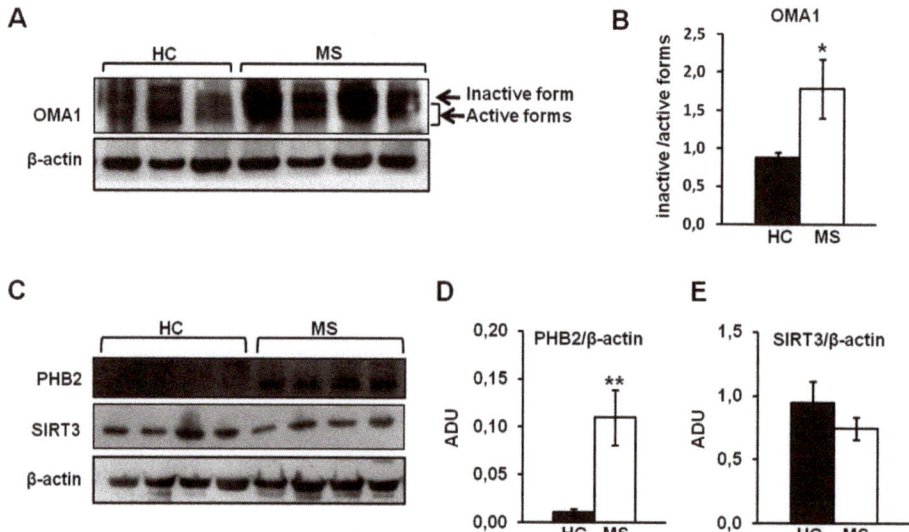

Figure 3. OMA1, SIRT3, and PHB2 in PBMCs of HC and MS patients. (**A,C**) Representative images of Western blotting analysis. Proteins from PBMC from HC and MS were loaded on 7.5% SDS-PAGE. After separation, the proteins were transferred on nitrocellulose membranes and immunoblotted with the antibodies against OMA1, SIRT3, and PHB2. Protein loading was assessed with β-actin antibody. The immunoblotting against β-actin in panel C is the same shown in the Figure 1A, belonging to the same experiment series (**B,D**). (**B**) The histograms represent the means of ratio values ± SEM between the ADU of inactive and active forms of OMA1 in HC and MS subjects. (**D,E**) The ADU of PHB2 and SIRT3 were normalized to ADU of β-actin. The histograms represent the means of values of ADU ± SEM of samples. (* $p < 0.05$, ** $p < 0.01$; Student's t-test).

To explore whether the alterations in the analyzed molecular parameters can cross correlate with each other, a correlation analysis was performed for HC and MS groups. The results in HC indicated a remarkable positive correlation of SIRT3 changes with changes of L- and S-OPA1 balance. This correlation was lost in MS group. In addition, in MS group, a significant positive correlation was observed between H_2O_2 level and PHB2 (Figure 4B), and negative correlations between H_2O_2 and L- and S-OPA1 balance (Figure 4C) and between PHB2 and L- and S-OPA1 balance (Figure 4D).

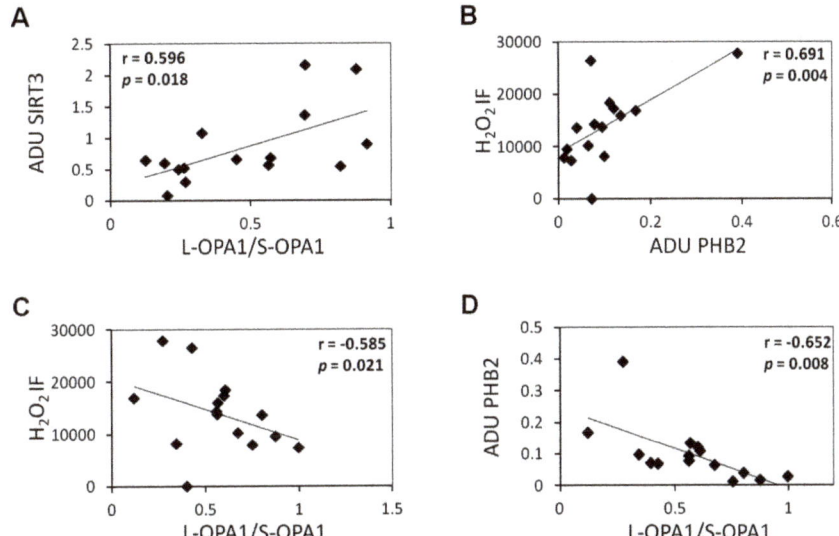

Figure 4. Correlation plots. Empty squares indicates HC group, full squares indicates MS group (**A**) Scatter plot and linear regression of data of relationship between SIRT3 protein level, expressed in ADU, and L-OPA1/S-OPA1 balance in HC group (correlation coefficient, r = 0.596; P, 0.021). (**B**) Scatter plot and linear regression of data of relationship between H_2O_2, expressed in intensity of fluorescence (IF), and PHB2 protein level, expressed in ADU in MS group (correlation coefficient, r = −0.691; P, 0.004). (**C**) Scatter plot and linear regression of data of relationship between H_2O_2 and L-OPA1/S-OPA1 balance in MS group (correlation coefficient r = −0.585, P,0.021). (**D**) Scatter plot and linear regression of data of relationship between PHB2 protein expression and cleaved long OPA1 (L-OPA1)/cleaved short OPA1 (S-OPA1) balance in MS group (correlation coefficient, r = −0.652; P = 0.008). Degree of freedom 13.

4. Discussion

The pathogenesis of MS involves autoreactive T lymphocytes that have the capacity to invade the CNS causing demyelization and axonal damage [4]. The deletion of autoreactive lymphocytes is normally mediated by apoptosis, however, an escape from mitochondria-mediated apoptosis has been reported in lymphocytes of MS patients [12]. Mitochondria from MS lymphocytes also show a decrease of mitochondrial respiration [13] associated with a specific decrease of complex I and complex IV activities [28], and, of note, mitochondria have been found to range in shape and size and showed thickened cristae [29]. Mitochondrial dependent apoptosis is also depending on mitochondrial respiration, shape and structure. A growing body of evidence suggests that OPA1 participates through several mechanisms in defining mitochondrial shape and structure of cristae [14] and modulating mitochondrial respiration [17]. This modulates cell susceptibility towards apoptotic stimuli [14]. Augmented level of OPA1, formation of OPA1 oligomers and a correct balance of L and S forms are considered anti-apoptotic factors [17]. In light of this and the data reporting that OPA1 mutations are associated with multiple sclerosis-like symptoms [18], in this work, we analyzed OPA1 and its modulators in PBMCs of MS patients compared to HC. Fifteen healthy controls and fifteen subjects affected by MS were enrolled in the study. The patients group included 12 females and 3 males and 11 RR forms and 4 SP forms of MS (see Table 1). No significant difference was observed between males and females subjects as well as between RR and SP forms.

Our results showed the same level of OPA1 total protein (L+S) in HC and SM samples and no differences were observed in the balance between L and S forms of OPA1 in PBMC of HC and MS patients. Interesting the analysis of the electrophoretic migration of immune-revealed bands of OPA1 in lymphocytes of MS samples showed only one S-form at a higher molecular weight in MS with respect to the two S forms observed in HC, thus suggesting a characteristic processing of OPA1 in MS samples. The functions of OPA1 are regulated, under stress conditions, by OMA1-dependent proteolytic cleavage. As expected PBMCs of MS patients show increased level of ROS that, anyway, not results in the activation of stress-induced OMA1 [22], as shown by the accumulation of inactive form of OMA1, thus suggesting an adaptation to exposure at chronic OS. Of note, it was reported that suppression of OMA1 activity strongly prevented cytochrome c release into the cytosol [30] and cells lacking the protease OMA1 showed an increased resistance to external apoptotic stimuli [31,32]. OPA1, beyond the proteolytic control, is also under the control of alternative splicing. Eight different OPA1 isoforms, generated by alternative splicing of four exons near the amino terminus (Figure S1), are characterized for the presence, or absence, of at least three different proteolytic cleavage sites, named S1, S2, and S3 [33]. The S1 site is cleaved by OMA1 while S2 and S3 by Ymel1 protease. The presence of isoform 3, which contains S3 and S1 cleavage sites (see Figure S1), together with the inactivation of OMA1 protease (see also [32]), could explain the shift of electrophoretic mobility observed in MS patients. Although YME1L and OMA1 constitutively control OPA1, the proteolytic processing of OPA1 is more complex, in fact, other proteases can act on OPA1 under particular stress condition or metabolic demands [33,34], thus, the involvement of other mitochondrial proteases cannot be ruled out. In this contest, should be noted that, in MS, several proteases are involved [35,36] and that mitochondrial proteases are often involved in the pathogenesis of neurological diseases [37].

It has been reported that SIRT3 has an important role in a variety of oxidative stress-mediated cellular responses [38], in the regulation of bioenergetic function and antioxidant defense of mitochondria under OS conditions [39]. OS regulated SIRT3 protein level that, in turn, is involved in mitochondrial apoptosis by modulating OPA1 acetylation/processing [20]. In particular, sustained level of SIRT3 protein favors the apoptosis resistance, while a decrease promotes cell death [20]. We have also investigated on SIRT3 protein level; however, despite the increased ROS production in MS, no difference has been observed in MS lymphocytes compared to HC samples. Although the SIRT3 protein level was unchanged, this could be interpreted as a loss of response of lymphocytes of MS patients to OS. The data on SIRT3 and OMA1 suggest a deregulation of normally stress response mechanisms of these proteins in PBMCs of MS patients.

Furthermore, OPA1 processing and stability is also controlled by PHB2 protein. In mitochondrial inner membrane, PHB2 protein forms with PHB1 a large membrane-bound complex [40,41]. This complex is required for OPA1 stability [42], indeed the deletion of PHB2 leads to the impaired cellular proliferation, aberrant mitochondrial cristae morphogenesis, and apoptosis [24,42], while an over-expression of PHB2 is reported to protect cells from apoptosis [43]. We show, according with others [26] and as response to OS [25], a strong increase of PHB2 protein level in MS samples, thus representing another element of resistance to apoptosis. It worth mentioning that an elevated autophagic flux has been reported in autoreactive T cells, both in patients and in the mouse model of experimental autoimmune encephalomyelitis [44]. It has been found that PHB2 participates in the mitophagy process (selective autophagy) by functioning as mitochondrial receptor in autophagosome formation [45].

Interestingly, using Pearson's correlation analysis, we found a positive correlation in HC group between SIRT3 changes and changes of L- and S-OPA1 balance. This is in agreement with the findings showing that the SIRT3-dependent deacetylation of L-OPA1 inhibits its proteolytic processing to form S-OPA1 [20]. This correlation was lost in the MS group, while changes of L- and S-OPA1 balance, PHB2 protein level and H_2O_2 correlated each other. In facts, under condition of oxidative stress, an increased cleavage of L-OPA1 to produce S-OPA1 has been observed [20] as well as an increase of PHB2 expression [25]. The over expression of PHB2 has been found to protect the cell from oxidative stress-dependent apoptosis [43].

5. Conclusions

Our data showed that, in PBMCs of MS patients, oxidative stress is associated with increased level of PHB2 and stabilization of OMA1. We propose that the alteration of PHB2, OMA1, and OPA1 is involved in the apoptosis resistance. We hypothesize involvement of specific proteolytic processing of OPA1 in lymphocytes of MS patients. Other investigations will be needed to define the mechanisms at the bases of this deregulations and the possible proteases involved in the characteristic processing of OPA1 in MS samples. The specific OPA1 electrophoretic profile and an increased level of PHB2 in MS patients could also be taken in account to assess disease activity. Understanding of the molecular mechanisms underlying these deregulations could shed light on new therapeutic interventions.

Supplementary Materials: The following are available online at http://www.mdpi.com/2227-9059/8/4/85/s1.

Author Contributions: Conceptualization, A.S. and D.D.R.; methodology, A.S. and D.D.R.; software, A.S. and D.D.R.; validation, A.S. and D.D.R.; formal analysis, A.S. and D.D.R.; resources, M.R., P.L., D.P., M.T.; data curation, A.S., D.D.R., A.F., S.R., M.R., D.P.; writing—original draft preparation, A.S. and D.D.R.; writing—review and editing, A.S., D.D.R., M.T., A.F., S.R., M.R., D.P.; supervision, A.S. and D.D.R.; project administration, A.S. and D.D.R.; funding acquisition, A.S. All authors have read and agreed to the published version of the manuscript.

Funding: This research was funded by University of Bari to Anna Signorile, project title "Regolazione dei sistemi redox e bioenergetici cellulari in condizioni fisio-patologiche".

Conflicts of Interest: The authors declare no conflict of interest.

References

1. Tobore, T.O. Towards a comprehensive etiopathogenetic and pathophysiological theory of multiple sclerosis. *Int. J. Neurosci.* **2020**, *130*, 279–300. [CrossRef]
2. Lassmann, H.; Brück, W.; Lucchinetti, C.F. The immunopathology of multiple sclerosis: An overview. *Brain Pathol.* **2007**, *17*, 210–218. [CrossRef]
3. Loma, I.; Heyman, R. Multiple sclerosis: Pathogenesis and treatment. *Curr. Neuropharmacol.* **2011**, *9*, 409–416. [CrossRef]
4. Sospedra, M.; Martin, R. Immunology of multiple sclerosis. *Annu. Rev. Immunol.* **2005**, *23*, 683–747. [CrossRef]
5. Gonzalo, H.; Nogueras, L.; Gil-Sánchez, A.; Hervás, J.V.; Valcheva, P.; González-Mingot, C.; Martin-Gari, M.; Canudes, M.; Peralta, S.; Solana, M.J.; et al. Impairment of Mitochondrial Redox Status in Peripheral Lymphocytes of Multiple Sclerosis Patients. *Front. Neurosci.* **2019**, *13*, 938. [CrossRef]
6. Gilgun-Sherki, Y.; Melamed, E.; Offen, D. The role of oxidative stress in the pathogenesis of multiple sclerosis: The need for effective antioxidant therapy. *J. Neurol.* **2004**, *251*, 261–268.
7. Ohl, K.; Tenbrock, K.; Kipp, M. Oxidative stress in multiple sclerosis: Central and peripheral mode of action. *Exp. Neurol.* **2016**, *277*, 58–67. [CrossRef] [PubMed]
8. Comabella, M.; Khoury, S.J. Immunopathogenesis of multiple sclerosis. *Clin. Immunol.* **2012**, *142*, 2–8. [CrossRef] [PubMed]
9. McFarland, H.F.; Martin, R. Multiple sclerosis: A complicated picture of autoimmunity. *Nat. Immunol.* **2007**, *8*, 913–919. [CrossRef] [PubMed]
10. Segal, B.M.; Cross, A.H. Fas(t) track to apoptosis in MS: TNF receptors may suppress or potentiate CNS demyelination. *Neurology* **2000**, *55*, 906–907. [CrossRef] [PubMed]
11. Ruggieri, M.; Avolio, C.; Scacco, S.; Pica, C.; Lia, A.; Zimatore, G.B.; Papa, S.; Livrea, P.; Trojano, M. Glatiramer acetate induces pro-apoptotic mechanisms involving Bcl-2, Bax and Cyt-c in peripheral lymphocytes from multiple sclerosis patients. *J. Neurol.* **2006**, *253*, 231–236. [CrossRef]
12. Julià, E.; Edo, M.C.; Horga, A.; Montalban, X.; Comabella, M. Differential susceptibility to apoptosis of CD4+T cells expressing CCR5 and CXCR3 in patients with MS. *Clin. Immunol.* **2009**, *133*, 364–374. [CrossRef]
13. La Rocca, C.; Carbone, F.; De Rosa, V.; Colamatteo, A.; Galgani, M.; Perna, F.; Lanzillo, R.; Brescia Morra, V.; Orefice, G.; Cerillo, I.; et al. Immunometabolic profiling of T cells from patients with relapsing-remitting multiple sclerosis reveals an impairment in glycolysis and mitochondrial respiration. *Metabolism* **2017**, *77*, 39–46. [CrossRef]

14. Benard, G.; Rossignol, R. Ultrastructure of the mitochondrion and its bearing on function and bioenergetics. *Antioxid. Redox Signal.* **2008**, *10*, 1313–1342. [CrossRef]
15. Kalkavan, H.; Green, D.R. MOMP, cell suicide as a BCL-2 family business. *Cell Death Differ.* **2018**, *25*, 46–55. [CrossRef]
16. Wai, T.; Langer, T. Mitochondrial Dynamics and Metabolic Regulation. *Trends Endocrinol. Metab.* **2016**, *27*, 105–117. [CrossRef]
17. Pernas, L.; Scorrano, L. Mito-Morphosis: Mitochondrial Fusion, Fission, and Cristae Remodeling as Key Mediators of Cellular Function. *Annu. Rev. Physiol.* **2016**, *78*, 505–531. [CrossRef]
18. Yu-Wai-Man, P.; Spyropoulos, A.; Duncan, H.J.; Guadagno, J.V.; Chinnery, P.F. A multiple sclerosis-like disorder in patients with OPA1 mutations. *Ann. Clin. Trans. Neurol.* **2016**, *3*, 723–729. [CrossRef]
19. Patten, D.A.; Wong, J.; Khacho, M.; Soubannier, V.; Mailloux, R.J.; Pilon-Larose, K.; MacLaurin, J.G.; Park, D.S.; McBride, H.M.; Trinkle-Mulcahy, L.; et al. OPA1-dependent cristae modulation is essential for cellular adaptation to metabolic demand. *EMBO J.* **2014**, *33*, 2676–2691. [CrossRef]
20. Signorile, A.; Santeramo, A.; Tamma, G.; Pellegrino, T.; D'Oria, S.; Lattanzio, P.; De Rasmo, D. Mitochondrial cAMP prevents apoptosis modulating Sirt3 protein level and OPA1 processing in cardiac myoblast cells. Biochim. Biophys. *Acta Mol. Cell. Res.* **2017**, *1864*, 355–366. [CrossRef]
21. MacVicar, T.; Langer, T. OPA1 processing in cell death and disease—The long and short of it. *J. Cell Sci.* **2016**, *129*, 2297–2306. [CrossRef]
22. Baker, M.J.; Lampe, P.A.; Stojanovski, D.; Korwitz, A.; Anand, R.; Tatsuta, T.; Langer, T. Stress-induced OMA1 activation and autocatalytic turnover regulate OPA1-dependent mitochondrial dynamics. *EMBO J.* **2014**, *33*, 578–593. [CrossRef]
23. Rainbolt, T.K.; Lebeau, J.; Puchades, C.; Wiseman, R.L. Reciprocal Degradation of YME1L and OMA1 Adapts Mitochondrial Proteolytic Activity during Stress. *Cell Rep.* **2016**, *14*, 2041–2049. [CrossRef]
24. Merkwirth, C.; Dargazanli, S.; Tatsuta, T.; Geimer, S.; Löwer, B.; Wunderlich, F.T.; von Kleist-Retzow, J.C.; Waisman, A.; Westermann, B.; Langer, T. Prohibitins control cell proliferation and apoptosis by regulating OPA1-dependent cristae morphogenesis in mitochondria. *Genes Dev.* **2008**, *22*, 476–488. [CrossRef]
25. Ross, J.A.; Robles-Escajeda, E.; Oaxaca, D.M.; Padilla, D.L.; Kirken, R.A. The prohibitin protein complex promotes mitochondrial stabilization and cell survival in hematologic malignancies. *Oncotarget* **2017**, *8*, 65445–65456. [CrossRef]
26. Kumar, M.K.S.; Nair, S.; Mony, U.; Kalingavarman, S.; Venkat, R.; Sivanarayanan, T.B.; Unni, A.K.K.; Rajeshkannan, R.; Anandakuttan, A.; Radhakrishnan, S.; et al. Significance of elevated Prohibitin 1 levels in Multiple Sclerosis patients lymphocytes towards the assessment of subclinical disease activity and its role in the central nervous system pathology of disease. *Int. J. Biol. Macromol.* **2018**, *110*, 573–581. [CrossRef]
27. Polman, C.H.; Reingold, S.C.; Banwell, B.; Clanet, M.; Cohen, J.A.; Filippi, M.; Fujihara, K.; Havrdova, E.; Hutchinson, M.; Kappos, L.; et al. Diagnostic criteria for multiple sclerosis: 2010 revisions to the McDonaldcriteria. *Ann. Neurol.* **2011**, *69*, 292–302. [CrossRef]
28. De Riccardis, L.; Rizzello, A.; Ferramosca, A.; Urso, E.; De Robertis, F.; Danieli, A.; Giudetti, A.M.; Trianni, G.; Zara, V.; Maffia, M. Bioenergetics profile of CD4+T cells in relapsing remittingmultiple sclerosissubjects. *J. Biotechnol.* **2015**, *202*, 31–39. [CrossRef]
29. Djaldetti, R.; Achiron, A.; Ziv, I.; Djaldetti, M. Lymphocyte ultrastructure in patients with multiple sclerosis. *Biomed. Pharmacother.* **1995**, *49*, 300–303. [CrossRef]
30. Jiang, X.; Jiang, H.; Shen, Z.; Wang, X. Activation of mitochondrial protease OMA1 by Bax and Bak promotes cytochrome c release during apoptosis. *Proc. Natl. Acad. Sci. USA* **2014**, *111*, 14782–14787. [CrossRef]
31. Anand, R.; Wai, T.; Baker, M.J.; Kladt, N.; Schauss, A.C.; Rugarli, E.; Langer, T. The i-AAA protease YME1L and OMA1 cleave OPA1 to balance mitochondrial fusion and fission. *J. Cell Biol.* **2014**, *204*, 919–929. [CrossRef]
32. Quirós, P.M.; Ramsay, A.J.; Sala, D.; Fernández-Vizarra, E.; Rodríguez, F.; Peinado, J.R.; Fernández-García, M.S.; Vega, J.A.; Enríquez, J.A.; Zorzano, A.; et al. Loss of mitochondrial proteaseOMA1alters processing of the GTPase OPA1 and causes obesity and defective thermogenesis in mice. *EMBO J.* **2012**, *31*, 2117–2133. [CrossRef]
33. Van der Bliek, A.M.; Shen, Q.; Kawajiri, S. Mechanisms of mitochondrial fission and fusion. *Cold Spring Harb. Perspect. Biol.* **2013**, *5*, a011072. [CrossRef]

34. Sood, A.; Jeyaraju, D.V.; Prudent, J.; Caron, A.; Lemieux, P.; McBride, H.M.; Laplante, M.; Tóth, K.; Pellegrini, L. A Mitofusin-2-dependent inactivating cleavage of Opa1 links changes in mitochondria cristae and ER contacts in the postprandial liver. *Proc. Natl. Acad. Sci. USA* **2014**, *111*, 16017–16022. [CrossRef]
35. Scarisbrick, I.A. The multiple sclerosis degradome: Enzymatic cascades in development and progression of central nervous system inflammatory disease. In *Advances in Multiple Sclerosis and Experimental Demyelinating Diseases*; Springer: Berlin/Heidelberg, Germany, 2008; Volume 318, pp. 133–175.
36. Muri, L.; Leppert, D.; Grandgirard, D.; Leib, S.L. MMPs and ADAMs in neurological infectious diseases and multiple sclerosis. *Cell. Mol. Life Sci.* **2019**, *76*, 3097–3116. [CrossRef]
37. Kozin, M.S.; Kulakova, O.G.; Favorova, O.O. Involvement of Mitochondria in Neurodegeneration in Multiple Sclerosis. *Biochemistry* **2018**, *83*, 813–830. [CrossRef]
38. Singh, C.K.; Chhabra, G.; Ndiaye, M.A.; Garcia-Peterson, L.M.; Mack, N.J.; Ahmad, N. The Role of Sirtuins in Antioxidant and Redox Signaling. *Antioxid. Redox Signal.* **2018**, *28*, 643–661. [CrossRef]
39. Wu, Y.T.; Wu, S.B.; Wei, Y.H. Roles of sirtuins in the regulation of antioxidant defense and bioenergetic function of mitochondria under oxidative stress. *Free Radic. Res.* **2014**, *48*, 1070–1084. [CrossRef]
40. Nijtmans, L.G.; Artal, S.M.; Grivell, L.A.; Coates, P.J. The mitochondrial PHB complex: Roles in mitochondrial respiratory complex assembly, ageing and degenerative disease. *Cell. Mol. Life Sci.* **2002**, *59*, 143–155. [CrossRef]
41. Signorile, A.; Sgaramella, G.; Bellomo, F.; De Rasmo, D. Prohibitins: A Critical Role in Mitochondrial Functions and Implication in Diseases. *Cells* **2019**, *8*, E71. [CrossRef]
42. Merkwirth, C.; Langer, T. Prohibitin function within mitochondria: Essential roles for cell proliferation and cristae morphogenesis. *Biochim. Biophys. Acta* **2009**, *1793*, 27–32. [CrossRef]
43. Muraguchi, T.; Kawawa, A.; Kubota, S. Prohibitin protects against hypoxia-induced H9c2 cardiomyocyte cell death. *Biomed. Res.* **2010**, *31*, 113–122. [CrossRef]
44. Alirezaei, M.; Fox, H.S.; Flynn, C.T.; Moore, C.S.; Hebb, A.L.; Frausto, R.F.; Bhan, V.; Kiosses, W.B.; Whitton, J.L.; Robertson, G.S.; et al. Elevated ATG5 expression in autoimmune demyelination and multiple sclerosis. *Autophagy* **2009**, *5*, 152–158. [CrossRef]
45. Wei, Y.; Chiang, W.C.; Sumpter, R., Jr.; Mishra, P.; Levine, B. Prohibitin 2 Is an Inner Mitochondrial Membrane Mitophagy Receptor. *Cell* **2017**, *168*, 224–238. [CrossRef]

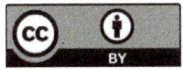

© 2020 by the authors. Licensee MDPI, Basel, Switzerland. This article is an open access article distributed under the terms and conditions of the Creative Commons Attribution (CC BY) license (http://creativecommons.org/licenses/by/4.0/).

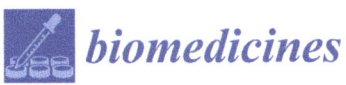

Article

Multiple Sclerosis in a Multi-Ethnic Population in Houston, Texas: A Retrospective Analysis

Vicki Mercado [1,2,3], Deepa Dongarwar [3], Kristen Fisher [4], Hamisu M. Salihu [5], George J. Hutton [6] and Fernando X. Cuascut [3,6,*]

1. Immunology and Microbiology Graduate Program, Baylor College of Medicine, Houston, TX 77030, USA; Vicki.Mercado@bcm.edu
2. Medical Scientist Training Program, Baylor College of Medicine, Houston, TX 77030, USA
3. Center of Excellence in Health Equity, Training and Research Program, Baylor College of Medicine, Houston, TX 77030, USA; deepa.dongarwar@bcm.edu
4. Texas Children Hospital, Blue Bird Circle Clinic for Multiple Sclerosis, Houston, TX 77030, USA; Kristen.Fisher@bcm.edu
5. Department of Family & Community Medicine, Baylor College of Medicine, Houston, TX 77030, USA; hamisu.salihu@bcm.edu
6. Baylor College of Medicine, Maxine Mesinger Multiple Sclerosis Center, Houston, TX 77030, USA; ghutton@bcm.edu
* Correspondence: Fernando.Cuascut@bcm.edu

Received: 21 October 2020; Accepted: 23 November 2020; Published: 25 November 2020

Abstract: Multiple Sclerosis (MS) is a progressive neurodegenerative disease that affects more than 2 million people worldwide. Increasing knowledge about MS in different populations has advanced our understanding of disease epidemiology and variation in the natural history of MS among White and minority populations. In addition to differences in incidence, African American (AA) and Hispanic patients have greater disease burden and disability in earlier stages of disease compared to White patients. To further characterize MS in AA and Hispanic populations, we conducted a retrospective chart analysis of 112 patients treated at an MS center in Houston, Texas. Here, we describe similarities and differences in clinical presentation, MRI findings, treatment regimens, disability progression, and relapse rate. While we found several similarities between the groups regarding mean age, disability severity, and degree of brain atrophy at diagnosis, we also describe a few divergences. Interestingly, we found that patients who were evaluated by a neurologist at symptom onset had significantly decreased odds of greater disability [defined as Expanded Disability Status Scale (EDSS) > 4.5] at last presentation compared to patients who were not evaluated by a neurologist (OR: 0.04, 95% CI: 0.16–0.9). We also found that active smokers had significantly increased odds of greater disability both at diagnosis and at last clinical encounter compared to nonsmokers (OR: 2.44, 95% CI: 1.10–7.10, OR= 2.44, 95% CI: 1.35–6.12, $p = 0.01$, respectively). Additionally, we observed significant differences in treatment adherence between groups. Assessment of the degree of brain atrophy and progression over time, along with an enumeration of T1, T2, and gadolinium-enhancing brain lesions, did not reveal differences across groups.

Keywords: multiple sclerosis; MS; disparities; minority populations

---

1. Introduction

Multiple Sclerosis (MS) is an autoimmune inflammatory demyelinating condition that affects more than 2 million people worldwide [1,2]. A recent study estimates that in 2017, nearly 1 million adults had MS in the United States [1]. MS leads to an accumulation of disability over time, although disease-modifying therapies (DMT) may lessen long-term disability severity in most patients [3]. MS is considered a heterogeneous disease thought to result from a complex interaction among genetic predisposition, sex, and environment [4]. Increasing evidence suggests that racial disparities are important factors that may explain differences in the disease course, prevalence, incidence, and outcomes [5–8]. Despite comprising 13.4% and 18.3% of the American population, African-Americans (AA) and Hispanics, respectively, remain largely underrepresented and understudied in clinical trials [9–11]. Fortunately, an accumulating body of work characterizes MS in diverse populations. This development could improve our understanding of disease course and epidemiology and uncover disparities across various racial/ethnic groups. Better understanding disparities in MS clinical course and outcomes will allow for the development of more effective disease management in patients of diverse backgrounds.

Historically, it had been widely accepted that MS incidence was higher in the White population compared to the AA population [12]. However, population-based cohort studies have challenged this paradigm. A 2013 retrospective cohort study found that AA had a 47% increased risk of MS compared to Whites [13]. Disparities in MS clinical course in minority populations also encompass disability progression, disease burden, symptom presentation, and relapse rates. AA and Hispanics with MS have a higher disease burden and more severe disability in earlier stages of disease than White patients [10,14–16]. Additionally, AA patients commonly have multi-symptomatic presentation and early motor system involvement [14,17]. AA also experience inadequate recovery from symptoms and have shorter intervals between clinical attacks [7,8]. Furthermore, amongst MS individuals admitted to US nursing homes, AA patients are younger and more disabled than White patients [18]. Studies comparing MRI findings between AA and White patients revealed that the former show an increased degree of T2 hyperintense lesions and T1 hypointense lesions, which correlate with greater MS-related disability [19].

Clinical data for MS in the Hispanic population is comparatively limited. The few studies on Hispanics suggest a more rapid disability accumulation over time compared to White patients [20–22]. Interestingly, Hispanics were found to have a 50% decreased risk of developing MS compared to Whites [13]. However, several studies concur that Hispanics may have an earlier age of disease onset compared with other patient cohorts [13,20]. Hispanics and AA with MS are less likely than their White counterparts to visit a neurologist or MS specialist for disease management and have decreased rates of DMT usage due to noncompliance or inappropriate understanding of the treatment plan [23,24]. DMTs are critical for effective management and reduction of long-term disability in MS patients. In assessing these data, it is essential to consider that the Hispanic population is multiethnic and diverse. Other compounding factors that should be considered include socioeconomic status, place of birth, age of migration to the US, health literacy, systemic biases and systematic racism in healthcare, and access to care [5,20,25].

Much of our understanding of MS manifestation and clinical course in minority populations have come from a limited set of studies. Clinical trials on DMTs mostly lack data for minorities despite mounting evidence that these groups are at higher risk for a more aggressive disease course [26]. Approximately only 1% of the MS literature focuses on minority populations [10]. The purpose of this study was to address this lack of information by describing the clinical presentation, MRI findings, treatment regimens, disability progression, and relapse patterns in a racially and ethnically diverse population of MS patients in Houston, Texas. Given that the data for this study were collected from a clinic that predominantly serves patients of low socioeconomic status (SES), this study captures ethnic and racial disparities in MS among patients with a similar SES, potentially decreasing the possible effects of confounding factors. This study is critical and timely because it adds to an emerging literature that explores disparity in MS disease progression in AA and Hispanic MS patients compared to their White counterparts.

2. Patients and Methods

2.1. Study Design and Setting

Subjects were identified by a retrospective chart review of patients treated at the Smith Clinic Multiple Sclerosis Center. Smith clinic is a unique center that is part of a network that specifically cares for underserved and low socio-economic groups in Harris County, which includes the city of Houston. Additionally, Harris County is the third most populous county in the US. The majority of the patient population seen in the clinic are Non-Hispanic Black (NH-Black) or of Hispanic descent, and Mexicans constitute the majority of the Hispanic population served at the clinic. There is also a small percentage of Non-Hispanic White (NH-White) patients seen in the clinic. For the purposes of this study we are using the terms NH-Black and NH-White to account for the racial diversity of Hispanics seen in our clinic. Patients are attended to irrespective of insurance status or ability to pay.

2.2. Cohort Identification and Selection

Information from all patients who visited Smith clinic from March 2019 to March 2020 was identified through chart review and included in this retrospective study. All patients with a diagnosis of Relapsing Remitting MS (RRMS), Secondary Progressive MS (SPMS), or Primary Progressive MS (PPMS) were included.

2.3. Outcome Measurements

The following pre-selected information was abstracted for each patient: year and age of first symptoms, age at diagnosis, the amount of time that elapsed between onset of symptoms and diagnosis, disease subtype, estimated Expanded Disability Status Scale (EDSS) at diagnosis and last encounter, Disease Modifying Therapy (DMT) history (adverse reactions, relapses, and changes in immunomodulatory therapy), radiological findings, number of clinical relapses, smoking status, and autoimmune comorbidities. Escalation therapies included Glatiramer Acetate, Interferons, Teriflunomide, Dimethyl Fumarate and Fingolimod. High efficacy therapies included Rituximab, Ocrelizumab, Alemtuzumab and Natalizumab. Symptoms at disease onset were recorded and included motor, sensory, cerebellar, brainstem, bowel, and bladder function among others.

2.4. Data Collection and Management

Two neurologists extracted patient data from medical records and the study protocol was approved by an Institutional Review Board. Information from the most recent clinical encounter and from the clinical encounter at diagnosis was included. The EDSS at presentation was estimated based on the first documented neurologic examination by a neurologist and was not indicative of the maximal neurologic deficit during the demyelinating episode that led to the diagnosis. Severe disability was defined as an estimated EDSS score > 4.5. MRI interpretations were collected from radiology reports. Lesion quantification and atrophy scoring were extracted directly from radiology reports and raw images were not independently interpreted by the neurologists gathering the data. A relapse was defined as a new, documented, neurological complaint lasting more than 24 h with objective findings in the documented neurological exam, or a follow-up MRI showing new enhancing lesions.

2.5. Statistical Analysis

The statistical analyses were performed using R (version 3·6·1, Vienna, Austria) and RStudio (Version 1·2·5001, Boston, MA, USA). Based on the race and ethnicity information of the patients, we created a composite variable called 'race/ethnicity' and categorized the responses as Non-Hispanic (NH) White, NH-Black, Hispanic and 'others'. We conducted descriptive statistics on patient socio-demographic and disease characteristics stratified by race/ethnicity. We conducted Fisher's exact tests (for categorical variables) and ANOVA (for continuous variables). We examined the usage and impact of DMTs across racial/ethnic groups. We also examined various markers of disease progression including lesions and atrophy in the brain as well as the thoracic and cervical spine stratified by race/ethnicity using Fisher's exact test. Applying adjusted Exact logistic regression models, we evaluated the association between various patient characteristics and a high EDSS score (EDSS > 4.5). Models were adjusted for different covariates based on the literature and context, along with experts' recommendations. All analyses were based on two-tailed probabilities with a type 1 error rate set at 5%.

3. Results

Data from a total of 114 patients were analyzed in this study. Two patients were excluded due to a substantial amount of missing information. Of the included 112 patients, most were diagnosed with Relapsing Remitting MS (RRMS). About 73% of NH-White, 92% of NH-Black, and 95% of Hispanic patients had RRMS, whereas only 18% of NH-White, 5% of NH-Black, and 2.5% of Hispanic patients were diagnosed with Primary Progressive MS (PPMS) (Table 1). One Hispanic patient had a diagnosis of SPMS. There were no significant differences among the groups with regard to MS type at diagnosis ($p = 0.1859$), or smoking status ($p = 0.3079$). All groups had a similar female to male ratio, with a greater proportion of female MS patients (Table 1, $p = 0.3675$). Average age at diagnosis ($p = 0.9918$) and mean time to diagnosis ($p = 0.9934$) were also similar across all groups (Table 1). Interestingly, between the groups, we found significant differences in the percentage of patients who were adherent or experienced relapse while on escalation or high efficacy therapies. Specifically, 63.2% of NH-White, 73% of NH-Black, and 61.8% of Hispanic patients were adherent to escalation therapy (Table 1, $p = 0.0252$). 100% of NH-White, 84.2% of NH-Black, and 50% of Hispanic patients were adherent to high efficacy therapy (Table 1, $p = 0.0252$). 26.3% of NH-White, 31.1% of NH-Black, and 36.4% of Hispanic patients relapsed while on escalation therapy (Table 1, $p = 0.000151$). 0% of NH-White, 10.5% of NH-Black, and 0% of Hispanic patients relapsed while on high efficacy therapy (Table 1, $p = 0.00015$). Of note, one of the reasons for relapse includes non-adherence; thus interpretation of relapse data must consider the adherence percentages presented.

Notably, only 28% of the NH-Black population had received an evaluation by a neurologist at symptom onset, whereas 53% of Hispanic and 45% of NH-White patients had, although this was not statistically significant (Table 1, $p = 0.1778$). In this cohort, there were no statistically significant differences in receipt of a medical evaluation at symptom onset; 63–70% of patients from all groups were able to access medical evaluation. Additionally, NH-White, NH-Black and Hispanic patients exhibited no differences in symptoms at diagnosis or mean EDSS score at diagnosis and last encounter (Table 2). There was a significant difference in the percentage of patients with severe disability (EDSS score > 4.5) at diagnosis and at last encounter; 14.3% of NH-White MS patients had severe disability at diagnosis compared to 50% of NH-Black and 31.6% of Hispanic patients (Table 2, $p < 0.001$). This was also true at last encounter with 32.5% of NH-White, 45.5% of NH-Black and 41% of Hispanic MS patients with severe disability at their most recent clinical visit (Table 2, $p < 0.001$).

Assessment of degree of brain atrophy and progression over time revealed that NH-White, NH-Black and Hispanic patients in this cohort had a similar degree of brain atrophy at diagnosis and over time (Figure 1). Enumeration of T1, T2, and gadolinium-enhancing brain lesions at diagnosis also showed no significant differences between the groups (data not shown). Spinal atrophy and quantity of T2 and gadolinium-enhancing lesions in the spine at diagnosis and at last presentation were also similar between groups (Figure 2).

Table 1. Diagnosis Characteristics of patients with MS stratified by race/ethnicity.

Characteristics	NH-White (n = 11)	NH-Black (n = 61)	Hispanic (n = 40)	p Value
Multiple Sclerosis (MS) type at diagnosis				p = 0.1859
Relapsing remitting MS	82%	95%	95%	
Primary progressive MS	18%	5%	2.5%	
Secondary progressive MS	0%	0%	2.5%	
Mean Age at diagnosis (years)	39.9 (11.3)	36.7 (11.4)	32.4 (11.5)	p = 0.9918
Female/Male ratio	1.70/1	2.33/1	1.22/1	p = 0.3765
Active smokers	55%	44%	30%	p = 0.3079
Mean time from symptom onset to diagnosis (months)	30.8 (38.9)	32.9 (32.1)	13.7 (15.4)	p = 0.9934
Medical Evaluation at symptom onset	64%	63%	70%	p = 0.8597
Neurological Evaluation at symptom onset	45%	28%	53%	p = 0.1778
Adherence (Adherence/Ever used)				p = 0.0252
Escalation therapy	63.2%	73%	61.8%	
High efficacy therapy	100%	84.2%	50%	
Relapse (Relapse/Ever used)				p = 0.00015
Escalation therapy	26.3%	31.1%	36.4%	
High efficacy therapy	0%	10.5%	0%	

EDSS score at diagnosis and EDSS score at last clinical visit were compared within each group. Standard deviation is shown in parentheses. $p = 0.4253$ (NH-Black), $p = 0.1757$ (Hispanic), $p = 0.0324$ (NH-White), (paired sample t-test). For adherence and relapse data, chi-squared test and Fisher's-exact test were used respectively. Escalation therapies included Glatiramer Acetate, Interferons, Teriflunomide, Dimethyl Fumarate and Fingolimod. High efficacy therapies included Rituximab, Ocrelizumab, Alemtuzumab and Natalizumab.

Table 2. Clinical characteristics of MS patients by race/ethnicity.

Clinical Characteristics	NH-White (n = 11)	NH-Black (n = 61)	Hispanic (n = 40)	p Value
EDSS scores				
Mean EDSS score at diagnosis (SD)	2.6 (2.1)	2.2 (1.1)	3.8 (1.9)	p = 0.9328
Mean EDSS score at last presentation (SD)	2.9 (2.8)	4.2 (2.9)	3.8 (2.3)	p = 0.9950
Severe disability at diagnosis (EDSS > 4.5)	14.3%	50%	31.6%	p = < 0.001
Severe disability at last presentation (EDSS > 4.5)	32.5%	45.5%	41%	p = < 0.001
Symptoms at Presentation				p = 0.1473
Motor	72.7%	57.4%	47.5%	
Brainstem	27.3%	24.9%	25%	
Cerebellar	27.3%	37.7%	37.5%	
Gait	27.3%	26.2%	15%	
Sensory	72.7%	37.7%	52.5%	
Visual	9.1%	27.9%	30%	
Cognitive	9.1%	9.8%	5%	
Other or unknown	36.4%	18.1%	15%	

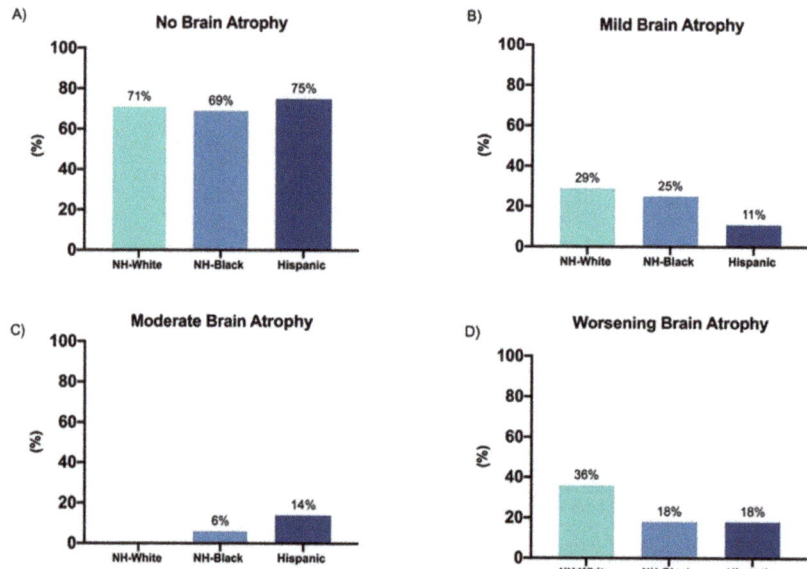

Figure 1. Degree of brain atrophy at diagnosis and worsening of brain atrophy from diagnosis to most recent MRI scan. Presented as the total percentage of each group, is the proportion of patients who had none (**A**), mild (**B**), or moderate (**C**) brain atrophy at the time of diagnosis, as well as the proportion of patients who had increased brain atrophy in their most recent MRI scan compared to diagnosis (**D**). Only patients who had MRI scans on file were included in this analysis. $p = 0.5155$ for comparison between degree of brain atrophy (none, mild, moderate) (Fisher's exact). $p = 0.3387$ for comparison of total percentage of patients who had worsening brain atrophy on most recent MRI compared to diagnosis (Fisher's exact).

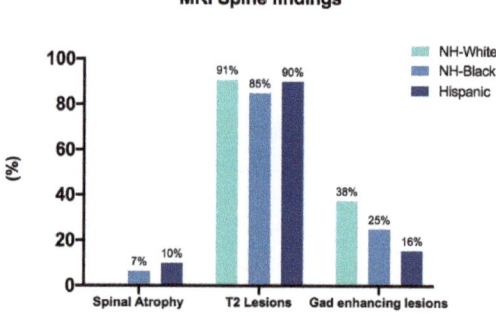

Figure 2. The total percentage of patients in each group who had spinal atrophy, T2, or gadolinium-enhancing lesions in the spine as determined by MRI findings at diagnosis. Only patients who had MRI scans on file were included in this analysis. $p = 0.6974$, $p = 0.5128$, $p = 0.2957$ for comparison of total percentage of patients in each group that had spinal atrophy, spinal T2 lesions, and spinal gadolinium-enhancing lesions respectively (Fisher's exact).

Patient usage of escalation or high efficacy therapies did not significantly impact the patient's likelihood of having an EDSS score > 4.5 at last clinical encounter after adjustment for adherence, smoking, race, age, prior exposure to escalation therapies, and EDSS at diagnosis (Table 3). Active smokers were 2.44 times as likely to have an EDSS score > 4.5 at their last clinical encounter compared to non-smokers after adjustment for age and race (OR: 2.44, 95% CI: 1.36–6.12, $p = 0.01$) (Table 3).

Interestingly, after adjustment for race and age, patients who were evaluated by a neurologist at diagnosis had significantly lower adjusted odds of an EDSS score > 4.5 at last presentation compared to patients who were not evaluated by a neurologist (OR: 0.40, 95% CI: 0.16–0.90, $p = 0.04$) (Table 3).

Table 3. Association between various patient characteristics and high EDSS score (>4.5) at last presentation.

	High EDSS Score at Last Presentation	
	OR	p-Value
Usage of escalation therapies [a]		
No	reference	
Yes	1.60 (0.45–6.14)	0.48
Usage of high efficacy therapies [b]		
No	reference	
Yes	2.64 (0.87–8.33)	0.09
Smoker [c]		
No	reference	
Yes	2.44 (1.36–6.12)	0.01
Medical evaluation by Neurologist [c]		
No	reference	
Yes	0.40 (0.16–0.90)	0.04
Adherence to DMT [c]		
Yes	reference	
No	0.73 (0.31–1.62)	0.43
Time to diagnosis [c]		
<=12 months	reference	
>12 months	1.73 (0.75–4.01)	0.2

[a] adjusted for adherence, smoking, race and age and EDSS at diagnosis; [b] adjusted for prior exposure to escalation therapies, adherence, smoking, race, age and EDSS at diagnosis; [c] adjusted for age and race.

Active smokers were 2.79 times as likely to have an EDSS score > 4.5 at diagnosis compared to non-smokers after adjustment for age and race (OR: 2.79, 95% CI: 1.10–7.10, $p = 0.01$) (Table 4). There was no significant association between time to diagnosis and having a high EDSS score at diagnosis (Table 4). There were no significant differences in total relapse occurrence for patients on escalation therapy vs. high efficacy therapy for each racial/ethnic group (data not shown). Of 24 NH-white patients, 19 had ever used escalation therapy, and 5 had used high efficacy therapy. Of 93 NH-Black patients, 74 had used escalation therapy, and 19 had used high efficacy therapy. For the Hispanic patients group of 63 patients, 55 had ever used escalation therapy while 18 had documented high efficacy therapy use. We found no differences between the groups concerning the usage of escalation vs. high efficacy therapies.

Table 4. Association between various patient characteristics and high EDSS score at diagnosis (>4.5).

	High EDSS Score at Diagnosis	
	OR	p-Value
Smoker [c]		
No	reference	
Yes	2.79 (1.10–7.10)	0.01
Time to diagnosis [c]		
<=12 months	reference	
>12 months	1.15 (0.46–2.83)	0.77

[c] adjusted for age and race.

4. Discussion

The goal of this retrospective cohort study was to describe MS patient characteristics in a multi-ethnic population in Houston and compare findings between racial/ethnic groups. Our study demonstrates several racial/ethnic similarities and a few differences in multiple sclerosis presentation and disease course. We found that the groups had a similar mean age at diagnosis, mean EDSS score at diagnosis and last presentation, and a similar degree of brain and spinal atrophy at diagnosis as well. MRI spinal findings were also comparable between NH-White, Black and Hispanic groups. The average time from symptom onset to diagnosis, and overall symptom presentation, were also similar between the groups. The clinic that these patients were treated at is a hub for the underserved and low socioeconomic communities. Thus, we suspect that many of the patients in this cohort were of a similar socioeconomic background, which undoubtedly can influence disease manifestation and outcomes. It is plausible that these similar environmental factors, along with the small sample size may explain the many similarities detected between the groups. However, further studies are required to evaluate this hypothesis.

Interestingly, after adjustment for race and age, patients who were evaluated by a neurologist at diagnosis had 60% lower odds (OR = 0.40, 95% CI: 0.16–0.90) of an EDSS score > 4.5 at last presentation compared to patients who were evaluated by a non-neurology specialist. This suggests a logical protective effect of treatment by a neurologist at symptom onset and highlights the importance of access to treatment for all patients. Indeed, a national descriptive study found that people with MS who saw a neurologist were more likely to receive appropriate DMT treatment and see rehabilitation and urologist specialists compared to people who saw other providers [27]. A 2017 study on racial disparities in neurologic health care access revealed that Black patients were 30% less likely to see an outpatient neurologist and were more likely to be cared for in the emergency department compared to their White counterparts [23]. Similarly, Hispanic patients were 40% less likely to see an outpatient neurologist compared to NH-Whites [23].

We found that actively smoking patients were 2.44 times as likely (95% CI: 1.36–6.12) to have severe disability at diagnosis and at the last clinic follow up. A recent systematic review and meta-analysis found evidence supporting the causal involvement of smoking in the development and progression of MS [28]. Altogether, these data suggest that smoking prevention and cessation education programs and early intervention by a neurologist should be implemented to achieve optimal MS care in diverse patient populations.

Consistent with published reports, a greater proportion of NH-Black patients had early severe disability (defined in our study as an estimated EDSS score > 4.5) when compared to NH-White and Hispanic patients [29,30]. In our present study, treatment modality did not impact the risk of having an estimated EDSS score > 4.5 at the last visit. Nonetheless, we observed a trend towards a higher relapse rate in escalation therapies vs. high efficacy therapies, especially in NH-Blacks. We also observed significant differences in adherence between the groups. Interestingly, a greater percentage of NH-Black patients relapsed while on high efficacy therapy compared to Hispanic patients, despite having greater adherence. Other studies have found that NH-Black patients treated with interferons experienced more relapses and new MS lesions on T2-weighted brain magnetic imaging than NH-Whites [31]. However, further studies on the interaction between race/ethnicity and DMT response for MS are necessary.

Several studies have shown that African Americans have significantly higher CNS lesion burden, more frequent relapses, worse ambulatory disability, worse post-relapse recoveries, and higher overall disability at diagnosis [5,10,19,29]. Overall, our findings did not confirm these prior observations and we believe that the similar socioeconomic background of this patient cohort, along with the small sample size, may have contributed to this. Nevertheless, it is evident that further studies are needed to investigate the various environmental and social factors contributing to divergent MS clinical course outcomes between diverse populations.

Limitations of this study include its retrospective nature, the variable periods of follow-up and the selection of therapy by the treating physician (nonrandomized). The study was also constrained by a small sample size, which could have induced a type 2 error leading to the inability to reject the null hypothesis in some of our comparisons. Additionally, our interpretation of the relapse data is limited because one of the possible reasons for relapse is non-adherence. Thus, relapse data are not corrected for the degree of non-adherence and should be assessed accordingly. Lastly, it is important to note that we did not analyze the imaging data ourselves. Instead, we collected information from MRI reports. Often, the number of lesions was documented as a range, thereby limiting data precision. Moreover, the atrophy measurements were subjective rather than objective quantification, and some patients were missing MRI information at diagnosis (e.g., performed at a different institution). These limitations may have impacted the capability to show radiological differences at presentation between groups.

Our study is important because it adds to emerging literature describing disease characteristics in minority populations with MS. The disparities in MS progression, onset, and disease course warrants further study. Of 60,000 published articles on MS, only 113 focused on NH-Black and only 23 focused on Hispanic American patients with MS as of 2014 [10]. This demonstrates a need for studies that are intentionally inclusive of these populations. Since 2014, there has been a modest but steady increase in studies focused on these populations. There is a clear disparity in MS treatment access for patients from different racial and ethnic backgrounds. Drivers of disparity are often comprised of complex interactions among factors such as socioeconomic status, access to healthcare and wellness resources (clinics, hospitals, grocery stores, fitness centers), systemic racism and biases in healthcare, and limited health literacy. This systemic web of disparity can be challenging to disentangle, but understanding it is necessary for improving the care of minority patients with MS.

Future prospective randomized controlled trials in different racial/ethnic groups with MS are essential to better understand the disease progression, management and treatment outcomes for diverse patient populations.

Author Contributions: Conceptualization, F.X.C. and G.J.H.; methodology D.D.; software, D.D.; validation, F.X.C. and V.M.; formal analysis, D.D.; writing—original draft preparation, V.M., D.D., K.F. and F.X.C.; writing—review and editing, H.M.S and G.J.H.; supervision, H.M.S. All authors have read and agreed to the published version of the manuscript.

Funding: This research was funded by U.S. Department of Health and Human Services and Health Resources and Services Administration, grant number D34HP31024.

Conflicts of Interest: The authors declare no conflict of interest.

References

1. Wallin, M.T.; Culpepper, W.J.; Campbell, J.D.; Nelson, L.M.; Langer-Gould, A.; Marrie, R.A.; Cutter, G.R.; Kaye, W.E.; Wagner, L.; Tremlett, H.; et al. The prevalence of MS in the United States: A population-based estimate using health claims data. *Neurology* **2019**, *92*, 1029–1040. [CrossRef] [PubMed]
2. Wallin, M.T.; Culpepper, W.J.; Nichols, E.; Bhutta, Z.A.; Gebrehiwot, T.T.; Hay, S.I.; Khalil, I.A.; Krohn, K.J.; Liang, X.; Naghavi, M.; et al. Global, regional, and national burden of multiple sclerosis 1990–2016: A systematic analysis for the Global Burden of Disease Study 2016. *Lancet Neurol.* **2019**, *18*, 269–285. [CrossRef]
3. Freedman, M.S. Present and emerging therapies for multiple sclerosis. *Contin. Lifelong Learn. Neurol.* **2013**, *19*, 968–991. [CrossRef] [PubMed]
4. Muñoz-Culla, M.; Irizar, H.; Otaegui, D. The genetics of multiple sclerosis: Review of current and emerging candidates. *Appl. Clin. Genet.* **2013**, *6*, 63–73. [CrossRef]
5. Amezcua, L.; McCauley, J.L. Race and ethnicity on MS presentation and disease course. *Mult. Scler. J.* **2020**, *26*, 561–567. [CrossRef]
6. Wallin, M.T.; Culpepper, W.J.; Coffman, P.; Pulaski, S.; Maloni, H.; Mahan, C.M.; Haselkorn, J.K.; Kurtzke, J.F.; Veterans Affairs Multiple Sclerosis Centres of Excellence Epidemiology Group. The Gulf War era multiple sclerosis cohort: Age and incidence rates by race, sex and service. *Brain* **2012**, *135*, 1778–1785. [CrossRef]
7. Amezcua, L.; Rivas, E.; Joseph, S.; Zhang, J.; Liu, L. Multiple Sclerosis Mortality by Race/Ethnicity, Age, Sex, and Time Period in the United States, 1999–2015. *Neuroepidemiology* **2018**, *50*, 35–40. [CrossRef]

8. Rivas-Rodríguez, E.; Amezcua, L. Ethnic Considerations and Multiple Sclerosis Disease Variability in the United States. *Neurol. Clin.* **2018**, *36*, 151–162. [CrossRef]
9. U.S. Census Bureau QuickFacts: United States. Available online: https://www.census.gov/quickfacts/fact/table/US/PST045219#qf-headnote-a (accessed on 4 September 2020).
10. Khan, O.; Williams, M.J.; Amezcua, L.; Javed, A.; Larsen, K.E.; Smrtka, J.M. Multiple Sclerosis in US Minority Populations Clinical Practice Insights. *Neurol Clin Pr.* **2015**, *5*, 132–142. [CrossRef]
11. Diaz, V. Encouraging participation of minorities in research studies. *Ann. Fam. Med.* **2012**, *10*, 372–373. [CrossRef]
12. Rosati, G. The prevalence of multiple sclerosis in the world: An update. *Neurol. Sci.* **2001**, *22*, 117–139. [CrossRef] [PubMed]
13. Langer-Gould, A.; Brara, S.M.; Beaber, B.E.; Zhang, J.L. Incidence of multiple sclerosis in multiple racial and ethnic groups. *Neurology* **2013**, *80*, 1734–1739. [CrossRef] [PubMed]
14. Kister, I.; Chamot, E.; Bacon, J.H.; Niewczyk, P.M.; De Guzman, R.A.; Apatoff, B.; Coyle, P.; Goodman, A.D.; Gottesman, M.; Granger, C.; et al. Rapid disease course in African Americans with multiple sclerosis. *Neurology* **2010**, *75*, 217–223. [CrossRef] [PubMed]
15. Marrie, R.A.; Cutter, G.; Tyry, T.; Vollmer, T.; Campagnolo, D. Does multiple sclerosis-associated disability differ between races? *Neurology* **2006**, *66*, 1235–1240. [CrossRef] [PubMed]
16. Weinstock-Guttman, B.; Jacobs, L.D.; Brownscheidle, C.M.; Baier, M.; Rea, D.F.; Apatoff, B.R.; Blitz, K.M.; Coyle, P.K.; Frontera, A.T.; Goodman, A.D.; et al. Multiple sclerosis characteristics in African American patients in the New York State Multiple Sclerosis Consortium. *Mult. Scler.* **2003**, *9*, 293–298. [CrossRef] [PubMed]
17. Cree, B.A.C.; Khan, O.; Bourdette, D.; Goodin, D.S.; Cohen, J.A.; Marrie, R.A.; Glidden, D.; Weinstock-Guttman, B.; Reich, D.; Patterson, N.; et al. Clinical Characteristics of African Americans vs Caucasian Americans with Multiple Sclerosis. *Neurology* **2004**, *63*, 2039–2045. [CrossRef] [PubMed]
18. Buchanan, R.J.; Wang, S.; Huang, C.; Graber, D. Profiles of nursing home residents with multiple sclerosis using the minimum data set. *Mult. Scler.* **2001**, *7*, 189–200. [CrossRef]
19. Howard, J.; Battaglini, M.; Babb, J.S.; Arienzo, D.; Holst, B. MRI Correlates of Disability in African-Americans with Multiple Sclerosis. *PLoS ONE* **2012**, *7*, e43061. [CrossRef]
20. Amezcua, L.; Lund, B.T.; Weiner, L.P.; Islam, T. Multiple sclerosis in Hispanics: A study of clinical disease expression. *Mult. Scler.* **2011**, *17*, 1010–1016. [CrossRef]
21. Hadjixenofontos, A.; Beecham, A.H.; Manrique, C.P.; Pericak-Vance, M.A.; Tornes, L.; Ortega, M.; Rammohan, K.W.; McCauley, J.L.; Delgado, S.R. Clinical expression of multiple sclerosis in Hispanic whites of primarily Caribbean ancestry. *Neuroepidemiology* **2015**, *44*, 62–268. [CrossRef]
22. Ventura, R.E.; Antezana, A.O.; Bacon, T.; Kister, I. Hispanic Americans and African Americans with multiple sclerosis have more severe disease course than Caucasian Americans. *Mult. Scler.* **2017**, *23*, 1554–1557. [CrossRef] [PubMed]
23. Saadi, A.; Himmelstein, D.U.; Woolhandler, S.; Mejia, N.I. Racial disparities in neurologic health care access and utilization in the United States. *Neurology* **2017**, *88*, 2268–2275. [CrossRef] [PubMed]
24. Shabas, D.; Heffner, M. Multiple sclerosis management for low-income minorities. *Mult. Scler. J.* **2005**, *11*, 635–640. [CrossRef] [PubMed]
25. Langille, M.M.; Islam, T.; Burnett, M.; Amezcua, L. Clinical Characteristics of Pediatric-Onset and Adult-Onset Multiple Sclerosis in Hispanic Americans. *J. Child Neurol.* **2016**, *31*, 1068–1073. [CrossRef]
26. Avasarala, J. FDA-approved drugs for multiple sclerosis have no efficacy or disability data in non-Caucasian patients. *CNS Spectr.* **2019**, *24*, 279–280. [CrossRef]
27. Minden, S.L.; Hoaglin, D.C.; Hadden, L.; Frankel, D.; Robbins, T.; Perloff, J. Access to and utilization of neurologists by people with multiple sclerosis. *Neurology* **2008**, *70*, 1141–1149. [CrossRef]
28. Degelman, M.L.; Herman, K.M. Smoking and multiple sclerosis: A systematic review and meta-analysis using the Bradford Hill criteria for causation. *Mult. Scler. Relat. Disord.* **2017**, *17*, 207–216. [CrossRef]
29. Dong, D.; Carlson, J.; Ruberwa, J.; Snihur, T.; Al-Obaidi, N.; Bustillo, J. Unmasking the Masquerader: A Delayed Diagnosis of MS and Its 4.5 Years of Implications in an Older African American Male. *Case Rep. Med.* **2019**. [CrossRef]

30. Naismith, R.T.; Trinkaus, K.; Cross, A.H. Phenotype and prognosis in African-Americans with multiple sclerosis: A retrospective chart review. *Mult. Scler.* **2006**, *12*, 775–781. [CrossRef]
31. Cree, B.A.C.; Al-Sabbagh, A.; Bennett, R.; Goodin, D. Response to interferon beta-1a treatment in African American multiple sclerosis patients. *Arch. Neurol.* **2005**, *62*, 1681–1683. [CrossRef]

Publisher's Note: MDPI stays neutral with regard to jurisdictional claims in published maps and institutional affiliations.

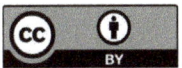

© 2020 by the authors. Licensee MDPI, Basel, Switzerland. This article is an open access article distributed under the terms and conditions of the Creative Commons Attribution (CC BY) license (http://creativecommons.org/licenses/by/4.0/).

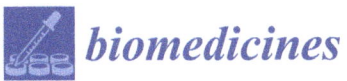

Review

Blood Neurofilament Light Chain: The Neurologist's Troponin?

Simon Thebault [1,*], Ronald A. Booth [2] and Mark S. Freedman [1,*]

1. Department of Medicine and the Ottawa Hospital Research Institute, The University of Ottawa, Ottawa, ON K1H8L6, Canada
2. Department of Pathology and Laboratory Medicine, Eastern Ontario Regional Laboratory Association and Ottawa Hospital Research Institute, University of Ottawa & The Ottawa Hospital, Ottawa, ON K1H8L6, Canada; rbooth@eorla.ca
* Correspondence: sthebault@toh.ca (S.T.); mfreedman@toh.ca (M.S.F.)

Received: 4 November 2020; Accepted: 18 November 2020; Published: 21 November 2020

Abstract: Blood neurofilament light chain (NfL) is a marker of neuro-axonal injury showing promising associations with outcomes of interest in several neurological conditions. Although initially discovered and investigated in the cerebrospinal fluid (CSF), the recent development of ultrasensitive digital immunoassay technologies has enabled reliable detection in serum/plasma, obviating the need for invasive lumbar punctures for longitudinal assessment. The most evidence for utility relates to multiple sclerosis (MS) where it serves as an objective measure of both the inflammatory and degenerative pathologies that characterise this disease. In this review, we summarise the physiology and pathophysiology of neurofilaments before focusing on the technological advancements that have enabled reliable quantification of NfL in blood. As the test case for clinical translation, we then highlight important recent developments linking blood NfL levels to outcomes in MS and the next steps to be overcome before this test is adopted on a routine clinical basis.

Keywords: neurofilament light chain; biomarkers; multiple sclerosis

---

1. Neurofilament Structure and Function

Neurofilaments are neuronal-specific heteropolymers conventionally considered to consist of a triplet of light (NfL), medium (NfM) and heavy (NfH) chains according to their molecular mass [1]. More recent discoveries show that α-Internexin in the central nervous system [2] and peripherin in the peripheral nervous system [3] can also be included in neurofilament heteropolymers. These five proteins co-assemble into the 10 nM intermediate filaments in different combinations and concentrations depending on the type of neuron, location in the axon and stage of development [4].

Each of the neurofilament proteins consists of an amino-terminal domain that is thought to regulate the formation of oligomers [5], a central helical rod domain, and a variable carboxy-terminal domain. The chain-specific C-terminal domains are the main determinants of differences in molecular mass and phosphorylation between subunits. Following synthesis and assembly in the neuron cell body, tetramers of neurofilament proteins are transported bidirectionally along axons by the microtubular apparatus prior to forming a continuously overlapping array that runs parallel to axons. Once formed, in the healthy state, they are remarkably stable for months to years [6].

In mature myelinated axons, neurofilaments are the single most abundant protein [7]. They perform key roles as part of the neuroaxonal scaffold to resist external pressures, determine axonal diameter, indirectly moderate conduction velocity, and act as an attachment for organelles and other proteins [4]. Beyond their primary structural role in axons, mounting evidence indicates that a unique pool of synaptic neurofilament proteins serves dynamic functions beyond static structural support [8].

Changes in neurofilament phosphorylation may be involved in long term potentiation that underpins memory [9] and NMDA receptor stability is dependent on a synaptic scaffold of neurofilament proteins.

2. Neurofilament Pathophysiology

Damage to central nervous system (CNS) neurons and physiologic turnover causes neurofilament release. This translates to elevated levels in the cerebrospinal fluid (CSF) and eventually blood, where the concentration reflects the rate of release from neurons (Figure 1, where we focus on NfL). Physiologic degradation of neurofilaments within neurons is proposed to be a combination of ubiquitin-mediated proteasomal and apophagocytotic pathways [10]. Based on the trafficking of other proteins degraded in the CNS, it is likely that partially degraded fragments of neurofilaments drain directly into CSF and blood via multiple routes. These include direct drainage into CSF and blood via arachnoid granulations as well as lymphatic drainage into the subarachnoid spaces and perivascular spaces [11,12]. Several studies have demonstrated strong correlations between blood and CSF NfL, with r values typically ranging from 0.7 to 8 (e.g., [13]). However, our understanding of the kinetics of neurofilament release, distribution and metabolism is incomplete.

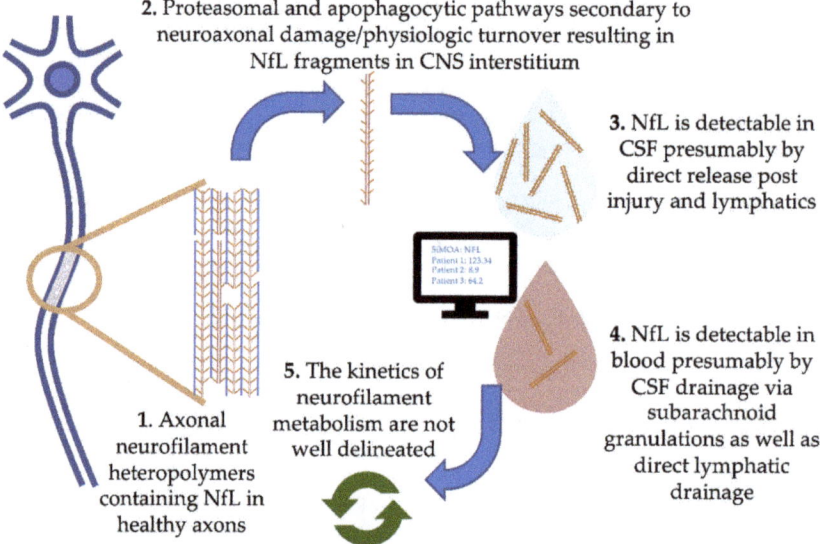

Figure 1. Pathophysiology of neurofilament light chain in blood and cerebrospinal fluid (CSF).

Blood–brain barrier permeability itself may be a confounder; neurofilament quotient in blood compared to CSF could be selectively increased following periods of inflammation such as that seen in MS relapse, positively skewing blood NfL levels. Two recent studies on this topic in MS patients present conflicting results [14,15].

Once NfL enters the blood, the half-life is a key consideration with implications on the frequency of disease activity monitoring. In a longitudinal study of NfL levels before and after intrathecal catheter insertion, NfL in both CSF and serum peaked at 1-month post-surgery, returning to baseline after 6 to 9 months [16]. In longitudinally sampled MS patients around the time of relapse, levels increasing 5 months before, peaking at clinical onset, and recovery within 4–5 months [17]. Therefore, quarterly measurement is likely sufficient, a frequency that our group is currently investigating in longitudinal prospective studies of serum NfL.

Age is the principal physiologic covariate of NfL levels. Levels in healthy controls increase by 2.2% per year [18,19]. Furthermore, an inflection point is observable above the age of 60, after which both sNfL levels, as well as the inter-individual variability in levels, increase greatly [20]. It is speculated that these changes are attributable to both aging itself as well as the accumulation of subclinical comorbidities. Other factors outside of neurological disease itself that may alter neurofilament levels include BMI [21] as well as vascular risk factors [22].

Although the primary focus of this review is the pathophysiologic relevance of NfL concentrations as they relate to neurological diseases such as MS, the vital role of neurofilaments is underlined by various human mutations that interfere with their function and homeostasis. Mutations of gigaxonin, a key component in the ubiquitin-dependent intermediate filament degradation, results in the pathological aggregation of neurofilaments in neurons and a severe neurodegenerative condition called giant axonal neuropathy [23]. Mutations in the neurofilament light chain gene itself result in axonal forms of hereditary motor sensory polyneuropathy [24] and variants of the heavy neurofilament subunit are associated with the development of amyotrophic lateral sclerosis [25].

Intriguingly there is evidence that autoimmunity can be directed against neurofilament proteins themselves [26–30]. CSF from MS patients contain anti-NfL antibodies [26] and these antibodies co-localise with neurons in human MS pathological lesions [27]. The pathogenic potential of anti-NfL antibodies is a topic of debate as the neurofilament light chain is intracellular and presumably not amenable to immune surveillance or targeting in the healthy state. However, intrathecally transferred anti-NfL antibodies in rodent models of experimental autoimmune encephalomyelitis (EAE) results in disability progression [28]. Anti-NfL antibody concentration also appears to correlate with MRI tissue damage, particularly lower brain volumes [29]. Following effective treatment of MS with natalizumab, anti-NfL antibody concentrations decrease [30]. Although the pathogenic potential of antibodies directed against an intracellular antigen such as NfL remains debatable, these circulating antibodies could also have important and unexplored implications on neurofilament metabolism in the periphery as well as interference in NfL assays which are antibody-based immunoassays.

3. Measurement of Blood Levels of Neurofilament Light Chain

Of the family of neurofilament proteins, neurofilament light chain (NfL) has gained the most interest as a candidate marker of outcomes in neurological diseases. This was not without contention. While the neurofilament light chain is the most abundant and soluble of the neurofilament proteins, phosphorylated neurofilament heavy chain (NfH) was initially thought to be more resistant to protease activity [31–33]. NfL was thought to be unstable in vitro [34] and initial research focused on NfH quantified by enzyme-linked immunosorbent assay (ELISA) or electrochemiluminescence (ECL) as a biomarker of axonal damage in MS [35,36]. However, in 2013, a comparative study of NfL and NfH found both proteins showed equivalent stability after several days at room temperature and through freeze–thaw cycles [37]. Moreover, although some of the differences observed may correspond to analytical methodologies, this study found that NfL levels were higher than NfH and NfL was a better discriminator of MS patients from controls.

Initial studies looking at NfL in association with neurological disease outcomes focused on CSF measurements. Although CSF is "closer" to the CNS pathologies (e.g., MS) and NfL concentration is approximately 500-fold higher, the inconvenient and invasive lumbar puncture required severely limits its clinical utility as a frequent serial biomarker. Concentrations in the blood however were too low to be reliably measured with conventional immunoassays such as ELISA or ECL assays. It was not until recently, with the development of the Single-Molecule Assay (SiMoA), that analytical methods become sufficiently sensitive to measure the single-digit picogram per milliliter levels present in blood [38]. This SiMoA technology, similar to other immunoassays, is based on fluorescent microbeads coated with high-affinity capture antibodies that bind NfL followed secondly by a fluorescently labelled detector antibody [39]. The increased analytical sensitivity of the SiMoA assay is due to its unique method of detection. Assay beads with captured NfL and fluorescent detector antibody, are loaded onto an assay disk containing >200,000 microwells capable of holding only a single bead. At high analyte concentration, the total fluorescence can be captured in the traditional manner (analog) and correlated to the analyte concentration. At low analyte concentrations, rather than detecting total fluorescence, a digital image is captured that enumerates individual fluorescent microwells in a binary fashion, effectively lowering the limit of quantitation to the femtomolar range. Although there are several neurofilament assays in development based on other technologies, including widely used chemiluminescent-based assay [40], the data we present here were exclusively generated using the SiMoA platform.

4. Blood NfL in Neurological Diseases

As a neuron-specific marker of neurological injury, elevated NfL levels can be found in a variety of conditions that involve neuroaxonal injury in both the central and peripheral nervous system (reviewed by Khalil et al., 2018 [41]). In purely neurodegenerative diseases, NfL could serve as both a prognostic marker of decline but also an efficacy biomarker of experimental therapies. In a meta-analysis of Alzheimer's disease, frontotemporal and amyotrophic lateral sclerosis [42], plasma NfL levels were elevated in patients compared to controls with utility in differentiating neurodegenerative conditions from non-neurodegenerative mimics. However, due to a lack of specificity to any particular flavor of neurodegeneration, its role as a diagnostic marker is limited. The exception to this is in amyotrophic lateral sclerosis where the uniquely rapid neurodegeneration that characterises this condition results in blood NfL levels several times higher than both controls and other forms of neurodegeneration, and hence may play are role in diagnosis.

In more indolent neurodegenerative processes, early prognostication is an important clinical role. In a study of carriers and non-carriers of autosomal dominant Alzheimer's disease, the trajectory of NfL in affected individuals compared to controls became segregated during their 30's, long before clinical onset [43]. Conversely, in Parkinson's, a condition characterised by particularly slow neurodegeneration, differences between controls and patients are especially small, and the separation NfL trajectories only become apparent after the age of 70 [44] at which point marked disability is usually apparent. Meanwhile, for more acute neuronal injury, neurofilament may also have utility in stroke and traumatic brain injury prognostication. Following a stroke, blood NfL takes several hours to rise, limiting their utility in the hyperacute setting, however, the presence of elevated NfL may have utility in diagnosing subacute strokes as well as in the prognostication of outcomes [45,46]. Similarly, following traumatic brain injury, the extent of NfL increase acutely is predictive of the severity of injury, and while NfL decreases over time, it remains elevated relative to controls several years after the injury. Of recent topical interest, NfL was found to be subtly elevated in the serum of mild-moderate COVID-19 patients [47]. While some have used this evidence to bolster theories of direct neuronal invasion by the virus, these subtle differences could also be attributed to cerebral hypoxia induced by the respiratory virus.

5. Blood NfL in MS

Multiple sclerosis is the most common neurological autoimmune disease, known for its varied clinical presentations and unpredictable clinical course [48]. Over the last few decades, there has been a dramatic expansion in the number of immunosuppressive therapies on offer to prevent damaging bouts of focal inflammation and demyelination that characterise this condition. However, a victim of its own success, objective disease monitoring biomarkers are lacking, and adjuncts that can help neurologists track and personalise treatments are sorely needed. Regular MRI scanning remains the gold standard means of detecting sub-clinical inflammatory lesions [49,50], but this costly and inconvenient test has a number of shortcomings. It is poorly predictive of future activity (Ontaneda and Fox, 2017), lacks sensitivity [51], tends to be focused mainly on the brain (leaving out the spinal cord and optic nerves) and entails a large degree of technical variation and subjective interpretation. Notable examples of fluid biomarkers that are already in clinical use in MS include oligoclonal bands [52] (now part of MS diagnostic criteria), antibodies against aquaporin-4 [53] and myelin oligodendrocyte protein [54] (which define pathologically discrete disease entities which previously fell under the umbrella of MS), as well as serological assays for JC virus [55] (pre-immunosuppression risk stratification). However, as of yet, no fluid biomarker has established clinical use in routine disease monitoring and prediction. As a result of this unmet need, associations of blood neurofilament have been intensely studied in MS. In the last two years, more than 200 studies have contributed to a groundswell of evidence associating NfL with outcomes related to disease activity, progression, treatment response and prognosis.

As a cross-sectional measure in groups of MS patients, the strongest evidence links high NfL levels with inflammatory endpoints such as relapses and MRI lesions [19,56–61]. This is perhaps counter-intuitive, as one might expect this neuroaxonal protein to associate most strongly with outcomes to neurodegeneration and disease progression. However, axonal damage and loss are hallmarks of demyelinating MS lesions even early-on [62], presumably reflected in a transient marked elevation of NfL.

Other than inflammatory disease activity, an interrelated facet of MS pathology is neurodegeneration and progressive disability accrual. Conveniently, this facet of MS pathology is also objectified with NfL measurement. Patients with progressive MS have higher levels than age and sex matched patients with relapsing disease [63]. Associations can be found between high blood NfL levels and poorer disease progression outcomes including disability scores, conversion to a secondary progressive phenotype, MRI atrophy, and measures of cognitive function [13,18,57,61,64–69].

Several groups have also studied the longitudinal significance of blood NfL as a serial disease monitoring/treatment response measure in prospective cohorts from clinical trials. Studies exploring the relationship of NfL kinetics with clinical relapse showed elevations beginning approximately 5 months prior to relapse with a peak at clinical onset and recovery within 4–5 months of remission [17]. When profiled longitudinally, "peaks" of NfL (more than three standard deviations above steady-state) were associated with nearly 80% of MRI and clinical disease activity.

In response to treatment, often related to the availability of retrospective sample sets from well-characterised groups of patients involved in seminal studies, longitudinal NfL reductions have been reported for most established treatments for relapsing MS. These include injectable therapies [18,56,59,70], dimethyl fumarate [71], fingolimod [61,70,72], natalizumab [73], rituximab [74], ocrelizumab [75], ofatumumab [76], alemtuzumab [17] and hematopoietic stem cell transplantation [13]. Encouragingly, reductions in NfL seen after different treatments broadly fall in line with the perceived hierarchy of treatment efficacies, with the greatest reductions seen following the most intensive treatments. Accordingly, in a recent Swedish cohort study of more than 1000 patients receiving one of 6 treatments, the largest reductions in plasma levels were seen following alemtuzumab (48%), and the smallest reduction for teriflunomide (7%), with the other agents falling in the middle [56].

For secondary progressive MS, reductions in NfL have been shown following siponimod [77], ocrelizumab [78] and natalizumab [79]. In primary progressive disease, reductions were seen following fingolimod [80] and ocrelizumab [78]. Given the lack of useful biomarkers otherwise for progressive types of MS, NfL is increasingly seen as an important secondary endpoint in phase 2 and 3 studies of treatments [81].

Many groups have shown the value of NfL in the prediction of future relapses, MRI disease activity, disability worsening, MRI brain and spine atrophy and poorer cognitive outcomes [18,19,59,60,82–84]. In a 5-year longitudinal study of more than 1200 Swiss MS patients, high age-adjusted NfL was associated with increased risk of relapse and new MRI activity in the following year [63]. Even in patients who met criteria for "no evidence of disease activity" [85], higher NfL was independently associated with increased risk of clinical and/or MRI disease activity in the next year, indicating that NfL is capable of predicting subclinical disease activity otherwise not captured. NfL may also have utility in long term prediction, with 2 separate studies finding an association of early NfL measurements with clinical and MRI disease outcomes more than a decade later [86,87].

While NfL is the closest blood-based disease monitoring marker to clinical translation in MS, there are also other promising candidates that may provide additional information. For instance, glial fibrillary acidic protein (GFAP) is a marker of astrocytic turnover or damage that may serve more as a marker of disease progression [88]. Although not a fluid biomarker, ocular coherence tomography (OCT) peripapillary retinal nerve fibre layer thickness also seems to be useful as a biomarker for the prediction of disability progression [89]. Thus, NfL may represent the first of several fluid biomarkers with relevance in MS monitoring and prediction; one-day multimodal composite indices could be used to most accurately objectify different components of an individual patient's disease and inform treatment decisions.

6. Conclusions

Measurement of a convenient objective blood marker of neuronal injury in patients is an appealing prospect for neurologists. Analogous to the cardiologist's troponin, neurofilament light chain is a structural axonal protein that can be detected in the blood at elevated levels in a variety of neurological disease states which can be followed longitudinally. Enabled by recent advancements in assay technologies, many consider this test to be on the verge of clinical translation in a number of different settings. Given its neuron-specific nature, but lack of disease specificity, on its own it is not a helpful diagnostic marker. However, in defined neurological conditions that require monitoring, in particular MS where we have treatments to offer, NfL is rapidly gaining traction.

It seems likely that MS will represent the test case for the clinical translation of blood NfL, where it will be a greatly-needed adjunct to clinical and MRI assessment. While we already know that elevated NfL is concerning and low NfL is reassuring, a number of challenges remain before this test is ready for widespread adoption. Foremost amongst them is the need for age-adjusted normative datasets and cutoff values so that physicians can better interpret individual patient results. Key elements of neurofilament kinetics in the blood, such as blood half-life, need to be delineated to inform optimal testing frequency in clinical practice. Additionally, the ongoing efforts of multisite validation efforts will be important in standardising measurement between clinical laboratories and ensuring that any concerns of analytical validity are allayed. Nonetheless, many are optimistic that NfL could represent the first of its kind in neurology: a broadly-applicable protein biomarker that objectively reflects underlying pathology which can be harnessed to improve patient outcomes.

Author Contributions: S.T.: conceptualization, literature review and writing—original draft preparation, reviewing and editing, R.A.B. and M.S.F.: conceptualization, writing—reviewing and editing, supervision. All authors have read and agreed to the published version of the manuscript.

Funding: This research received no external funding.

Conflicts of Interest: The authors declare no conflict of interest.

References

1. Fuchs, E.; Cleveland, D.W. A structural scaffolding of intermediate filaments in health and disease. *Science* **1998**, *279*, 514–519. [CrossRef] [PubMed]
2. Yuan, A.; Rao, M.V.; Sasaki, T.; Chen, Y.; Kumar, A.; Veeranna; Liem, R.K.H.; Eyer, J.; Peterson, A.C.; Julien, J.P.; et al. α-internexin is structurally and functionally associated with the neurofilament triplet proteins in the mature CNS. *J. Neurosci.* **2006**, *26*, 10006–10019. [CrossRef] [PubMed]
3. Yuan, A.; Sasaki, T.; Kumar, A.; Peterhoff, C.M.; Rao, M.V.; Liem, R.K.; Julien, J.P.; Nixon, R.A. Peripherin is a subunit of peripheral nerve neurofilaments: Implications for differential vulnerability of cns and peripheral nervous system axons. *J. Neurosci.* **2012**, *32*, 8501–8508. [CrossRef] [PubMed]
4. Yuan, A.; Rao, M.V.; Veeranna; Nixon, R.A. Neurofilaments and neurofilament proteins in health and disease. *Cold Spring Harb. Perspect. Biol.* **2017**, *9*, a018309. [CrossRef] [PubMed]
5. Ching, G.Y.; Liem, R.K.H. Roles of head and tail domains in α-internexin's self-assembly and coassembly with the neurofilament triplet proteins. *J. Cell Sci.* **1998**, *111*, 321–333.
6. Millecamps, S.; Gowing, G.; Corti, O.; Mallet, J.; Julien, J.P. Conditional NF-L transgene expression in mice for in vivo analysis of turnover and transport rate of neurofilaments. *J. Neurosci.* **2007**, *27*, 4947–4956. [CrossRef]
7. Fliegner, K.H.; Liem, R.K.H. Cellular and Molecular Biology of Neuronal Intermediate Filaments. *Int. Rev. Cytol.* **1991**, *131*, 109–167. [CrossRef]

8. Bragina, L.; Conti, F. Expression of Neurofilament Subunits at Neocortical Glutamatergic and GABAergic Synapses. *Front. Neuroanat.* **2018**, *12*, 74. [CrossRef]
9. Hashimoto, R.; Nakamura, Y.; Komai, S.; Kashiwagi, Y.; Tamura, K.; Goto, T.; Aimoto, S.; Kaibuchi, K.; Shiosaka, S.; Takeda, M. Site-specific phosphorylation of neurofilament-L is mediated by calcium/calmodulin-dependent protein kinase II in the apical dendrites during long-term potentiation. *J. Neurochem.* **2000**, *75*, 373–382. [CrossRef]
10. Bomont, P. Degradation of the Intermediate Filament Family by Gigaxonin. *Methods Enzymol.* **2016**, *569*, 215–231. [CrossRef]
11. Carare, R.O.; Bernardes-Silva, M.; Newman, T.A.; Page, A.M.; Nicoll, J.A.R.; Perry, V.H.; Weller, R.O. Solutes, but not cells, drain from the brain parenchyma along basement membranes of capillaries and arteries: Significance for cerebral amyloid angiopathy and neuroimmunology. *Neuropathol. Appl. Neurobiol.* **2008**, *34*, 131–144. [CrossRef] [PubMed]
12. Gafson, A.R.; Barthélemy, N.R.; Bomont, P.; Carare, R.O.; Durham, H.D.; Julien, J.-P.; Kuhle, J.; Leppert, D.; Nixon, R.A.; Weller, R.O.; et al. Neurofilaments: Neurobiological foundations for biomarker applications. *Brain* **2020**, *143*, 1975–1998. [CrossRef] [PubMed]
13. Thebault, S.; Tessier, D.; Lee, H.; Bowman, M.; Bar-Or, A.; Arnold, D.L.; Atkins, H.; Tabard-Cossa, V.; Freedman, M.S. High Serum Neurofilament Light Chain normalises after Haematopoietic Stem Cell Transplant for MS. *Neurol. Neuroimmunol. Neuroinflamm.* **2019**, *6*, e598. [CrossRef] [PubMed]
14. Kalm, M.; Boström, M.; Sandelius, Å.; Eriksson, Y.; Ek, C.J.; Blennow, K.; Björk-Eriksson, T.; Zetterberg, H. Serum concentrations of the axonal injury marker neurofilament light protein are not influenced by blood-brain barrier permeability. *Brain Res.* **2017**, *1668*, 12–19. [CrossRef]
15. Uher, T.; McComb, M.; Galkin, S.; Srpova, B.; Oechtering, J.; Barro, C.; Tyblova, M.; Bergsland, N.; Krasensky, J.; Dwyer, M.; et al. Neurofilament levels are associated with blood–brain barrier integrity, lymphocyte extravasation, and risk factors following the first demyelinating event in multiple sclerosis. *Mult. Scler. J.* **2020**, 1–12. [CrossRef]
16. Bergman, J.; Dring, A.; Zetterberg, H.; Blennow, K.; Norgren, N.; Gilthorpe, J.; Bergenheim, T.; Svenningsson, A. Neurofilament light in CSF and serum is a sensitive marker for axonal white matter injury in MS. *Neurol. Neuroimmunol. Neuroinflamm.* **2016**, *3*, e271. [CrossRef]
17. Akgün, K.; Kretschmann, N.; Haase, R.; Proschmann, U.; Kitzler, H.H.; Reichmann, H.; Ziemssen, T. Profiling individual clinical responses by high-frequency serum neurofilament assessment in MS. *Neurol. Neuroimmunol. NeuroInflamm.* **2019**, *6*, 1–12. [CrossRef]
18. Disanto, G.; Barro, C.; Benkert, P.; Naegelin, Y.; Schädelin, S.; Giardiello, A.; Zecca, C.; Blennow, K.; Zetterberg, H.; Leppert, D.; et al. Serum Neurofilament light: A biomarker of neuronal damage in multiple sclerosis. *Ann. Neurol.* **2017**, *81*, 857–870. [CrossRef]
19. Barro, C.; Benkert, P.; Disanto, G.; Tsagkas, C.; Amann, M.; Naegelin, Y.; Leppert, D.; Gobbi, C.; Granziera, C.; Yaldizli, Ö.; et al. Serum neurofilament as a predictor of disease worsening and brain and spinal cord atrophy in multiple sclerosis. *Brain* **2018**, *141*, 2382–2391. [CrossRef]
20. Khalil, M.; Pirpamer, L.; Hofer, E.; Voortman, M.M.; Barro, C.; Leppert, D.; Benkert, P.; Ropele, S.; Enzinger, C.; Fazekas, F.; et al. Serum neurofilament light levels in normal aging and their association with morphologic brain changes. *Nat. Commun.* **2020**, *11*, 1–9. [CrossRef]
21. Manouchehrinia, A.; Piehl, F.; Hillert, J.; Kuhle, J.; Alfredsson, L.; Olsson, T.; Kockum, I. Confounding effect of blood volume and body mass index on blood neurofilament light chain levels. *Ann. Clin. Transl. Neurol.* **2020**, *7*, 139–143. [CrossRef] [PubMed]
22. Korley, F.K.; Goldstick, J.; Mastali, M.; Van Eyk, J.E.; Barsan, W.; Meurer, W.J.; Sussman, J.; Falk, H.; Levine, D. Serum NfL (Neurofilament Light Chain) Levels and Incident Stroke in Adults with Diabetes Mellitus. *Stroke* **2019**, *50*, 1669–1675. [CrossRef] [PubMed]
23. Bomont, P.; Cavalier, L.; Blondeau, F.; Hamida, C. Ben; Belal, S.; Tazir, M.; Demir, E.; Topaloglu, H.; Korinthenberg, R.; Tüysüz, B.; et al. The gene encoding gigaxonin, a new member of the cytoskeletal BTB/kelch repeat family, is mutated in giant axonal neuropathy. *Nat. Genet.* **2000**, *26*, 370–374. [CrossRef] [PubMed]
24. Mersiyanova, I.V.; Perepelov, A.V.; Polyakov, A.V.; Sitnikov, V.F.; Dadali, E.L.; Oparin, R.B.; Petrin, A.N.; Evgrafov, O.V. A new variant of Charcot-Marie-Tooth disease type 2 is probably the result of a mutation in the neurofilament-light gene. *Am. J. Hum. Genet.* **2000**, *67*, 37–46. [CrossRef] [PubMed]

25. Figlewicz, D.A.; Krizus, A.; Martinoli, M.G.; Meininger, V.; Dib, M.; Rouleau, G.A.; Julien, J.P. Variants of the heavy neurofilament subunit are associated with the development of amyotrophic lateral sclerosis. *Hum. Mol. Genet.* **1994**, *3*, 1757–1761. [CrossRef]
26. Silber, E.; Semra, Y.K.; Gregson, N.A.; Sharief, M.K. Patients with progressive multiple sclerosis have elevated antibodies to neurofilament subunit. *Neurology* **2002**, *58*, 1372–1381. [CrossRef]
27. Sádaba, M.C.; Tzartos, J.; Paíno, C.; García-Villanueva, M.; Álvarez-Cermeño, J.C.; Villar, L.M.; Esiri, M.M. Axonal and oligodendrocyte-localized IgM and IgG deposits in MS lesions. *J. Neuroimmunol.* **2012**, *247*, 86–94. [CrossRef]
28. Puentes, F.; van der Star, B.J.; Boomkamp, S.D.; Kipp, M.; Boon, L.; Bosca, I.; Raffel, J.; Gnanapavan, S.; van der Valk, P.; Stephenson, J.; et al. Neurofilament light as an immune target for pathogenic antibodies. *Immunology* **2017**, *152*, 580–588. [CrossRef]
29. Eikelenboom, M.J.; Petzold, A.; Lazeron, R.H.C.; Silber, E.; Sharief, M.; Thompson, E.J.; Barkhof, F.; Giovannoni, G.; Polman, C.H.; Uitdehaag, B.M.J. Multiple sclerosis: Neurofilament light chain antibodies are correlated to cerebral atrophy. *Neurology* **2003**, *60*, 219–223. [CrossRef]
30. Amor, S.; van der Star, B.J.; Bosca, I.; Raffel, J.; Gnanapavan, S.; Watchorn, J.; Kuhle, J.; Giovannoni, G.; Baker, D.; Malaspina, A.; et al. Neurofilament light antibodies in serum reflect response to natalizumab treatment in multiple sclerosis. *Mult. Scler. J.* **2014**, *20*, 1355–1362. [CrossRef]
31. Schlaepfer, W.W.; Lee, C.; Lee, V.M.; Zimmerman, U.-J.P. An Immunoblot Study of Neurofilament Degradation In Situ and During Calcium-Activated Proteolysis. *J. Neurochem.* **1985**, *44*, 502–509. [CrossRef] [PubMed]
32. Goldstein, M.E.; Sternberger, N.H.; Sternberger, L.A. Phosphorylation protects neurofilaments against proteolysis. *J. Neuroimmunol.* **1987**, *14*, 149–160. [CrossRef]
33. Pant, H.C. Dephosphorylation of neurofilament proteins enhances their susceptibility to degradation by calpain. *Biochem. J.* **1988**, *256*, 665–668. [CrossRef] [PubMed]
34. Koel-Simmelink, M.J.A.; Teunissen, C.E.; Behradkia, P.; Blankenstein, M.A.; Petzold, A. The neurofilament light chain is not stable in vitro. *Ann. Neurol.* **2011**, *69*, 1065–1066. [CrossRef] [PubMed]
35. Petzold, A.; Keir, G.; Green, A.J.E.; Giovannoni, G.; Thompson, E.J. A specific ELISA for measuring neurofilament heavy chain phosphoforms. *J. Immunol. Methods* **2003**, *278*, 179–190. [CrossRef]
36. Leppert, D.; Petzold, A.; Regeniter, A.; Schindler, C.; Mehling, M.; Anthony, D.C.; Kappos, L.; Lindberg, R.L.P. Neurofilament heavy chain in CSF correlates with relapses and disability in multiple sclerosis. *Neurology* **2011**, *76*, 1206–1213.
37. Kuhle, J.; Plattner, K.; Bestwick, J.P.; Lindberg, R.L.; Ramagopalan, S.V.; Norgren, N.; Nissim, A.; Malaspina, A.; Leppert, D.; Giovannoni, G.; et al. A comparative study of CSF neurofilament light and heavy chain protein in MS. *Mult. Scler. J.* **2013**, *19*, 1597–1603. [CrossRef]
38. Kuhle, J.; Barro, C.; Andreasson, U.; Derfuss, T.; Lindberg, R.; Sandelius, Å.; Liman, V.; Norgren, N.; Blennow, K.; Zetterberg, H. Comparison of three analytical platforms for quantification of the neurofilament light chain in blood samples: ELISA, electrochemiluminescence immunoassay and Simoa. *Clin. Chem. Lab. Med.* **2016**, *54*, 1655–1661. [CrossRef]
39. Wilson, D.H.; Rissin, D.M.; Kan, C.W.; Fournier, D.R.; Piech, T.; Campbell, T.G.; Meyer, R.E.; Fishburn, M.W.; Cabrera, C.; Patel, P.P.; et al. The Simoa HD-1 Analyzer: A Novel Fully Automated Digital Immunoassay Analyzer with Single-Molecule Sensitivity and Multiplexing. *J. Lab. Autom.* **2016**, *21*, 533–547. [CrossRef]
40. Carvalho, T. Siemens Healthineers, Novartis Partner to Develop NfL Diagnostic Test. 2020. Available online: https://multiplesclerosisnewstoday.com/news-posts/2020/09/21/siemens-healthineers-novartis-partner-to-develop-new-nfl-diagnostic-test-for-ms/ (accessed on 28 October 2020).
41. Khalil, M.; Teunissen, C.E.; Otto, M.; Piehl, F.; Sormani, M.P.; Gattringer, T.; Barro, C.; Kappos, L.; Comabella, M.; Fazekas, F.; et al. Neurofilaments as biomarkers in neurological disorders. *Nat. Rev. Neurol.* **2018**, *14*, 577–589. [CrossRef]
42. Forgrave, L.M.; Ma, M.; Best, J.R.; DeMarco, M. The diagnostic performance of neurofilament light chain in CSF and blood for Alzheimer's disease, frontotemporal dementia, and amyotrophic lateral sclerosis: A systematic review and meta-analysis. *Alzheimer's Dement. Diagnosis Assess. Dis. Monit.* **2019**, *11*, 730–743. [CrossRef] [PubMed]

43. Quiroz, Y.T.; Zetterberg, H.; Reiman, E.M.; Chen, Y.; Su, Y.; Fox-Fuller, J.T.; Garcia, G.; Villegas, A.; Sepulveda-Falla, D.; Villada, M.; et al. Plasma neurofilament light chain in the presenilin 1 E280A autosomal dominant Alzheimer's disease kindred: A cross-sectional and longitudinal cohort study. *Lancet Neurol.* **2020**, *19*, 513–521. [CrossRef]
44. Wilke, C.; dos Santos, M.C.T.; Schulte, C.; Deuschle, C.; Scheller, D.; Verbelen, M.; Brockmann, K.; von Thaler, A.K.; Sünkel, U.; Roeben, B.; et al. Intraindividual Neurofilament Dynamics in Serum Mark the Conversion to Sporadic Parkinson's Disease. *Mov. Disord.* **2020**, *35*, 1233–1238. [CrossRef] [PubMed]
45. Nielsen, H.H.; Soares, C.B.; Høgedal, S.S.; Madsen, J.S.; Hansen, R.B.; Christensen, A.A.; Madsen, C.; Clausen, B.H.; Frich, L.H.; Degn, M.; et al. Acute Neurofilament Light Chain Plasma Levels Correlate With Stroke Severity and Clinical Outcome in Ischemic Stroke Patients. *Front. Neurol.* **2020**, *11*. [CrossRef] [PubMed]
46. O'Connell, G.C.; Alder, M.L.; Smothers, C.G.; Still, C.H.; Webel, A.R.; Moore, S.M. Diagnosis of ischemic stroke using circulating levels of brain-specific proteins measured via high-sensitivity digital ELISA. *Brain Res.* **2020**, *1739*. [CrossRef]
47. Ameres, M.; Brandstetter, S.; Toncheva, A.A.; Kabesch, M.; Leppert, D.; Kuhle, J.; Wellmann, S. Association of neuronal injury blood marker neurofilament light chain with mild-to-moderate COVID-19. *J. Neurol.* **2020**. [CrossRef]
48. Confavreux, C.; Vukusic, S. The clinical course of multiple sclerosis. *Handb. Clin. Neurol.* **2014**, *122*, 343–369. [CrossRef]
49. Igra, M.S.; Paling, D.; Wattjes, M.P.; Connolly, D.J.A.; Hoggard, N. Multiple sclerosis update: Use of MRI for early diagnosis, disease monitoring and assessment of treatment related complications. *Br. J. Radiol.* **2017**, *90*, 20160721. [CrossRef]
50. Wattjes, M.P.; Steenwijk, M.D.; Stangel, M. MRI in the Diagnosis and Monitoring of Multiple Sclerosis: An Update. *Clin. Neuroradiol.* **2015**, *25*, 157–165. [CrossRef]
51. Wattjes, M.P.; Rovira, À.; Miller, D.; Yousry, T.A.; Sormani, M.P.; De Stefano, N.; Tintoré, M.; Auger, C.; Tur, C.; Filippi, M.; et al. Evidence-based guidelines: MAGNIMS consensus guidelines on the use of MRI in multiple sclerosis—Establishing disease prognosis and monitoring patients. *Nat. Rev. Neurol.* **2015**, *11*, 597–606. [CrossRef]
52. Freedman, M.S.; Thompson, E.J.; Deisenhammer, F.; Giovannoni, G.; Grimsley, G.; Keir, G.; Öhman, S.; Racke, M.K.; Sharief, M.; Sindic, C.J.M.; et al. Recommended standard of cerebrospinal fluid analysis in the diagnosis of multiple sclerosis: A consensus statement. *Arch. Neurol.* **2005**, *62*, 865–870. [CrossRef] [PubMed]
53. Lennon, V.A.; Wingerchuk, D.M.; Kryzer, T.J.; Pittock, S.J.; Lucchinetti, C.F.; Fujihara, K.; Nakashima, I.; Weinshenker, B.G. A serum autoantibody marker of neuromyelitis optica: Distinction from multiple sclerosis. *Lancet* **2004**, *364*, 2106–2112. [CrossRef]
54. Waters, P.; Woodhall, M.; O'Connor, K.C.; Reindl, M.; Lang, B.; Sato, D.K.; Jurynczyk, M.; Tackley, G.; Rocha, J.; Takahashi, T.; et al. MOG cell-based assay detects non-MS patients with inflammatory neurologic disease. *Neurol. Neuroimmunol. NeuroInflamm.* **2015**, *2*, e89. [CrossRef] [PubMed]
55. Subramanyam, M.; Goelz, S.; Natarajan, A.; Lee, S.; Plavina, T.; Scanlon, J.V.; Sandrock, A.; Bozic, C. Risk of Natalizumab-Associated Progressive Multifocal Leukoencephalopathy. *N. Engl. J. Med.* **2012**, *366*, 1870–1880.
56. Delcoigne, B.; Manouchehrinia, A.; Barro, C.; Benkert, P.; Michalak, Z.; Kappos, L.; Leppert, D.; Tsai, J.A.; Plavina, T.; Kieseier, B.C.; et al. Blood neurofilament light levels segregate treatment effects in multiple sclerosis. *Neurology* **2020**, *94*, e1201–e1212. [CrossRef]
57. Novakova, L.; Zetterberg, H.; Sundström, P.; Axelsson, M.; Khademi, M.; Gunnarsson, M.; Malmeström, C.; Svenningsson, A.; Olsson, T.; Piehl, F.; et al. Monitoring disease activity in multiple sclerosis using serum neurofilament light protein. *Neurology* **2017**, *89*, 2230–2237. [CrossRef]
58. Bittner, S.; Steffen, F.; Uphaus, T.; Muthuraman, M.; Fleischer, V.; Salmen, A.; Luessi, F.; Berthele, A.; Klotz, L.; Meuth, S.G.; et al. Clinical implications of serum neurofilament in newly diagnosed MS patients: A longitudinal multicentre cohort study. *EBioMedicine* **2020**, *56*, 1–13. [CrossRef]
59. Varhaug, K.N.; Barro, C.; Bjørnevik, K.; Myhr, K.M.; Torkildsen, Ø.; Wergeland, S.; Bindoff, L.A.; Kuhle, J.; Vedeler, C. Neurofilament light chain predicts disease activity in relapsing-remitting MS. *Neurol. Neuroimmunol. NeuroInflamm.* **2018**, *5*, e422. [CrossRef]

60. Siller, N.; Kuhle, J.; Muthuraman, M.; Barro, C.; Uphaus, T.; Groppa, S.; Kappos, L.; Zipp, F.; Bittner, S. Serum neurofilament light chain is a biomarker of acute and chronic neuronal damage in early multiple sclerosis. *Mult. Scler. J.* **2018**. [CrossRef]
61. Kuhle, J.; Kropshofer, H.; Haering, D.A.; Kundu, U.; Meinert, R.; Barro, C.; Dahlke, F.; Tomic, D.; Leppert, D.; Kappos, L. Blood neurofilament light chain as a biomarker of MS disease activity and treatment response. *Neurology* **2019**, *92*, E1007–E1015. [CrossRef]
62. Bitsch, A.; Schuchardt, J.; Bunkowski, S.; Kuhlmann, T.; Brück, W. Acute axonal injury in multiple sclerosis. Correlation with demyelination and inflammation. *Brain* **2000**, *123*, 1174–1183. [CrossRef] [PubMed]
63. Yaldizli, O. Value of serum neurofilament light chain levels as a biomarker of suboptimal treatment response in MS clinical practice. *ECTRIMS Online Library*, 10 December 2018.
64. Ferraro, D.; Guicciardi, C.; De Biasi, S.; Pinti, M.; Bedin, R.; Camera, V.; Vitetta, F.; Nasi, M.; Meletti, S.; Sola, P. Plasma neurofilaments correlate with disability in progressive multiple sclerosis patients. *Acta Neurol. Scand.* **2020**, *141*, 16–21. [CrossRef] [PubMed]
65. Högel, H.; Rissanen, E.; Barro, C.; Matilainen, M.; Nylund, M.; Kuhle, J.; Airas, L. Serum glial fibrillary acidic protein correlates with multiple sclerosis disease severity. *Mult. Scler. J.* **2020**, *26*, 210–219. [CrossRef] [PubMed]
66. Filippi, P.; Vestenická, V.; Siarnik, P.; Sivakova, M.; Čopíková-Cudráková, D.; Belan, V.; Hanes, J.; Novák, M.; Kollar, B.; Turcani, P. Neurofilament light chain and MRI volume parameters as markers of neurodegeneration in multiple sclerosis. *Neuro Endocrinol. Lett.* **2020**, *41*, 17–26. [PubMed]
67. Mattioli, F.; Bellomi, F.; Stampatori, C.; Mariotto, S.; Ferrari, S.; Monaco, S.; Mancinelli, C.; Capra, R. Longitudinal serum neurofilament light chain (sNfL) concentration relates to cognitive function in multiple sclerosis patients. *J. Neurol.* **2020**. [CrossRef]
68. Bridel, C.; van Wieringen, W.N.; Zetterberg, H.; Tijms, B.M.; Teunissen, C.E.; Alvarez-Cermeño, J.C.; Andreasson, U.; Axelsson, M.; Bäckström, D.C.; Bartos, A.; et al. Diagnostic Value of Cerebrospinal Fluid Neurofilament Light Protein in Neurology. *JAMA Neurol.* **2019**, *76*, 1035. [CrossRef]
69. Jakimovski, D.; Zivadinov, R.; Ramanthan, M.; Hagemeier, J.; Weinstock-Guttman, B.; Tomic, D.; Kropshofer, H.; Fuchs, T.A.; Barro, C.; Leppert, D.; et al. Serum neurofilament light chain level associations with clinical and cognitive performance in multiple sclerosis: A longitudinal retrospective 5-year study. *Mult. Scler. J.* **2019**. [CrossRef]
70. Reinert, M.C.; Benkert, P.; Wuerfel, J.; Michalak, Z.; Ruberte, E.; Barro, C.; Huppke, P.; Stark, W.; Kropshofer, H.; Tomic, D.; et al. Serum neurofilament light chain is a useful biomarker in pediatric multiple sclerosis. *Neurol. Neuroimmunol. Neuroinflamm.* **2020**, *7*. [CrossRef]
71. Sejbaek, T.; Nielsen, H.H.; Penner, N.; Plavina, T.; Mendoza, J.P.; Martin, N.A.; Elkjaer, M.L.; Ravnborg, M.H.; Illes, Z. Dimethyl fumarate decreases neurofilament light chain in CSF and blood of treatment naïve relapsing MS patients. *J. Neurol. Neurosurg. Psychiatry* **2019**, *90*, 1324–1330. [CrossRef]
72. Piehl, F.; Kockum, I.; Khademi, M.; Blennow, K.; Lycke, J.; Zetterberg, H.; Olsson, T. Plasma neurofilament light chain levels in patients with MS switching from injectable therapies to fingolimod. *Mult. Scler. J.* **2017**. [CrossRef]
73. Gunnarsson, M.; Malmeström, C.; Axelsson, M.; Sundström, P.; Dahle, C.; Vrethem, M.; Olsson, T.; Piehl, F.; Norgren, N.; Rosengren, L.; et al. Axonal damage in relapsing multiple sclerosis is markedly reduced by natalizumab. *Ann. Neurol.* **2011**, *69*, 83–89. [CrossRef] [PubMed]
74. de Flon, P.; Laurell, K.; Sundström, P.; Blennow, K.; Söderström, L.; Zetterberg, H.; Gunnarsson, M.; Svenningsson, A. Comparison of plasma and cerebrospinal fluid neurofilament light in a multiple sclerosis trial. *Acta Neurol. Scand.* **2019**, *139*, 462–468. [CrossRef] [PubMed]
75. Cross, A. Ocrelizumab treatment reduced levels of neurofilament light chain and numbers of B cells in the cerebrospinal fluid of patients with relapsing multiple sclerosis in the OBOE study S56.008. *Neurology* **2019**, *92*, 52.
76. Hauser, S.L.; Bar-Or, A.; Cohen, J.A.; Comi, G.; Correale, J.; Coyle, P.K.; Cross, A.H.; de Seze, J.; Leppert, D.; Montalban, X.; et al. Ofatumumab versus Teriflunomide in Multiple Sclerosis. *N. Engl. J. Med.* **2020**, *383*, 546–557. [CrossRef]
77. Kuhle, J.; Kropshofer, H.; Barro, C.; Meinert, R.; Haring, D.A.; Leppert, D.; Tomic, D.; Dahlke, F.; Kuhle, J.; Kropshofer, H.; et al. Siponimod Reduces Neurofilament Light Chain Blood Levels in Secondary Progressive Multiple Sclerosis Patients. *Neurology* **2018**, *90* (Suppl. 15), S8.006.

78. Bar-Or, A. Blood neurofilament light levels are lowered to a healthy donor range in patients with RMS and PPMS following ocrelizumab treatment. *ECTRIMS Online Library*, 9 December 2019.
79. Kapoor, R.; Sellebjerg, F.; Hartung, H.-P.; Arnold, D.L.; Freedman, M.S.; Jeffery, D.; Miller, A.; Edwards, K.R.; Singh, C.M.; Chang, I.; et al. Natalizumab reduced serum levels of neurofilament light chain in secondary progressive multiple sclerosis patients from the phase 3 ASCEND study. *Mult. Scler. J.* **2018**, *24*, 988. [CrossRef]
80. Kuhle, J.; Kropshofer, H.; Haring, D.A.; Barro, C.; Dahlke, F.; Leppert, D.; Tomic, D. Neurofilament light levels in the blood of patients with secondary progressive MS are higher than in primary progressive MS and may predict brain atrophy in both MS subtypes. *Mult. Scler. J.* **2018**, *24*, 111. [CrossRef]
81. Kapoor, R.; Smith, K.E.; Allegretta, M.; Arnold, D.L.; Carroll, W.; Comabella, M.; Furlan, R.; Harp, C.; Kuhle, J.; Leppert, D.; et al. Serum neurofilament light as a biomarker in progressive multiple sclerosis. *Neurology* **2020**. [CrossRef]
82. Kuhle, J.; Nourbakhsh, B.; Grant, D.; Morant, S.; Barro, C.; Yaldizli, Ö.; Pelletier, D.; Giovannoni, G.; Waubant, E.; Gnanapavan, S. Serum neurofilament is associated with progression of brain atrophy and disability in early MS. *Neurology* **2017**, *88*, 826–831. [CrossRef]
83. Jakimovski, D.; Kuhle, J.; Ramanathan, M.; Barro, C.; Tomic, D.; Hagemeier, J.; Kropshofer, H.; Bergsland, N.; Leppert, D.; Dwyer, M.G.; et al. Serum neurofilament light chain levels associations with gray matter pathology: A 5-year longitudinal study. *Ann. Clin. Transl. Neurol.* **2019**, *6*, 1757–1770. [CrossRef]
84. Manouchehrinia, A.; Stridh, P.; Khademi, M.; Leppert, D.; Barro, C.; Michalak, Z.; Benkert, P.; Lycke, J.; Alfredsson, L.; Kappos, L.; et al. Plasma neurofilament light levels are associated with risk of disability in multiple sclerosis. *Neurology* **2020**, *94*, e2457–e2467. [CrossRef] [PubMed]
85. Lublin, F.D. Disease activity free status in MS. *Mult. Scler. Relat. Disord.* **2012**, *1*, 6–7. [CrossRef] [PubMed]
86. Thebault, S.; Abdoli, M.; Fereshtehnejad, S.M.; Tessier, D.; Tabard-Cossa, V.; Freedman, M.S. Serum neurofilament light chain predicts long term clinical outcomes in multiple sclerosis. *Sci. Rep.* **2020**, *10*, 1–11. [CrossRef] [PubMed]
87. Chitnis, T.; Gonzalez, C.; Healy, B.C.; Saxena, S.; Rosso, M.; Barro, C.; Michalak, Z.; Paul, A.; Kivisakk, P.; Diaz-Cruz, C.; et al. Neurofilament light chain serum levels correlate with 10-year MRI outcomes in multiple sclerosis. *Ann. Clin. Transl. Neurol.* **2018**, 1478–1491. [CrossRef]
88. Novakova, L.; Axelsson, M.; Khademi, M.; Zetterberg, H.; Blennow, K.; Malmeström, C.; Piehl, F.; Olsson, T.; Lycke, J. Cerebrospinal fluid biomarkers as a measure of disease activity and treatment efficacy in relapsing-remitting multiple sclerosis. *J. Neurochem.* **2017**, *141*, 296–304. [CrossRef]
89. Bsteh, G.; Hegen, H.; Teuchner, B.; Amprosi, M.; Berek, K.; Ladstätter, F.; Wurth, S.; Auer, M.; Di Pauli, F.; Deisenhammer, F.; et al. Peripapillary retinal nerve fibre layer as measured by optical coherence tomography is a prognostic biomarker not only for physical but also for cognitive disability progression in multiple sclerosis. *Mult. Scler. J.* **2019**, *25*, 196–203. [CrossRef]

Publisher's Note: MDPI stays neutral with regard to jurisdictional claims in published maps and institutional affiliations.

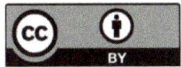

© 2020 by the authors. Licensee MDPI, Basel, Switzerland. This article is an open access article distributed under the terms and conditions of the Creative Commons Attribution (CC BY) license (http://creativecommons.org/licenses/by/4.0/).

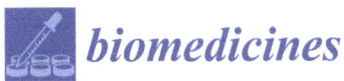

Review

Spinal Cord Involvement in MS and Other Demyelinating Diseases

Mariano Marrodan, María I. Gaitán and Jorge Correale *

Neurology Department, Fleni, C1428AQK Buenos Aires, Argentina; mmarrodan@fleni.org.ar (M.M.); migaitan@fleni.org.ar (M.I.G.)
* Correspondence: jcorreale@fleni.org.ar or jorge.correale@gmail.com; Tel.: +54-11-5777-3200 (ext. 2704/2456)

Received: 29 April 2020; Accepted: 20 May 2020; Published: 22 May 2020

Abstract: Diagnostic accuracy is poor in demyelinating myelopathies, and therefore a challenge for neurologists in daily practice, mainly because of the multiple underlying pathophysiologic mechanisms involved in each subtype. A systematic diagnostic approach combining data from the clinical setting and presentation with magnetic resonance imaging (MRI) lesion patterns, cerebrospinal fluid (CSF) findings, and autoantibody markers can help to better distinguish between subtypes. In this review, we describe spinal cord involvement, and summarize clinical findings, MRI and diagnostic characteristics, as well as treatment options and prognostic implications in different demyelinating disorders including: multiple sclerosis (MS), neuromyelitis optica spectrum disorder, acute disseminated encephalomyelitis, anti-myelin oligodendrocyte glycoprotein antibody-associated disease, and glial fibrillary acidic protein IgG-associated disease. Thorough understanding of individual case etiology is crucial, not only to provide valuable prognostic information on whether the disorder is likely to relapse, but also to make therapeutic decision-making easier and reduce treatment failures which may lead to new relapses and long-term disability. Identifying patients with monophasic disease who may only require acute management, symptomatic treatment, and subsequent rehabilitation, rather than immunosuppression, is also important.

Keywords: myelitis; spinal cord; multiple sclerosis; neuromyelitis optica; acute disseminated encephalomyelitis; myelin oligodendrocyte glycoprotein; glial fibrillary acidic protein

---

1. Introduction

Diagnostic accuracy in myelopathies is poor and therefore a challenge for neurologists in daily practice, mainly due to the multiple underlying pathophysiologic mechanisms observed in this group of disorders. In an initial approach, temporal profile (time to symptom nadir) contributes to differentiate vascular or traumatic causes from those of metabolic, neoplastic, and infectious or inflammatory etiology. To further assist in the identification of patients with acute vascular myelopathies for whom specific treatment strategies may be indicated, patients whose symptoms reach maximal severity in <4 h from onset are currently presumed to have an ischemic pathology unless proven otherwise [1]. By contrast, inflammatory processes affecting the spinal cord produce symptoms in a subacute manner, typically over hours or days. However, despite extensive patient work-up, a significant number of myelopathy cases are ultimately considered idiopathic [2]. Unfortunately, the term inflammatory myelitis is still applied to a complex and heterogeneous subgroup of post-infectious, rheumatologic, granulomatous, paraneoplastic, and demyelinating diseases, commonly affecting the spinal cord in which substantial overlap in clinical and imaging findings subsists. Identifying relapsing forms of disease has prognostic implications and can guide preventive treatment. Failure to indicate appropriate treatments may lead to new relapses and long-term disability. In contrast, patients in whom monophasic disease is suspected may only require acute management, symptomatic treatment, and subsequent rehabilitation rather than immunosuppression. In the case of demyelinating disorders, although multiple sclerosis (MS) is the main cause of inflammatory myelitis, other important differential diagnoses need to be ruled out to select the best treatment strategy in individual patients [3,4]. Thorough understanding of individual case etiology is therefore crucial, not only for correct treatment, but also to determine patient outcome.

In this review, we describe the epidemiologic characteristics, pathophysiology, clinical and (magnetic resonance imaging) MRI findings, treatment options and prognostic implications in MS and other demyelinating disorders including: neuromyelitis optica spectrum disorder (NMOSD), acute disseminated encephalomyelitis (ADEM), anti-myelin oligodendrocyte glycoprotein (MOG)-antibodies (ab) associated disease, and glial fibrillary acidic protein (GFAP)-IgG associated disease, to provide guidance in the diagnosis of these conditions.

A Pubmed search was conducted for articles published between 2000 and 2020, that included the terms: "acute disseminated encephalomyelitis; "demyelinating diseases"; "glial fibrillary acidic protein"; "multiple sclerosis"; "myelin oligodendrocyte glycoprotein"; "myelitis"; "neuromyelitis optica"; and "spinal cord diseases". Only those originally in English were considered. Earlier publications were identified from references cited in the articles reviewed.

2. Multiple Sclerosis

MS is a chronic inflammatory disease of the CNS leading to demyelination, neurodegeneration, and gliosis. It is by far the most common demyelinating disease, affecting over 2 million people worldwide [5]. Although its etiology remains elusive, environmental factors and susceptibility genes are now known to be involved in the pathogenesis [6]. Results from immunological, genetic, and histopathology studies of patients with MS support the concept that autoimmunity plays a major role in the disease [7]. In the majority of cases, the disease follows a relapsing remitting course (RRMS) from onset, which may later convert into a secondary progressive form (SPMS). Less often, patients show continued progression from disease debut (primary progressive MS, PPMS) [8].

Spinal cord abnormalities are common in MS and include a variety of pathological processes, such as demyelination, neuroaxonal loss and gliosis. Ultimately these result in motor weakness with accompanying difficulties in deambulation, spasticity, sensory disturbances, as well as bladder and bowel dysfunction [9]. Relapsing remitting MS can cause acute myelitis presenting with sensory loss, gait impairment, and incoordination, generally worsening over days to weeks, followed by stabilization or recovery [10]. During progressive phases of the disease however, especially in PPMS, slowly increasing or stuttering gait impairment due to demyelinating myelopathy is the most frequent presentation [11]. Once gait impairment has developed, cumulative disability increase will depend on patient age, clinical, and radiological disease activity and degree of spinal cord atrophy [12–15].

Histopathology findings in the spinal cord are characterized by significant decrease in axonal density in normal-appearing white matter (NAWM); perivascular T-cell infiltrates are rare, but robust, and diffuse inflammation is observed both in normal-appearing parenchyma and particularly in the meninges. Extent of diffuse axonal loss in NAWM correlates with both MHC class II$^+$ microglia cell density in NAWM, and significant increase in T cell density in the meninges. Interestingly, close interaction has been observed between T cells and MHC class II$^+$ macrophages in spinal cord meninges from MS patients, suggesting the meninges may form an immunological niche in which T lymphocytes become activated and proliferate in response to antigen presentation [16]. In support of this concept, similar findings have previously been described in experimental autoimmune encephalomyelitis [17], raising the possibility that activated meningeal T cells, through release of soluble factors such as IFN-γ, could instruct parenchymal macrophages/microglia to engage in neurotoxic activation programs [18].

Although spinal cord involvement has been difficult both to characterize and to quantify because current clinical and MRI parameters lack sensitivity and specificity [19], the spinal cord was one of four anatomical locations incorporated in a revision to McDonald diagnostic criteria for MS in 2017, to document spatial dissemination in patients presenting clinical isolated syndrome (CIS) suggestive of

MS. Likewise, new or gadolinium-enhancing spinal cord lesions can be used to document chronological progression [20].

Poor correlation between spinal cord injury load and clinical disability may be due to several different factors. Spinal cord MRI is more challenging than brain imaging in patients with MS. The spine is extremely thin and commonly subjected to ghosting artifacts (due to breathing, swallowing, and/or pulsation of blood and cerebrospinal fluid (CSF)) [21]. The amount of bone and fat may also produce significant artifacts, greater than those observed in brain imaging. Conventional, sagittal proton density (PD) and T2-weighted scans, with spatial resolution of 3 × 1 × 1 mm, should be considered the reference standard to detect MS spinal cord lesions [22,23]. Short-tau inversion recovery (STIR) sequences seem to be more sensitive to lesion detection than T2-weighted sequences and may be used to substitute PD sequences [24]. Contrast-enhanced T1-weighted images are recommended if T2 lesions are detected.

Conventional spine MRI has low sensitivity and specificity in relation to the pathological changes observed in MS [25]. Use of sagittal sections alone may underestimate lesion numbers [25]. Axial imaging may detect more lesions than sagittal imaging [26], especially smaller ones in the spinal cord periphery [27] and 2D or 3D T2-weighted sequences should be included in MRI protocols [21]. Axial multiple-echo recombined gradient echo (MERGE) seems to provide greater sensitivity for cord lesion detection and may represent a good alternative [28]. Ultimately, combined use of sagittal and axial images can facilitate identification and location of spinal lesions (Figure 1A–F) [26].

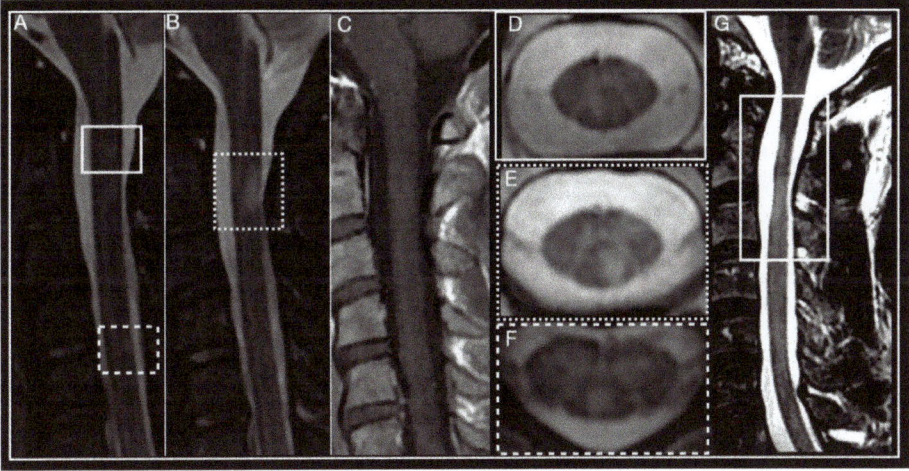

Figure 1. Multiple Sclerosis myelitis. (**A–F**) 32-year-old woman diagnosed with relapsing remitting course (RRMS) 2 years earlier, EDSS 0. (**A,B**) Sagittal short-tau inversion recovery (STIR) showing small, focal, chronic, peripheral lesions. (**C**) Sagittal post-contrast T1 weighted, absence of enhancement, T2 lesions are isointense. (**D–F**) axial T2 multiple-echo recombined gradient echo (MERGE). (**D**) right paramedian posterior lesion corresponds to lesion framed by a box in (**A**). (**E**) left paramedian posterior lesion corresponds to lesion framed by a dotted box in (**A**). (**F**) posterior lesion corresponds to lesion framed by a dotted line in (**A**). (**G**) 46-year-old man diagnosed with primary progressive multiple sclerosis (PPMS) in 2011, EDSS 6. Sagittal T2-weighted, framed area shows multiple sclerosis (MS) lesions and spinal cord atrophy.

Often more than one demyelinating plaque is present in spinal cord MRIs from patients with MS. The cervical spine (53–59%) is the most common location, followed by the thoracic region (20–47%) [10]. Lesions usually present as hyperintense on T2-weighted and isointense on T1-weighted sequences. Gadolinium enhancement is variable and depends mainly on acquisition timing, with acute lesions usually enhancing during 4–8 weeks [29,30]. Most MS lesions are small in size, wedge-shaped in axial and ovoid-shaped in sagittal views, and predominantly found in ascending sensory (i.e., posterior column), and descending motor (i.e., corticospinal) spinal cord tracts, because of the high myelin concentration within these fascicules [31]. Rarely, they may extend to involve central grey matter, occupying over half the cross-sectional area of the cord. Small focal lesions may coalesce to form more extensive ones, involving three or more segments, particularly in cases of progressive MS. High-resolution axial MRI demonstrates these images actually result from the confluence of multiple discrete lesions [25,32].

Spinal cord lesions, when present, are particularly helpful to discriminate MS from its radiological mimics, which include conditions such as migraine and cerebrovascular disorders. They can also present together with multifocal T2 lesions in brain white matter [33].

In addition to their diagnostic value, spine lesions contribute prognostic information in MS. Asymptomatic lesions are present in approximately 35% of patients with radiological isolated syndrome [34], in one-third of patients with CIS [35], and 83% of patients with early RRMS [36]. Interestingly, the number of asymptomatic lesions found in patients with CIS has been linked to risk of a second clinical event at 2 and 5 years [37,38], making spine MRI advisable in CIS patient workup. However, detection of asymptomatic spinal cord lesions during follow-up of RRMS patients was less common than detection of asymptomatic lesions in the brain, suggesting spinal cord MRI may be less useful than brain MRI for monitoring patients with RRMS [39]. Some authors have observed that greater number of spinal cord lesions at MS time of diagnosis and lesional topography at time of relapse were associated with increased relapse rates and higher risk of developing secondary progressive MS [10,11,39].

Spinal cord atrophy (Figure 1G) present in early stages of the disease may correlate with degree of disability and predict long term outcome [38,40]. Measuring changes in cross-sectional area at the cervical level yields the most reproducible results and shows closest correlation to clinical findings [41,42]. Grey matter atrophy on the other hand correlates more strongly with degree of physical disability than other MRI parameters of brain and cord atrophy [43–45]. Notably, a significant association between reduced cervical cord sectional diameter and disability progression has been demonstrated in different studies, independent of brain atrophy [46–48]. Cord atrophy has also been associated with reduction in retinal nerve layer thickness [48], suggesting it is probably part of a global pathological process and not just determined by local damage.

Rate of atrophy is more accelerated in the spinal cord than in the brain (1.5–2.2% per year vs. 0.5–1% per year) [49,50], and in patients with SPMS than in patients with CIS or RRMS. In RRMS, cord atrophy presents primarily in the posterior spinal cord, while in SPMS, atrophy is generalized [49]. Interestingly, regional atrophy does not seem to be influenced by focal lesion presence [51–53]. A recent study reported that a 1% increase in the annual rate of spinal cord volume loss was associated with a 28% risk of disability progression in the subsequent year [50]. Unfortunately, widespread use of this parameter has so far been limited by poor reproducibility and lack of sensitivity to small changes in the cord cross-sectional area. Since the rate of spinal atrophy over time appears to be associated with disability progression, atrophy has been considered a secondary outcome measure in phase 3 clinical trials of progressive MS [50,51]. When it was later analyzed more thoroughly, results were inconclusive [54–56]. This may have been due to lack of treatment efficacy, inadequate patient selection, poor reproducibility of cord atrophy quantification, or low sensitivity of MRI techniques used to detect small changes in cord cross-sectional area [30]. Eventually, spinal cord atrophy could also be considered a primary outcome in phase 2 clinical trials of progressive MS. However, this will require adequate patient selection and more precise MR imaging techniques for exact assessment.

It should be noted that neuronal loss in MS is not limited to white matter only, post mortem studies have also shown extensive neuronal loss in gray matter of the spinal cord as well, generating considerable interest in detection of gray matter abnormalities in MS [57]. The use of a combination of axial fast-field echo (FFE) and phase-sensitive inversion recovery (PSIR) sequences has been proposed to identify gray matter abnormalities in the upper cervical spinal cord [58]. However, further studies are still necessary to verify the sensitivity of this technique. Although both double inversion recovery (DIR) and PSIR can help distinguish focal gray matter lesions from normal-appearing tissue on sagittal views [59,60], these are often confounded by artifacts [61,62]. Use of 3T and higher field-strength (4.7 T) scanners as well as dedicated imaging sequences have increased MRI sensitivity for MS-associated gray matter lesion detection in the spinal cord [63,64]. Nevertheless, greater knowledge of spinal cord lesion pathogenesis, as well as its relationship to disability progression, still need to be established to better define the role of spinal cord assessment in MS diagnosis and follow-up [30].

More sensitive and better standardized methods are needed to assess clinical manifestations related to spinal cord atrophy over time, as well as monitor disease course and response to therapy. Promising MRI techniques to study the spinal cord include myelin water imaging, magnetization transfer imaging, diffusion tensor imaging, and magnetic resonance spectroscopy. At present however, use of these modalities is mostly restricted to research. Automated image-acquisition techniques, increased precision, and reduced quantification variability over time still need to be developed, and application in the clinical setting will likely be limited to select sites with experience using advanced imaging techniques.

Several studies have demonstrated that residual deficits persist after MS relapses affecting the spinal cord, contributing to stepwise progression of disability. For this reason, prompt and adequate treatment of relapses is key, although optimal regimens have to be better defined [65,66]. Unfortunately, despite significant advances in disease-modifying treatment, management of acute MS relapses with intravenous or oral corticosteroids has remained largely unchanged for the past 20 years [67].

Since the first prospective trial demonstrated superiority of high-dose intravenous methylprednisolone use (IVMPS; up to 1000 mg daily) over placebo, acute MS relapses are initially treated with IVMPS during three to five days [68]. Although faster recovery of relapses has been documented, clinical improvement is insufficient in approximately 25% of patients after the first course of IVMPS [69]. Aside from increasing steroid treatment dose and prolonging treatment (up to 2000 mg daily for five additional days), use of plasma exchange (PLEX) has also been considered an alternative option [70]. One recent study in a group of patients receiving PLEX within 6 weeks of a relapse showed not only significantly better response rates than those of patients receiving extended IVMPS treatment, but also lower risk deterioration 3 months after discharge [71,72]. For long-term treatment of MS, the last 2 decades have seen the development of numerous drugs aimed at correcting the different pathogenic mechanisms proposed in multiple sclerosis, most of which have been compounds targeting immune system dysfunction. Several clinical trials are currently ongoing, some using neuroprotective therapies to halt progression, others aimed at reversing neurological disability, at least in part, by repairing damaged brain and spinal cord tissue. Discussion of particular disease-modifying therapies for MS is beyond the scope of this manuscript, however, several comprehensive reviews on the subject have recently been published [73–76].

3. Acute Disseminated Encephalomyelitis

Acute disseminated encephalomyelitis (ADEM) is an autoimmune demyelinating disorder of the CNS, commonly affecting brain and spinal cord white matter, although deep grey matter nuclei (e.g., thalamus and basal ganglia) may also be involved [77,78]. ADEM is more common in children (mean age 5 to 8 years), but can occur at any age [79] with an estimated annual incidence of 0.23 to 0.40/100,000 children [80–82]. Although no clear gender predominance has been identified, slight male preponderance has been described in some pediatric ADEM cohorts [79]. Most pediatric ADEM cases appear to be preceded by symptoms of viral or bacterial infection, usually of the upper-respiratory tract. Vaccination has also been reported to precede ADEM, although at much lower rates [83]. Some cases have been linked to specific vaccines produced in neural tissue cultures (rabies and Japanese B encephalitis). However, a marked drop in post vaccination ADEM has occurred since CNS tissue culture-derived production was replaced by recombinant protein-based vaccines. Nevertheless in up to 26% of patients, no triggering event can be observed [84].

Histopathology findings in ADEM show perivenular inflammatory infiltrates consisting of T cells and macrophages, associated with perivenular demyelination and relative preservation of axons in most cases. In hemorrhagic variants, demyelination is often more widespread through the CNS, with important neutrophilic infiltrates [79].

The pathogenesis of ADEM is still unclear. Two main hypotheses have been proposed. One, the molecular mimicry hypothesis, suggests partial structural or amino-acid sequence homology may exist between certain pathogens or vaccines and host CNS myelin antigens, which in turn may activate myelin-reactive T cells, thereby eliciting a CNS-specific autoimmune response [85]. The second hypothesis proposes CNS infection may directly prompt a secondary inflammatory cascade, leading to blood-brain barrier rupture, exposure of CNS-antigens, and breakdown of tolerance resulting in an autoimmune attack driven mainly by T cells [86].

Criteria for ADEM diagnosis, established in 2013 by the International Multiple Sclerosis Study Group (IPMSSG), require the following to be present: (1) an initial polyfocal clinical CNS event of presumed inflammatory demyelinating cause; (2) encephalopathy (alteration in consciousness or behavior unexplained by fever, systemic illness, or post ictal symptoms); (3) brain MRI abnormalities consistent with demyelination during the acute phase (first 3 months); (4) no new clinical or MRI findings 3 months or more after onset [87].

Depending on the series, spinal cord involvement has been described in 20% to 54% of ADEM patients, predominantly affecting the thoracic region [88]. Coincident brain and spinal cord lesions are more common; isolated spinal cord ADEM is exceptional [89] and typically extends over multiple segments, cause cord swelling, and showing variable enhancement in the acute phase. In most ADEM patients, partial or complete resolution of MRI abnormalities occurs within a few months of treatment [84,90]. Interestingly, ADEM patients with anti-MOG antibodies show large, more widespread brain lesions with ill-defined borders and longitudinally extensive spinal cord lesions on MRI [91]. Lesions involving more than two segments are more frequent in adults than in children (50% vs. 27%, respectively) [92].

No specific studies on CSF have been conducted in ADEM. Pleocytosis is typically mild, with a high percentage of lymphocytes and monocytes [92,93] and increased protein levels (up to 1.1 g/L) in 23% to 62% of pediatric patients [94–96]. OCBs are only present in 0% to 29% of cases [79]. However, they are usually transient as opposed to those observed in MS.

Although ADEM usually has a monophasic course, multiphasic forms have been reported in 10–31% of patients [84,97], making differential diagnosis with MS more difficult in these cases. Multiphasic forms are defined as new encephalopathic events consistent with ADEM, separated by a 3-month interval from the initial illness but not followed by any further event [98]. Relapsing disease following ADEM occurring beyond a second encephalopathic event is no longer consistent with multiphasic ADEM, but rather indicates a chronic disorder such as MS, NMOSD, or ADEM-optic neuritis [98,99], and should prompt testing for anti-MOG ab. It is worth highlighting that progression from ADEM to MS is relatively low, estimated at 0% to 17% in studies with follow-up periods lasting several years [88].

Clinical presentation and outcome of ADEM in adults differs from that of children. Disease course is worse in adults, with more than one-third of patients requiring admission to an ICU, and duration of hospitalization can be twice as long. Outcome is also less favorable, complete motor recovery is observed in only 15% of adults compared to 58% of children and more adult patients die, although no difference in the occurrence of relapses or conversion to MS has been reported [92,100]. Poorer outcomes in adults cannot be explained by differences in clinical presentation (preceding factors, symptoms, blood and CSF parameters or radiological features are all similar). Perhaps reduced plasticity in ageing CNS tissue is the cause, rather than a difference in pathophysiology from onset [92].

No randomized-controlled studies have been conducted on ADEM treatment. Despite the lack of conclusive evidence, a widely accepted regimen in use today is administration of IV methylprednisolone (30 mg/kg/day in children or 1000 mg/day in adults) for 5 days, followed by oral taper with dexamethasone at a starting dose of 1–2 mg/kg/day, for 4–6 weeks [101,102]. Plasma exchange is recommended for therapy-refractory patients with fulminant disease [103,104]. Beyond treatment of the initial event, it is important to have a plan for long term follow-up to exclude a multiphasic disorder, which would warrant further diagnostic evaluation and a different therapeutic approach.

4. Neuromyelitis Optica Spectrum-Disorder

Neuromyelitis optica (NMO) is an inflammatory disorder, traditionally considered monophasic, although relapsing cases have been described in which patients present optic neuritis and transverse myelitis [105]. NMO had been considered a variant of MS until an autoantibody against the water channel protein aquaporin-4 (AQP4), expressed abundantly on astrocyte end-feet, called AQP4-IgG (also called NMO-IgG), was discovered in patients with NMO, and found to be absent in patients with MS [106,107]. Incorporation of AQP4-IgG serology to revised NMO diagnostic criteria broadened the clinical and radiological spectrum of NMO [108]. The term NMO spectrum disorders (NMOSD) was introduced to include AQP4-IgG seropositive patients with limited forms of NMO, and at risk of future attacks, as well as patients with cerebral, diencephalic, and brainstem lesions, or coexisting autoimmune disease (e.g., systemic lupus erythematosus [SLE] or Sjögren syndrome [SS]) [109]. Accordingly, NMOSD was recognized as a humoral disease entity distinct from MS, and diagnostic criteria were revised in 2015 unifying the terms NMO and NMOSD [110].

Evidence supporting a pathogenic role of AQP4-IgG comes from different sources. Complement- as well as ab-dependent cytotoxicity [101,102] has been associated to AQP4-IgG, which when administered along with complement and/or pathogenic T cells, promotes development of NMOSD-like CNS lesions in rodents [111,112]. Inflammatory damage is characterized by astrocyte loss and deposition of both immunoglobulins and complement, followed by neutrophil, monocyte, phagocyte and eosinophil infiltration [113]. Importantly, AQP4 distribution coincides with deposition patterns of IgG, IgM, and products of complement activation present in active NMO tissue [114,115], and MRI lesions of patients with NMO overlap with sites of high AQP4 expression [116]. AQP4-IgG is believed to determine internalization of the glutamate transporter EAAT2, limiting glutamate uptake from the extracellular space into astrocytes, also resulting in oligodendrocyte damage and myelin loss [117]. Although most strongly expressed in the CNS, AQP4 is also present in the collecting duct of the kidney, parietal cells of the stomach, as well as in airways, salivary glands, and skeletal muscle [118]. However, peripheral organ damage does not typically occur, probably due to the presence of complement inhibitory proteins in these secondary target organs [119].

Despite caveats in knowledge on NMOSD epidemiology, prevalence has been estimated depending on the study population at 0.1–4.4 cases/100,000 individuals, and annual incidence at 0.20–4.0 per 1,000,000 [120,121]. Initial clinical manifestations occur at around 40 years of age, although children and the elderly account for 18% of cases. Female/male predominance is around 9:1, but not in children, where equal gender distribution has been observed [32,122].

According to the most recent diagnostic criteria, core clinical characteristics can involve 1 of 6 CNS regions, namely: optic nerve, spinal cord, area postrema of the dorsal medulla, brainstem, diencephalon, or cerebrum [110]. Clinical presentation particularly suggestive of NMOSD diagnosis includes: bilateral ON involving the optic chiasm with poor recovery compared to MS-ON, complete spinal cord syndrome determining paroxysmal spasms, and area postrema clinical syndrome characterized by intractable hiccups, or nausea and vomiting. No single clinical characteristic is pathognomonic of NMOSD, however [110]. In AQP4-IgG seronegative patients, diagnostic criteria are more rigorous. Patients must present at least 2 of the core clinical characteristics, and at least one of these must be: ON, longitudinally extensive transverse myelitis (LETM), or area postrema syndrome.

Given the focus of this review, in the following sections, only aspects related to NMOSD-related to spinal cord involvement will be addressed.

Acute transverse myelitis symptoms in NMOSD patients (motor, sensitive, and frequently sphincter) are usually severe and bilateral, and recovery is incomplete compared to MS. Although overlap of clinical characteristics in MS and NMOSD myelitis does occur, symptom magnitude and disease history frequently contribute to establish differential diagnosis [30,32,120], as do certain MRI findings. LETM is the most specific neuroimaging characteristic found in NMOSD, and is uncommon in MS (Figure 2) [108]. Mirroring severe underlying tissue damage, lesions are generally hyperintense on T2-weighted, and hypointense on T1-weighted sequences [30]. Extending over three or more complete vertebral segments, they tend to localize in the center of the cord, because of the abundant AQP4 channel expression in grey matter. Lesions will usually occupy over 50% of the cross-sectional surface area of the spine, representing a complete, rather than incomplete, form of transverse myelitis which is more characteristic in MS. However, they also may be lateral, anterior, or posterior over the length of the lesion and be accompanied by cord swelling. The latter, when present, can generate concern over presence of a spinal cord tumor [123]. Chronic necrosis caused by NMOSD can in some cases result in spinal cord cavitation and cystic myelomalacia. Small areas of strong hyperintensity, higher than that of the surrounding cerebrospinal fluid (CSF), so-called bright spotty lesions, may be observed and could be useful to distinguish NMOSD from MS [124]. Acute NMO lesions extensively enhance following IV gadolinium administration. Lens-shaped ring-enhancement is detected in up to 32% of NMOSD patients [29,125,126]. Rostral extension of cervical lesions to the area postrema is another characteristic of NMOSD and can be helpful to distinguish it from other causes of longitudinal extensive myelopathy such as sarcoidosis, spondylotic myelopathy with enhancement, dural arteriovenous fistula, spinal cord infarct, and paraneoplastic myelopathy [127]. Although LETM is the most frequent form, 7–14% of NMO-myelitis involve <3 vertebral segments. However, short forms of NMO-myelitis are followed by LETM in ninety percent of cases. Short cord lesions should be suspected in patients with tonic spasm, coexistence of autoimmune disease, grey matter involvement and absence of OCB. As in MS, in 7–14% of cases, variation in presentation will be linked to time at which MRI scans are obtained [128–130]. Lesions limited to less than three segments will be detected at the beginning of disease or during remission [131]. In contrast, patients with longstanding disease may present short but coalescing lesions suggesting a LETM pattern [22]. Presence of a longitudinally extensive segment of cord atrophy is another characteristic finding in support of prior NMOSD myelitis [131].

Although in NMOSD the relationship between spinal cord atrophy, disease activity and disability is not fully known, two observations deserve mention. First, NMOSD patients predominantly show spinal cord atrophy with only mild brain atrophy, while MS patients demonstrate more brain atrophy, especially in gray matter, suggesting a different underlying pathogenic mechanism [132]. Second, spinal cord atrophy can occur in patients without a clinical history of myelitis or visible spinal cord lesions on MRI, suggesting cord atrophy may be due to a diffuse underlying process. Alternatively, or perhaps in co-contributory fashion, patients may have experienced transient or subclinical inflammatory events not evident on conventional MRI [133].

Serum AQP4-IgG assay is the most useful test for NMOSD diagnosis. Based on criteria proposed by the International Panel for NMOSD, approximately 73–90% of patients with NMOSD express AQP4-IgG [134,135]. A cell-based assay (CBA) is recommended whenever possible because of its higher sensitivity (76.7%) and very low false-positive rate (0.1%) [136,137]. Indirect immunofluorescence assays and ELISA have less sensitivity (63–64% each), and can yield false-positive results (0.5–1.3% for ELISA) particularly at low titers [135,137]. Ultimately, 10–27% of patients with typical clinical and radiological features of NMOSD will not have detectable AQP4-IgG despite use of the best available assay. Lack of a diagnostic biomarker makes management of these patients more challenging especially of patients with monophasic disease [121,136]. Notably, using CBA, approximately 15–40% of AQP4-IgG seronegative NMOSD patients have been reported to have detectable antibodies against myelin oligodendrocyte glycoprotein (MOG) [137,138]. Aside from causing optico-spinal disease resembling NMOSD, anti-MOG antibodies have been identified in patients with clinical characteristics unlike those of patients with AQP4-IgG [32,137,139] (see below), suggesting a different underlying pathogenesis. Occasionally, patients without detectable serum AQP4-IgG are later found to be positive, possibly related to assay timing (antibody levels increase during exacerbations), or to impact of immunosuppressive treatment.

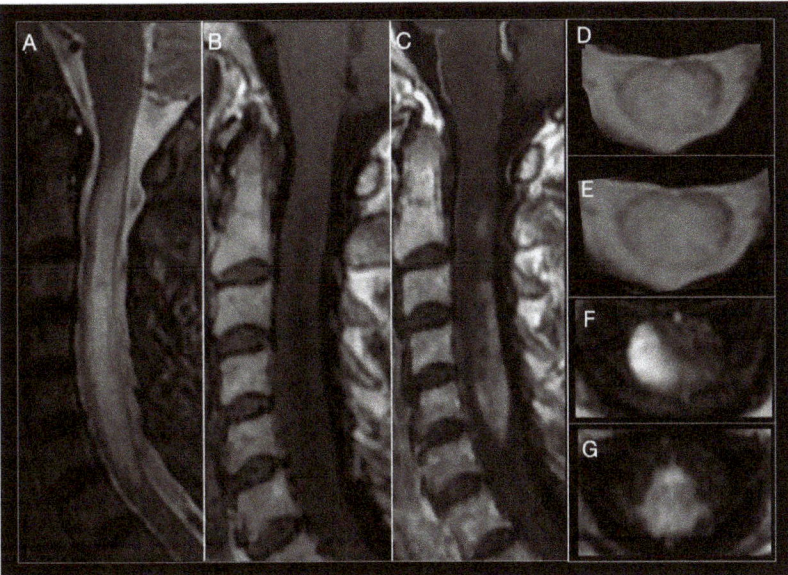

Figure 2. Neuromyelitis optica (NMO) myelitis. Images from a 58-year-old woman with acute longitudinally extensive myelitis (C1–C7). (**A**) Sagittal STIR showing an extensive lesion, involving more than 3 segments, that widens the cervical spinal cord. (**B**) Sagittal T1-weighted sequences show an extensive T1-hypointense lesion. (**C**) T1-weighted images after contrast administration, extensive enhancement of cervical lesion. (**D,E**) Axial T2-MERGE hyperintense area that involves more than half the diameter of the spinal cord. (**E,F**) Axial T1-weighted, intense contrast enhancement of lateral (**E**) and central-posterior (**F,G**) areas.

Serum AQP4-IgG concentration is much higher than that found in CSF. The hypothesis behind this is that most AQP4-IgG is produced in peripheral lymphoid tissues and that a favorable serum/CSF antibody gradient is needed for penetration into the CNS, a concept supported by the fact that commercial CBA and flow cytometry detection of AQP4-IgG is more sensitive in serum than in CSF. Serum is therefore the optimal specimen for AQP4-IgG testing [140].

Some patients with NMOSD produce other autoantibodies in addition to AQP4-IgG, as occurs in patients with SLE or SS [118]. Since LETM has also been described in patients with these conditions, the possibility exists that NMOSD symptoms arise secondary to SLE or SS. Limited existing data in this regard shows that in such patients, AQP4-IgG detection rates are similar to those observed in patients with NMOSD without associated rheumatic disease, suggesting LETM in NMOSD is not secondary to SLE or SS, and these patients suffer from two independent, coexisting autoimmune diseases [118,141–143].

CSF pleocytosis (>50 cells/μL) or presence of neutrophils or eosinophils during NMOSD attacks may help to distinguish NMOSD from MS [123,137].CSF OCBs are usually absent, although they may sometimes be transiently detectable during an attack [123,144].Given the high morbidity associated with NMOSD exacerbations, the goals of pharmacotherapy are to aggressively treat acute attacks, (including the initial episode) and prevent future relapses, minimizing CNS damage and long-term disability [145,146]. Different pathophysiologic mechanisms are known to characterize MS and NMOSD, a finding at least partially demonstrated by the fact that exacerbations can be precipitated by fingolimod, IFNβ and natalizumab, treatments that are effective in MS. Aside from the need for accurate diagnosis, evaluation of occult infection or metabolic disturbances should be carried out to identify pseudo-relapses Although there are no randomized controlled trials in large cohorts examining treatment of acute relapses, NMOSD exacerbations are typically treated with 1 g of IVMP for 3–5 consecutive days [147,148]. Severe NMOSD relapses or patients who do not respond to treatment with IVMP may benefit from plasma exchange (PLEX) [72,147–149]; which targets specific antibodies, complement and several pro-inflammatory proteins [150] Early (≤5 days), aggressive treatment with PLEX is linked to better outcome [151]. Interestingly, positive results of PLEX are obtained both in seropositive as well as seronegative NMOSD patients [152–154]. In order to avoid relapses, different immunosuppressive strategies are used in daily neurological practice including: oral corticosteroids, mycophenolate mofetil or azathioprine (both oral purine analog anti-metabolites), rituximab (IV anti-CD20 monoclonal antibody) and tocilizumab (anti-IL-6 receptor monoclonal antibody [146,147]. However, none of these agents have been specifically approved for NMOSD treatment, and off-label use has arisen based almost entirely on results from uncontrolled observational studies [146,147]. Recently, three new monoclonal antibodies with different mechanisms of action and routes of administration have shown efficacy in NMOSD patients: eculizumab (anti-complement protein C5) [155], inebilizumab (anti-CD19) [156], and satralizumab (anti-IL-6R) [157], significantly reducing risk of new relapses compared to placebo, particularly in AQP4-ab-positive patients, with clinical stabilization or improvement in most cases. All these drugs demonstrated good safety and tolerability profiles with limited side effects. Future evaluation in real-life studies will be needed though, to estimate annual relapse rates and compare results to those of older drugs.

5. Myelin Oligodendrocyte Glycoprotein Antibody-Associated Disease

Myelin oligodendrocyte glycoprotein, a member of the immunoglobulin superfamily, is exclusively expressed on the surface of oligodendrocytes and on the outermost lamellae of myelin sheaths in the CNS. Given its structure and location it could potentially function as a cell surface receptor, or cell adhesion molecule. Furthermore, its extracellular location makes it a target for autoimmune ab- and cell-mediated responses, in inflammatory demyelinating diseases. Interesting results from animal studies on MOG ab-associated demyelination lead to this antibody being considered a marker for MS [158,159]. However, subsequent studies in large populations of MS patients found seropositivity prevalence in this condition was similar to that detected in other inflammatory neurological diseases, as well as to levels in control subjects, generating skepticism over whether these ab could be considered a true biomarker of MS [160–162]. Seminal studies using murine anti-MOG ab have highlighted the fact that ab target epitopes of native MOG are biologically relevant in their conformational state, rather than in linearized or denatured MOG. Therefore, CBA, which maintains the native conformational form of the extracellular portion of MOG, is the most recommended technique to study ab levels.

There is current international consensus that anti-MOG ab are important in both pediatric and adult demyelination. Different research groups have identified seropositive MOG ab populations in children with ADEM, particularly in recurrent forms of the disease [163–166]. Other studies later confirmed presence of MOG ab in 25% to 30% of AQP4 seronegative NMOSD patients with recurrent ON. Substantial differences between both diseases in histopathology, as well as in vivo and vitro studies demonstrating a direct pathogenic role for MOG-IgG, suggest it represents a separate individual entity. Anti-MOG ab are already present at disease onset, both in serum and CSF, in some patients, persisting also during remission in the majority of patients, which argues against anti-MOG ab presence as a secondary epiphenomenon [167–170]. Notably, serum anti-MOG ab detection is more sensitive than CSF assay.

Since these observations, an increasing number of patients with diverse phenotypes related to these antibodies have been described. A comparison of patients with MOG ab disease to AQP4 NMOSD cases showed the former were younger [68,169–171], did not show significant female predominance [172], and were more commonly Caucasians; whereas AQP4-seropositive NMOSD was found predominantly in non-Caucasian populations [173,174].

The most commonly reported presentation of anti-MOG ab-associated disease is ON, which can be bilateral and recurrent in up to 61% of cases. Interesting, imaging of the optic nerve frequently shows peri-optic nerve sheath contrast enhancement, extending into the surrounding soft tissue, a radiological characteristic not observed in MS or AQP4 positive patients [175,176].

Approximately half the patients with MOG ab-associated disease present episodes involving the spinal cord [177,178]. The most common symptoms include paraparesis, and sensory and sphincter dysfunction. On MRI, LETM is frequent and short myelitis less common. Any segment of the spinal cord can be affected, although lesions are more frequent in the thoracolumbar and/or conus medullaris regions, as opposed to the more common cervicothoracic involvement observed in AQP4 ab positive and MS myelitis cases [178,179]. Anti-MOG ab associated myelitis is hyperintense on T2-weighted and iso-hypointense on T1-weighted sequences, showing contrast enhancement during acute phases in up to 70% of cases [172]; Figures 3 and 4. MOG ab-related disease does not commonly result in cord necrosis or cavitations as observed in AQP4-mediated cases [134,175,178]. Due to the predilection for conus localization, bladder, bowel, and erectile dysfunction is observed in approximately 70% of patients [167]. In comparison to AQP4-IgG$^+$ NMOSD, MOG ab disease myelitis appears to more focal and with better clinical outcome, although poor outcome with permanent disability has been described for both conditions [156]. Notably, anti-MOG ab serum titers follow disease activity levels, with significantly higher concentration during acute attacks than remission, further supporting the concept of their pathogenic role [172].

Although ON and myelitis are the two most frequent forms of presentation of anti-MOG ab disease, coexistence of brain, brainstem, or cerebellar involvement is frequent, and may even be extensive. Nausea, vomiting, and respiratory disturbances are some of the symptoms that can be present in cases of brainstem involvement [177].

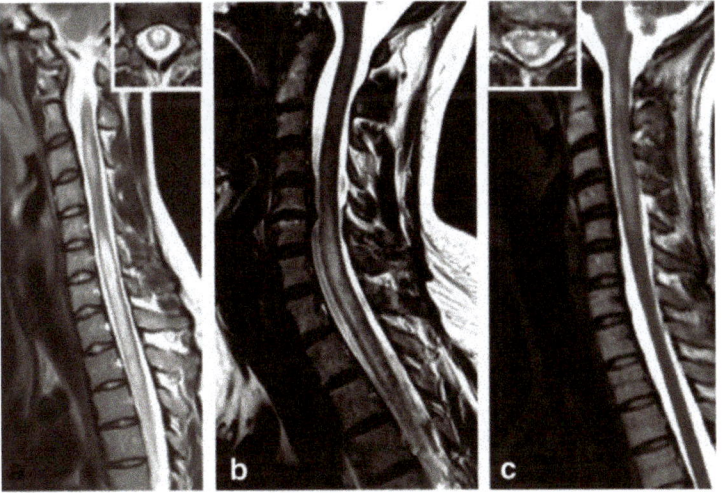

Figure 3. Anti-myelin oligodendrocyte glycoprotein (MOG) antibody myelitis. (**a**) Sagittal T2-weighted spinal MRI performed at disease onset revealed a large longitudinal centrally-located lesion extending over the entire spinal cord, as well as swelling of the cord. (**b**) Longitudinally extensive central spinal cord T2 lesion in another patient. (**c**) T2-hyperintense lesions extending from the pontomedullary junction throughout the cervical cord to C5, in a third patient. Insets in (**a**) and C show axial sections of the thoracic cord at lesion level [172]. Figure is extracted from Jarius, S. et al., *J Neuroinflammation* 2016, 13, 280 (http://creativecommons.org/licenses/by/4.0/).

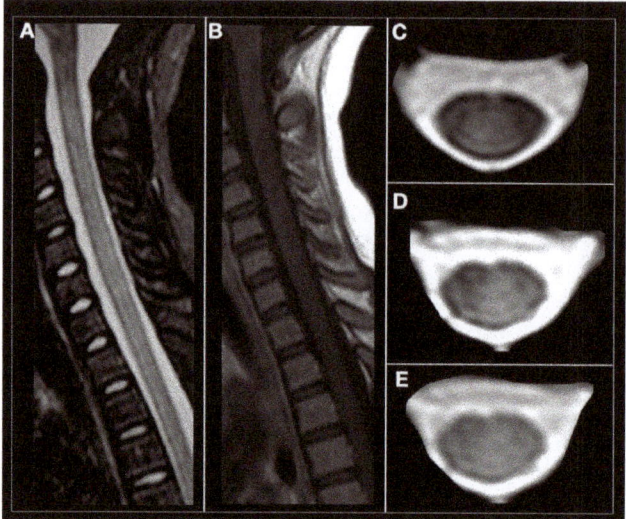

Figure 4. Anti-MOG antibody myelitis. A 12-year-old girl with relapse in the cervical spine. (**A**) sagittal STIR, subtle and diffuse hyperintensity of the cervical spinal cord. (**B**) Sagittal T1-weighted, spinal cord is isointense without contrast enhancement. (**C–E**) axial T2-weighted images showing subtle and diffuse spinal cord hyperintensity (Courtesy Dr. Angeles Schteinschnaider).

Different study groups have developed MRI diagnostic criteria to differentiate MS, from NMOSD and from anti-MOG ab-associated disease, showing 91% sensitivity distinguishing MS from AQP4+ NMOSD, and 95% from anti-MOG ab-associated disease [173,179]. More recently, the criteria were subtly modified to include spinal cord in the analysis, increasing sensitivity to 100% and specificity to 79%, reflecting the crucial importance of spinal cord findings in anti-MOG-ab disease. Interestingly, this radiological criterion was particularly useful in patients with ON, a clinical presentation common to all three diseases [180].

Patients with anti-MOG ab-associated disease were initially described as experiencing a monophasic disease [91,140,178]. However, recent studies found a high proportion of patients presenting relapsing disease [173,181]. Anti-MOG ab-positive patients exhibited better motor and visual outcome compared to AQP4-IgG positive patients after the first episode [170,181].

Anti-MOG ab are present in approximately 40% of children with ADEM. In this group, most patients develop LETM, and similar to patients without anti-MOG ab, show large, ill-defined, bilateral lesions in the brain, which typically resolve completely, in correlation with improved clinical outcome [165,177].

MOG ab-positive patients show rapid response to steroids and plasma exchange [177], but tend to relapse quickly after steroid withdrawal or cessation [182,183]. Therefore, slow steroid taper is recommended to minimize chances of early relapses. In adult patients, persistent seropositivity following initial treatment and clinical resolution is one of the main reasons to consider long term immunosuppression with steroid-sparing agents including mycophenolate, azathioprine or rituximab [135,169,170,184–186]. The significance of this finding is less clear in pediatric patients with ADEM and persistence of serum anti-MOG abs.

6. Glial Fibrillary Acid Protein Antibody-Associated Myelitis

A novel autoimmune CNS disorder characterized by the presence of antibodies specific for glial fibrillary acidic protein (GFAP) has recently been described. In the largest series published to date, median symptom onset age was around 40 years, with similar incidence in both women and men [187,188]. All patients with GFAP-IgGs reacted against the mature (α) GFAP isoform, with only a few patients showing immunoreactivity against the immature (ε) isoform [188]. GFAP is a cytoplasmic protein not accessible to IgG in intact cells, therefore, it is possible that immune cells also contribute to the tissue damage observed in this condition, for example GFAP peptide-specific $CD8^+$ T lymphocytes [189]. Eventually other immune cells sensitive to steroids, such as microglia and macrophages, can also play a role in the disease, acting directly, or through the release of molecules modulating the immune response such as cytokines or chemokines [187,190–192].

Clinical phenotype of GFAP-IgG astrocytopathy is heterogeneous and still poorly defined. The predominant clinical syndrome includes meningitis, encephalitis, and myelitis, or all three (meningoencephalomyelitis) with or without optic disc edema [188,193,194].

Myelitis occurs in up to 68% of patients with GFAP-IgG. However, its presentation as isolated clinical manifestation is infrequent. Despite the fact that autoimmune GFAP astrocytopathy and NMOSD-related myelitis share some clinical features, certain differences are worth mentioning [195]. Influenza-like prodromal symptoms and bowel/bladder dysfunction are common features in GFAP-IgG myelitis, while numbness and weakness followed by tonic spasms, frequent NMOSD symptoms, are rare. Notably, sensory level and Lhermitte's phenomenon are usually absent in GFAP-IgG myelitis, which is found in the cervical or thoracic spinal cord, in central location, usually involving at least three vertebral segments [195]. Lesions are hyperintense on T2-weighted sequences and may show a thin and linear pattern of contrast enhancement along the course of the central canal, different to the patchy or ring-like contrast uptake seen in NMOSD [187]. GFAP-IgG lesions have poorly-defined margins and less cord swelling compared to AQP4-IgG myelitis [195]. Short myelitis has also been reported in association with brain symptoms [187,194,195].

Notably, brain MRI findings significantly contribute to discriminate GFAP-IgG from other pathologies. A striking pattern of linear radial periventricular contrast enhancement is highly specific for GFAP-IgG-associated disease. Similar radial enhancement patterns have been described in the cerebellum in a lower percentage of patients [184,185,193].

Anti-GFAP abs can be detected in serum in 45% of patients, but sensitivity increases to 92% when ab are assayed in CSF [187]. Up to 50% of cases coexist with N-methyl-D-aspartate receptor (NMDAr) antibodies or anti-AQP4 ab, and up to 34% of patients may present concomitant neoplasms, with ovarian teratoma as the most prevalent [187]. These associations explain the diverse phenotypes reported [187,188,194]. Marked elevation of white cells and protein are common findings in CSF, and intrathecal oligoclonal bands may be present in 50% of patients [187].

Most reported GFAP-IgG cases show improvement in clinical, radiological, and CSF abnormalities after receiving high-dose intravenous methylprednisolone for 3–5 days [184,192]. Although nonresponsive-patients have been described, need for plasma exchange is significantly less frequent compared to patients with NMOSD [193,195,196]. In one study, 50% of patients with long-term follow-up (>24 months) had a relapsing course, 27% had a monophasic course and 23% had progressive disease in spite of adequate treatment. Clinical relapses were frequently associated with recurrent gadolinium enhancement on MRI and elevated CSF white cell count, with further remission observed after restarting steroids [187].

GFAP-IgG is unlikely to be directly pathogenic, as GFAP is an intracellular protein. However, it could be an excellent biomarker, identifying a neoplasm early on, leading to prompt and efficient treatment and prevention of long-term disability in GFAP-IgG myelitis cases.

7. Conclusions

Overall, demyelinating myelopathies belong to a complex and heterogeneous group of diseases, in which differential diagnosis can be difficult (Table 1). Clinical features, time-course, CSF characteristics, specific serum assays, and brain and spinal cord MRI findings all contribute to determine diagnosis, select the best treatment option and establish prognosis for each subtype. Early treatment with IV steroids and PLEX is accepted in all etiologies, but more specific treatment strategies may subsequently be adopted based on final diagnosis.

Table 1. Main features in demyelinating myelopathies of different etiology.

	MS	ADEM	NMOSD	MOG-IgG Disease	GFAP-IgG Disease
Estimated F:M ratio	3:1	1:1	9:1	1.3:1	1:1
Age * (yrs)	30	6	37	33	40
Myelitis clinical features	Sensory loss, gait impairment, weakness, sphincter involvement	Transverse myelitis	Transverse myelitis	Paraparesis, sensory symptoms and sphincter involvement	Sensory symptoms, sphincter dysfunction
Clinical course	Relapsing (85%) or progressive (15%)	Typically monophasic (69–90%)	Relapsing (90%)	Monophasic (58%) or relapsing (42%)	Relapsing (50%), monophasic (27%) or progressive (23%)
Serology findings	Not relevant	Not relevant	Serum AQP4-IgG. coexistence with other systemic disease antibodies (ANA, SSA or SSB).	Serum MOG-IgG	Anti-GFAP ab + in serum or CSF (Serum Anti-AQP4-IgG and/or anti-NMDAR ab coexistence,
Presence of OCB	80–95%	0% to 29% (usually transient)	Up to 30% (usually transient)	Up to 12%	Up to 50%
CSF	Generally normal or mild inflammatory changes	Mild pleocytosis and increased proteins up to 62%	Pleocytosis (neutrophils and eosinophils can be found) and mild elevated proteins	Normal or slightly inflammatory changes	Marked elevation of white blood cells and elevated protein levels
Brain MRI	Dawson fingers, lesions perpendicular to ventricles Cortical/yuxtacortical lesions Perivenular Nodular or ring/open-ring enhancing lesions Unilateral short optic nerve enhancement	Subcortical or deep gray matter bilateral, sometimes poorly-defined Simultaneous enhancement with gadolinium	Periependimal lesions Tumefactive lesions Involvement of corticospinal tract Marked enhancement, 'cloud like' Bilateral, long optic nerve enhancement	Non-specific supratentorial subcortical or small deep white matter foci. Occasionally T2 lesions in brainstem, and infratentorial regions Anterior bilateral ON with perineural optic nerved enhancement	Linear radial periventricular contrast enhancement pattern
Spinal cord MRI	Small, peripheral, posterolateral lesions Less than 3 segments Gadolinium enhancement during acute phase	LETM or multiple short segment myelitis Edematous lesions and gadolinium enhancement in acute phase	Central LETM Edematous Necrosis or cavitation Gadolinium enhancement in acute phase	LETM or short myelitis, frequent conus medullaris involvement Linear gadolinium enhancement of the ependymal canal	LETM Central lesions

Ab: antibodies, ADEM: acute disseminated encephalomyelitis, AQP4: Aquaporin 4, F: female, GFAP: glial fibrillary acid protein, LETM: longitudinally extensive transverse myelitis, M: male, MOG: myelin oligodendrocyte glycoprotein, MRI: magnetic resonance imaging, MS: multiple sclerosis, NMDAR: N-Methyl-D-aspartate receptor, NMOSD: neuromyelitis optica spectrum disorder, OCB: oligoclonal bands. * estimated media.

Author Contributions: M.M. contributed to draft the original manuscript, design the figures, revise the draft and provide important intellectual contributions. M.I.G. contributed to draft the original manuscript, design the figures, revise the draft and provide important intellectual contributions. J.C. contributed to the conception and design of the manuscript, draft the original manuscript, revise the draft, provide important intellectual contributions, and supervised the writing of the manuscript. All authors have read and agreed to the published version of the manuscript.

Funding: This study was supported by an internal grant from FLENI (J.C.).

Acknowledgments: We thank Angeles Schteinschnaider for providing Figure 4 and Ismael L. Calandri for providing the graphical abstract.

Conflicts of Interest: M.M. has nothing to disclose. M.I.G. has received reimbursement for developing educational presentations, from Merck Argentina, Biogen Argentina, Sanofi-Genzyme Argentina, Bayer Inc Argentina and Novartis Argentina, and has received travel/accommodations stipends from Merck Argentina, Biogen Argentina, Roche Argentina, Novartis Argentina, and TEVA Argentina. J.C. is a board member of Merck-Serono Argentina, Biogen-Idec LATAM, Merck-Serono. LATAM, Novartis and Genzyme global. Correale has received reimbursement for developing educational presentations for Merck-Serono Argentina, Merck-Serono LATAM, Biogen-Idec Argentina, Genzyme Argentina, and Novartis Argentina and Roche Argentina as well as professional travel/accommodations stipends. The funders had no role in the design of the study; in the collection, analysis, or interpretation of data; in the writing of the manuscript, or in the decision to publish the results.

References

1. Barreras, P.; Fitzgerald, K.C.; Mealy, M.A.; Jimenez, J.A.; Becker, D.; Newsome, S.D.; Levy, M.; Gailloud, P.; Pardo, C.A. Clinical biomarkers differentiate myelitis from vascular and other causes of myelopathy. *Neurology* **2018**, *90*, E12–E21. [CrossRef] [PubMed]
2. Transverse Myelitis Consortium Working Group. Proposed diagnostic criteria and nosology of acute transverse myelitis. *Neurology* **2002**, *59*, 499–505. [CrossRef] [PubMed]
3. de Seze, J.; Lanctin, C.; Lebrun, C.; Malikova, I.; Papeix, C.; Wiertlewski, S.; Pelletier, J.; Gout, O.; Clerc, C.; Moreau, C.; et al. Idiopathic acute transverse myelitis: Application of the recent diagnostic criteria. *Neurology* **2005**, *65*, 1950–1953. [CrossRef] [PubMed]
4. Jacob, A.; Weinshenker, B.G. An approach to the diagnosis of acute transverse myelitis. *Semin. Neurol.* **2008**, *28*, 105–120. [CrossRef] [PubMed]
5. GBD 2015 Neurological Disorders Collaborator Group. Global, regional, and national burden of neurological disorders during 1990–2015: A systematic analysis for the Global Burden of Disease Study 2015. *Lancet Neurol.* **2017**, *16*, 877–897. [CrossRef]
6. Dendrou, C.A.; Fugger, L.; Friese, M.A. Immunopathology of multiple sclerosis. *Nat. Rev. Immunol.* **2015**, *15*, 545–558. [CrossRef] [PubMed]
7. McFarland, H.F.; Martin, R. Multiple sclerosis: A complicated picture of autoimmunity. *Nat. Immunol.* **2007**, *8*, 913–919. [CrossRef]
8. Lublin, F.D.; Reingold, S.C.; Cohen, J.A.; Cutter, G.R.; Sørensen, P.S.; Thompson, A.J.; Wolinsky, J.S.; Balcer, L.J.; Banwell, B.; Barkhof, F.; et al. Defining the clinical course of multiple sclerosis: The 2013 revisions. *Neurology* **2014**, *83*, 278–286. [CrossRef]
9. Compston, A.; Mc Donald, I.; Noseworthy, J.; Lassmann, H.; Miller, D.; Smith, K.; Wekerle, H.; Confavreux, C. *McAlpine's Multiple Sclerosis*, 4th ed.; Churchill-Livingstone: London, UK, 2005.
10. Cordonnier, C.; De Seze, J.; Breteau, G.; Ferriby, D.; Michelin, E.; Stojkovic, T.; Pruvo, J.P.; Vermersch, P. Prospective study of patients presenting with acute partial transverse myelopathy. *J. Neurol.* **2003**, *250*, 1447–1452. [CrossRef]
11. Kantarci, O.H. Phases and Phenotypes of Multiple Sclerosis. *Continuum (Minneap Minn)* **2019**, *25*, 636–654. [CrossRef]
12. Ingle, G.T.; Sastre-Garriga, J.; Miller, D.H.; Thomson, A.J. Is inflammation important in early PPMS? A longitudinal MRI study. *J. Neurol. Neurosurg. Psychiatry* **2005**, *76*, 1255–1258. [CrossRef] [PubMed]
13. Koch, M.W.; Greenfield, J.; Javizian, O.; Deighton, S.; Wall, W.; Metz, L.M. The natural history of early versus late disability accumulation in primary progressive M.S. *J. Neurol. Neurosurg. Psychiatry* **2015**, *86*, 615–621. [CrossRef] [PubMed]
14. Vukusic, S.; Confavreux, C. Primary and secondary progressive multiple sclerosis. *J. Neurol. Sci.* **2003**, *206*, 153–155. [CrossRef]

15. Marrodan, M.; Bensi, C.; Pappolla, A.; Rojas, J.I.; Gaitán, M.I.; Ysrraelit, M.C.; Negrotto, L.; Fiol, M.P.; Patrucco, L.; Cristiano, E. Disease activity impacts disability progression in primary progressive multiple sclerosis. *Mult. Scler. Relat. Disord.* **2020**, *39*, 101892. [CrossRef] [PubMed]
16. Androdias, G.; Reynolds, R.; Chanal, M.; Ritleng, C.; Confavreux, C.; Nataf, S. Meningeal T cells associate with diffuse axonal loss in multiple sclerosis spinal cords. *Ann. Neurol.* **2010**, *68*, 465–476. [CrossRef] [PubMed]
17. Cross, A.H.; McCarron, R.; McFarlin, D.E.; Raine, C.S. Adoptively transferred acute and chronic relapsing autoimmune encephalomyelitis in the PL/J mouse and observations on altered pathology by intercurrent virus infection. *Lab. Investig.* **1987**, *57*, 499–512.
18. Schwartz, M.; Butovsky, O.; Brück, W.; Hanisch, U.K. Microglial phenotype: Is the commitment reversible? *Trends Neurosci.* **2006**, *29*, 68–74. [CrossRef]
19. Krieger, S.C.; Lublin, F.D. Location, location, location. *Mult. Scler. J.* **2018**, *24*, 1396–1398. [CrossRef]
20. Thompson, A.J.; Banwell, B.L.; Barkhof, F.; Carroll, W.M.; Coetzee, T.; Comi, G.; Correale, J.; Fazekas, F.; Filippi, M.; Freedman, M.S.; et al. Diagnosis of multiple sclerosis: 2017 revisions of the McDonald criteria. *Lancet Neurol.* **2018**, *17*, 162–173. [CrossRef]
21. Lycklama, G.; Thompson, A.; Filippi, M.; Miller, D.; Polman, C.; Fazekas, F.; Barkhof, F. Spinal-cord MRI in multiple sclerosis. *Lancet Neurol.* **2003**, *2*, 555–562. [CrossRef]
22. Lycklama, À.; Nijeholt, G.J.; Castelijns, J.A.; Weerts, J.; Adèr, H.; van Waesberghe, J.H.; Polman, C.; Barkhof, F. Sagittal MR of multiple sclerosis in the spinal cord: Fast versus conventional spin-echo imaging. *Am. J. Neuroradiol.* **1998**, *19*, 355–360.
23. Gass, A.; Rocca, M.A.; Agosta, F.; Ciccarelli, O.; Chard, D.; Valsasina, P.; Brooks, J.C.; Bischof, A.; Eisele, P.; Kappos, L.; et al. MRI monitoring of pathological changes in the spinal cord in patients with multiple sclerosis. *Lancet Neurol.* **2015**, *14*, 443–454. [CrossRef]
24. Rovira, Á.; Wattjes, M.P.; Tintoré, M.; Tur, C.; Yousry, T.A.; Sormani, M.P.; De Stefano, N.; Filippi, M.; Auger, C.; Rocca, M.A.; et al. Evidence-based guidelines: MAGNIMS consensus guidelines on the use of MRI in multiple sclerosis—Clinical implementation in the diagnostic process. *Nat. Rev. Neurol.* **2015**, *11*, 471–482. [CrossRef]
25. Bergers, E.; Bot, J.C.J.; De Groot, C.J.A.; Polman, C.H.; Lycklama, G.J.; Nijeholt, Á.; Castelijns, J.A.; van der Valk, P.; Barkhof, F. Axonal damage in the spinal cord of MS patients occurs largely independent of T2 MRI lesions. *Neurology* **2002**, *59*, 1766–1771. [CrossRef]
26. Weier, K.; Mazraeh, J.; Naegelin, Y.; Thoeni, A.; Hirsch, J.G.; Fabbro, T.; Bruni, N.; Duyar, H.; Bendfeldt, K.; Radue, E.W. Biplanar MRI for the assessment of the spinal cord in multiple sclerosis. *Mult. Scler. J.* **2012**, *18*, 1560–1569. [CrossRef] [PubMed]
27. Breckwoldt, M.O.; Gradl, J.; Hähnel, S.; Hielscher, T.; Wildemann, B.; Diem, R.; Platten, M.; Wick, W.; Heiland, S.; Bendszus, M. Increasing the sensitivity of MRI for the detection of multiple sclerosis lesions by long axial coverage of the spinal cord: A prospective study in 119 patients. *J. Neurol.* **2017**, *264*, 341–349. [CrossRef]
28. Martin, N.; Malfair, D.; Zhao, Y.; Li, D.; Traboulsee, A.; Lang, F.; Vertinsky, A.T. Comparison of MERGE and axial T2-weighted fast spin-echo sequences for detection of multiple sclerosis lesions in the cervical spinal cord. *Am. J. Roentgenol.* **2012**, *199*, 157–162. [CrossRef] [PubMed]
29. Zalewski, N.L.; Morris, P.P.; Weinshenker, B.G.; Lucchinetti, C.F.; Guo, Y.; Pittock, S.J.; Krecke, K.N.; Kaufmann, T.J.; Wingerchuk, D.M.; Kumar, N.; et al. Ring-enhancing spinal cord lesions in neuromyelitis optica spectrum disorders. *J. Neurol. Neurosurg. Psychiatry* **2017**, *88*, 218–225. [CrossRef] [PubMed]
30. Ciccarelli, O.; Cohen, J.A.; Reingold, S.C.; Weinshenker, B.G. Spinal cord involvement in multiple sclerosis and neuromyelitis optica spectrum disorders. *Lancet Neurol.* **2019**, *18*, 185–197. [CrossRef]
31. de Seze, J. Acute myelopathies: Clinical, laboratory and outcome profiles in 79 cases. *Brain* **2001**, *124*, 1509–1521. [CrossRef]
32. Kitley, J.L.; Leite, M.I.; George, J.S.; Palace, J.A. The differential diagnosis of longitudinally extensive transverse myelitis. *Mult. Scler. J.* **2012**, *18*, 271–285. [CrossRef] [PubMed]
33. Geraldes, R.; Ciccarelli, O.; Barkhof, F.; De Stefano, N.; Enzinger, C.; Filippi, M.; Hofer, M.; Paul, F.; Preziosa, P.; Rovira, A.; et al. The current role of MRI in differentiating multiple sclerosis from its imaging mimics. *Nat. Rev. Neurol.* **2018**, *14*, 199–213. [CrossRef] [PubMed]

34. Kantarci, O.H.; Lebrun, C.; Siva, A.; Keegan, M.B.; Azevedo, C.J.; Inglese, M.; Tintoré, M.; Newton, B.D.; Durand-Dubief, F.; Amato, M.P.; et al. Primary Progressive Multiple Sclerosis Evolving from Radiologically Isolated Syndrome. *Ann. Neurol.* **2016**, *79*, 288–294. [CrossRef]
35. O'Riordan, J.I.; Thompson, A.J.; Kingsley, D.P.E.; MacManus, D.G.; Kendall, B.E.; Rudge, P.; McDonald, W.I.; Miller, D.H. The prognostic value of brain MRI in clinically isolated syndromes of the CNS. A 10-year follow-up. *Brain* **1998**, *121*, 495–503. [CrossRef] [PubMed]
36. Bot, J.C.J.; Barkhof, F.; Polman, C.H.; Lycklama, Á.; Nijeholt, G.J.; de Groot, V.; Bergers, E.; Ader, H.J.; Castelijns, J.A. Spinal cord abnormalities in recently diagnosed MS patients: Added value of spinal MRI examination. *Neurology* **2004**, *62*, 226–233. [CrossRef] [PubMed]
37. Arrambide, G.; Tintore, M.; Auger, C.; Río, J.; Castilló, J.; Vidal-Jordana, A.; Galán, I.; Nos, C.; Comabella, M.; Mitjana, R.; et al. Lesion topographies in multiple sclerosis diagnosis: A reappraisal. *Neurology* **2017**, *89*, 2351–2356. [CrossRef] [PubMed]
38. Brownlee, W.J.; Altmann, D.R.; Alves Da Mota, P.; Swanton, J.K.; Miszkiel, K.A.; Wheeler-Kingshott, C.G.; Ciccarelli, O.; Miller, D.H. Association of asymptomatic spinal cord lesions and atrophy with disability 5 years after a clinically isolated syndrome. *Mult. Scler. J.* **2017**, *23*, 665–674. [CrossRef] [PubMed]
39. Zecca, C.; Disanto, G.; Sormani, M.P.; Riccitelli, G.C.; Cianfoni, A.; Del Grande, F.; Pravatà, E.; Gobbi, C. Relevance of asymptomatic spinal MRI lesions in patients with multiple sclerosis. *Mult. Scler. J.* **2016**, *22*, 782–791. [CrossRef]
40. Vukusic, S.; Confavreux, C. Prognostic factors for progression of disability in the secondary progressive phase of multiple sclerosis. *J. Neurol. Sci.* **2003**, *206*, 135–137. [CrossRef]
41. Biberacher, V.; Boucard, C.C.; Schmidt, P.; Engl, C.; Buck, D.; Berthele, A.; Hoshi, M.M.; Zimmer, C.; Hemmer, B.; Mühlau, M. Atrophy and structural variability of the upper cervical cord in early multiple sclerosis. *Mult. Scler. J.* **2015**, *21*, 875–884. [CrossRef]
42. Casserly, C.; Seyman, E.E.; Alcaide-Leon, P.; Guenette, M.; Lyons, C.; Sankar, S.; Svendrovski, A.; Baral, S.; Oh, J. Spinal Cord Atrophy in Multiple Sclerosis: A Systematic Review and Meta-Analysis. *J. Neuroimaging* **2018**, *28*, 556–586. [CrossRef] [PubMed]
43. Schlaeger, R.; Papinutto, N.; Zhu, A.H.; Lobach, I.V.; Bevan, C.J.; Bucci, M.; Castellano, A.; Gelfand, J.M.; Graves, J.S.; Green, A.J.; et al. Association Between Thoracic Spinal Cord Gray Matter Atrophy and Disability in Multiple Sclerosis. *JAMA Neurol.* **2015**, *72*, 897–904. [CrossRef] [PubMed]
44. Agosta, F.; Pagani, E.; Caputo, D.; Filippi, M. Associations between cervical cord gray matter damage and disability in patients with multiple sclerosis. *Arch. Neurol.* **2007**, *64*, 1302–1305. [CrossRef] [PubMed]
45. Schlaeger, R.; Papinutto, N.; Panara, V.; Bevan, C.; Lobach, I.V.; Bucci, M.; Caverzasi, E.; Gelfand, J.M.; Green, A.J.; Jordan, K.M.; et al. Spinal cord gray matter atrophy correlates with multiple sclerosis disability. *Ann. Neurol.* **2014**, *76*, 568–580. [CrossRef]
46. Tsagkas, C.; Magon, S.; Gaetano, L.; Pezold, S.; Naegelin, Y.; Amann, M.; Stippich, C.; Cattin, P.; Wuerfel, J.; Bieri, O.; et al. Spinal cord volume loss: A marker of disease progression in multiple sclerosis. *Neurology* **2018**, *91*, e349–e358. [CrossRef]
47. Kearney, H.; Rocca, M.A.; Valsasina, P.; Balk, L.; Sastre-Garriga, J.; Reinhardt, J.; Ruggieri, J.; Rovira, A.; Stippich, C.; Kappos, L.; et al. Magnetic resonance imaging correlates of physical disability in relapse onset multiple sclerosis of long disease duration. *Mult. Scler. J.* **2014**, *20*, 72–80. [CrossRef]
48. Oh, J.; Sotirchos, E.S.; Saidha, S.; Whetstone, A.; Chen, M.; Newsome, S.D.; Zackowski, K.; Balcer, L.J.; Frohman, E.; Prince, J.; et al. Relationships between quantitative spinal cord MRI and retinal layers in multiple sclerosis. *Neurology* **2015**, *84*, 720–728. [CrossRef]
49. Valsasina, P.; Agosta, F.; Absinta, M.; Sala, S.; Caputo, D.; Filippi, M. Cervical cord functional MRI changes in relapse-onset MS patients. *J. Neurol. Neurosurg. Psychiatry* **2010**, *81*, 405–408. [CrossRef]
50. Lukas, C.; Knol, D.L.; Sombekke, M.H.; Bellenberg, B.; Hahn, H.K.; Popescu, V.; Weier, K.; Radue, E.W.; Gass, A.; Kappos, L.; et al. Cervical spinal cord volume loss is related to clinical disability progression in multiple sclerosis. *J. Neurol. Neurosurg. Psychiatry* **2015**, *86*, 410–418. [CrossRef]
51. Rocca, M.A.; Valsasina, P.; Damjanovic, D.; Horsfield, M.A.; Mesaros, S.; Stosic-Opincal, T.; Drulovic, J.; Filippi, M. Voxel-wise mapping of cervical cord damage in multiple sclerosis patients with different clinical phenotypes. *J. Neurol. Neurosurg. Psychiatry* **2013**, *84*, 35–41. [CrossRef]

52. Lin, X.; Blumhardt, L.D.; Constantinescu, C.S. The relationship of brain and cervical cord volume to disability in clinical subtypes of multiple sclerosis: A three-dimensional MRI study. *Acta Neurol. Scand.* **2003**, *108*, 401–406. [CrossRef] [PubMed]
53. Gilmore, C.P.; Deluca, G.C.; Bö, L.; Owens, T.; Lowe, J.; Esiri, M.M.; Evangelou, N. Spinal cord neuronal pathology in multiple sclerosis. *Brain Pathol.* **2009**, *19*, 642–649. [CrossRef] [PubMed]
54. Montalban, X.; Sastre-Garriga, J.; Filippi, M.; Khaleeli, Z.; Téllez, N.; Vellinga, M.M.; Tur, C.; Brochet, B.; Barkhof, F.; Rovaris, M.; et al. Primary progressive multiple sclerosis diagnostic criteria: A reappraisal. *Mult. Scler.* **2009**, *15*, 1459–1465. [CrossRef] [PubMed]
55. Kapoor, R.; Furby, J.; Hayton, T.; Smith, K.J.; Altmann, D.R.; Brenner, R.; Chataway, J.; Hughes, R.A.; Miller, D.H. Lamotrigine for neuroprotection in secondary progressive multiple sclerosis: A randomised, double-blind, placebo-controlled, parallel-group trial. *Lancet Neurol.* **2010**, *9*, 681–688. [CrossRef]
56. Cawley, N.; Tur, C.; Prados, F.; Plantone, D.; Kearney, H.; Abdel-Aziz, K.; Ourselin, S.; Wheeler-Kingshott, C.A.G.; Miller, D.H.; Thompson, A.J.; et al. Spinal cord atrophy as a primary outcome measure in phase II trials of progressive multiple sclerosis. *Mult. Scler. J.* **2018**, *24*, 932–941. [CrossRef]
57. Evangelou, N.; DeLuca, G.C.; Owens, T.; Esiri, M.M. Pathological study of spinal cord atrophy in multiple sclerosis suggests limited role of local lesions. *Brain* **2005**, *128*, 29–34. [CrossRef]
58. Kearney, H.; Miszkiel, K.A.; Yiannakas, M.C.; Ciccarelli, O.; Miller, D.H. A pilot MRI study of white and grey matter involvement by multiple sclerosis spinal cord lesions. *Mult. Scler. Relat. Disord.* **2013**, *2*, 103–108. [CrossRef]
59. Philpott, C.; Brotchie, P. Comparison of MRI sequences for evaluation of multiple sclerosis of the cervical spinal cord at 3 T. *Eur. J. Radiol.* **2011**, *80*, 780–785. [CrossRef]
60. Calabrese, M.; De Stefano, N.; Atzori, M.; Bernardi, V.; Mattisi, I.; Barachino, L.; Rinaldi, L.; Morra, A.; McAuliffe, M.M.; Perini, P.; et al. Detection of cortical inflammatory lesions by double inversion recovery magnetic resonance imaging in patients with multiple sclerosis. *Arch. Neurol.* **2007**, *64*, 1416–1422. [CrossRef]
61. Bot, J.C.; Barkhof, F.; Lycklama à Nijeholt, G.J.; Bergers, E.; Polman, C.H.; Adèr, H.J.; Castelijns, J.A. Comparison of a conventional cardiac-triggered dual spin-echo and a fast STIR sequence in detection of spinal cord lesions in multiple sclerosis. *Eur. Radiol.* **2000**, *10*, 753–758. [CrossRef]
62. Sethi, V.; Yousry, T.A.; Muhlert, N.; Ron, M.; Golay, X.; Wheeler-Kingshott, C.; Miller, D.H.; Chard, D.T. Improved detection of cortical MS lesions with phase-sensitive inversion recovery MRI. *J. Neurol. Neurosurg. Psychiatry* **2012**, *83*, 877–882. [CrossRef] [PubMed]
63. Nair, G.; Absinta, M.; Reich, D.S. Optimized T1-MPRAGE sequence for better visualization of spinal cord multiple sclerosis lesions at 3T. *AJNR Am. J. Neuroradiol.* **2013**, *34*, 2215–2222. [CrossRef] [PubMed]
64. Gilmore, C.P.; Bö, L.; Owens, T.; Lowe, J.; Esiri, M.M.; Evangelou, N. Spinal cord gray matter demyelination in multiple sclerosis-a novel pattern of residual plaque morphology. *Brain Pathol.* **2006**, *16*, 202–208. [CrossRef] [PubMed]
65. Lublin, F.D.; Baier, M.; Cutter, G. Effect of relapses on development of residual deficit in multiple sclerosis. *Neurology* **2003**, *61*, 1528–1532. [CrossRef] [PubMed]
66. Koch-Henriksen, N.; Thygesen, L.C.; Sørensen, P.S.; Migyari, M. Worsening of disability caused by relapses in multiple sclerosis: A different approach. *Mult. Scler. Relat. Disord.* **2019**, *32*, 1–8. [CrossRef] [PubMed]
67. Berkovich, R.R. Acute Multiple Sclerosis Relapse. *Continuum (Minneap Minn)* **2016**, *22*, 799–814. [CrossRef]
68. Goodin, D.S. Glucocorticoid treatment of multiple sclerosis. *Handb. Clin. Neurol.* **2014**, *122*, 455–464.
69. Stoppe, M.; Busch, M.; Krizek, L.; Then Bergh, F. Outcome of MS relapses in the era of disease-modifying therapy. *BMC Neurol.* **2017**, *17*, 151. [CrossRef]
70. Schröder, A.; Linker, R.A.; Gold, R. Plasmapheresis for neurological disorders. *Expert Rev. Neurother.* **2009**, *9*, 1331–1339. [CrossRef]
71. Pfeuffer, S.; Rolfes, L.; Bormann, E.; Sauerland, C.; Ruck, T.; Schilling, M.; Melzer, N.; Brand, M.; Pul, R.; Kleinschnitz, C.; et al. Comparing Plasma Exchange to Escalated Methyl Prednisolone in Refractory Multiple Sclerosis Relapses. *J. Clin. Med.* **2019**, *9*, 35. [CrossRef]
72. Keegan, M.; Pineda, A.A.; McClelland, R.L.; Darby, C.H.; Rodriguez, M.; Weinshenker, B.G. Plasma exchange for severe attacks of CNS demyelination: Predictors of response. *Neurology* **2002**, *58*, 143–148. [CrossRef] [PubMed]
73. Derfuss, T.; Mehling, M.; Papadopoulou, A.; Bar-Or, A.; Cohen, J.A.; Kappos, L. Advances in oral immunomodulating therapies in relapsing multiple sclerosis. *Lancet Neurol.* **2020**, *19*, 336–347. [CrossRef]

74. Ontaneda, D.; Tallantyre, E.; Kalincik, T.; Planchon, S.M.; Evangelou, N. Early highly effective versus escalation treatment approaches in relapsing multiple sclerosis. *Lancet Neurol.* **2019**, *18*, 973–980. [CrossRef]
75. Reich, D.S.; Lucchinetti, C.F.; Calabresi, P.A. Multiple sclerosis. *N. Engl. J. Med.* **2018**, *378*, 169–180. [CrossRef] [PubMed]
76. Correale, J.; Gaitán, M.I.; Ysrraelit, M.C.; Fiol, M.P. Progressive multiple sclerosis: From pathogenic mechanisms to treatment. *Brain* **2017**, *140*, 527–546. [CrossRef]
77. Young, N.P.; Weinshenker, B.G.; Lucchinetti, C.F. Acute disseminated encephalomyelitis: Current understanding and controversies. *Semin. Neurol.* **2008**, *28*, 84–94. [CrossRef]
78. Tenembaum, S.; Chitnis, T.; Ness, J.; Hahn, J.S.; International Pediatric MS Study Group. Acute disseminated encephalomyelitis. *Neurology* **2007**, *68*, S23–S36. [CrossRef]
79. Tenembaum, S.N. Acute disseminated encephalomyelitis. *Handb. Clin. Neurol.* **2013**, *112*, 1253–1262.
80. de Mol, C.L.; Wong, Y.Y.M.; van Pelt, E.D.; Ketelslegers, I.A.; Bakker, D.P.; Boon, M.; Braun, K.P.J.; van Dijk, K.G.J.; Eikelenboom, M.J.; Engelen, M.; et al. Incidence and outcome of acquired demyelinating syndromes in Dutch children: Update of a nationwide and prospective study. *J. Neurol.* **2018**, *265*, 1310–1319. [CrossRef]
81. Yamaguchi, Y.; Torisu, H.; Kira, R.; Ishizaki, Y.; Sakai, Y.; Sanefuji, M.; Ichiyama, T.; Oka, A.; Kishi, T.; Kimura, S.; et al. A nationwide survey of pediatric acquired demyelinating syndromes in Japan. *Neurology* **2016**, *87*, 2006–2015. [CrossRef]
82. Xiong, C.H.; Yan, Y.; Liao, Z.; Peng, S.H.; Wen, H.R.; Zhang, Y.X.; Chen, S.H.; Li, J.; Chen, H.Y.; Feng, X.W.; et al. Epidemiological characteristics of acute disseminated encephalomyelitis in Nanchang, China: A retrospective study. *BMC Public Health* **2014**, *14*, 111. [CrossRef] [PubMed]
83. Karussis, D.; Petrou, P. The spectrum of post-vaccination inflammatory CNS demyelinating syndromes. *Autoimmun. Rev.* **2014**, *13*, 215–224. [CrossRef] [PubMed]
84. Tenembaum, S.; Chamoles, N.; Fejerman, N. Acute disseminated encephalomyelitis: A long-term follow-up study of 84 pediatric patients. *Neurology* **2002**, *59*, 1224–1231. [CrossRef] [PubMed]
85. Fujinami, R.S.; Oldstone, M.B. Amino acid homology between the encephalitogenic site of myelin basic protein and virus: Mechanism for autoimmunity. *Science* **1985**, *230*, 1043–1045. [CrossRef]
86. Smyk, D.S.; Alexander, A.K.; Walker, M.; Walker, M. Acute disseminated encephalomyelitis progressing to multiple sclerosis: Are infectious triggers involved? *Immunol. Res.* **2014**, *60*, 16–22. [CrossRef]
87. Krupp, L.B.; Tardieu, M.; Amato, M.P.; Banwell, B.; Chitnis, T.; Dale, R.C.; Ghezzi, A.; Hintzen, R.; Kornberg, A.; Poh, D.; et al. International Pediatric Multiple Sclerosis Study Group criteria for pediatric multiple sclerosis and immune-mediated central nervous system demyelinating disorders: Revisions to the 2007 definitions. *Mult. Scler. J.* **2013**, *19*, 1261–1267. [CrossRef]
88. Cole, J.; Evans, E.; Mwangi, M.; Mar, S. Acute Disseminated Encephalomyelitis in Children: An Updated Review Based on Current Diagnostic Criteria. *Pediatr. Neurol.* **2019**, *100*, 26–34. [CrossRef]
89. Flanagan, E.P. Autoimmune myelopathies. *Handb. Clin. Neurol.* **2016**, *133*, 327–351.
90. Callen, D.J.A.; Shroff, M.M.; Branson, H.M.; Li, D.K.; Lotze, T.; Stephens, D.; Banwell, B.L. Role of MRI in the differentiation of ADEM from MS in children. *Neurology* **2009**, *72*, 968–973. [CrossRef]
91. Baumann, M.; Sahin, K.; Lechner, C.; Wendel, E.M.; Lechner, C.; Behring, B.; Blaschek, A.; Diepold, K.; Eisenkölbl, A.; Fluss, J.; et al. Clinical and neuroradiological differences of paediatric acute disseminating encephalomyelitis with and without antibodies to the myelin oligodendrocyte glycoprotein. *J. Neurol. Neurosurg. Psychiatry* **2015**, *86*, 265–272. [CrossRef]
92. Ketelslegers, I.A.; Visser, I.; Neuteboom, R.F.; Boon, M.; Catsman-Berrevoets, C.E.; Hintzen, R.Q. Disease course and outcome of acute disseminated encephalomyelitis is more severe in adults than in children. *Mult. Scler. J.* **2011**, *17*, 441–448. [CrossRef] [PubMed]
93. Leake, J.A.D.; Albani, S.; Kao, A.S.; Senac, M.O.; Billman, G.F.; Nespeca, M.P.; Paulino, A.D.; Quintela, E.R.; Sawyer, M.H.; Bradley, J.S. Acute disseminated encephalomyelitis in childhood: Epidemiologic, clinical and laboratory features. *Pediatr. Infect. Dis. J.* **2004**, *23*, 756–764. [CrossRef] [PubMed]
94. Hung, P.C.; Wang, H.S.; Chou, M.L.; Lin, K.L.; Hsieh, M.Y.; Wong, A.M.C. Acute disseminated encephalomyelitis in children: A single institution experience of 28 patients. *Neuropediatrics* **2012**, *43*, 64–71. [CrossRef] [PubMed]

95. Pavone, P.; Pettoello-Mantovano, M.; Le Pira, A.; Giardino, I.; Pulvirenti, A.; Giugno, R.; Parano, E.; Polizzi, A.; Distefano, A.; Ferro, A.; et al. Acute disseminated encephalomyelitis: A long-term prospective study and meta-analysis. *Neuropediatrics* **2010**, *41*, 246–255. [CrossRef]
96. Erol, I.; Ozkale, Y.; Alkan, O.; Alehan, F. Acute disseminated encephalomyelitis in children and adolescents: A single center experience. *Pediatr. Neurol.* **2013**, *49*, 266–273. [CrossRef]
97. Mikaeloff, Y.; Caridade, G.; Husson, B.; Suissa, S.; Tardieu, M.; Neuropediatric KIDSEP Study Group of the French Neuropediatric Society. Acute disseminated encephalomyelitis cohort study: Prognostic factors for relapse. *Eur. J. Paediatr. Neurol.* **2007**, *11*, 90–95. [CrossRef]
98. Pohl, D.; Alper, G.; Van Haren, K.; Kornberg, A.J.; Lucchinetti, C.F.; Tenembaum, S.; Belman, A.L. Acute disseminated encephalomyelitis: Updates on an inflammatory CNS syndrome. *Neurology* **2016**, *87*, S38–S45. [CrossRef]
99. Verhey, L.H.; Branson, H.M.; Shroff, M.M.; Callen, D.J.; Sled, J.G.; Narayanan, S.; Sadovnick, A.D.; Bar-Or, A.; Arnold, D.L.; Marrie, R.A.; et al. MRI parameters for prediction of multiple sclerosis diagnosis in children with acute CNS demyelination: A prospective national cohort study. *Lancet Neurol.* **2011**, *10*, 1065–1073. [CrossRef]
100. Lin, C.H.; Jeng, J.S.; Hsieh, S.T.; Yip, P.K.; Wu, R.M. Acute disseminated encephalomyelitis: A follow-up study in Taiwan. *J. Neurol. Neurosurg. Psychiatry* **2007**, *78*, 162–167. [CrossRef]
101. Waldman, A.; Gorman, M.; Rensel, M.; Austin, T.E.; Hertz, D.P.; Kuntz, N.L. Network of Pediatric Multiple Sclerosis Centers of Excellence of the National Multiple Sclerosis Society. Management of Pediatric Central Nervous System Demyelinating Disorders: Consensus of United States Neurologists. *J. Child. Neurol.* **2011**, *26*, 675–682. [CrossRef]
102. Dale, R.C. Acute disseminated encephalomyelitis, multiphasic disseminated encephalomyelitis and multiple sclerosis in children. *Brain* **2000**, *123*, 2407–2422. [CrossRef] [PubMed]
103. Khurana, D.S.; Melvin, J.J.; Kothare, S.V.; Valencia, I.; Hardison, H.H.; Yum, S.; Faerber, E.N.; Legido, A. Acute disseminated encephalomyelitis in children: Discordant neurologic and neuroimaging abnormalities and response to plasmapheresis. *Pediatrics* **2005**, *116*, 431–436. [CrossRef] [PubMed]
104. Pohl, D.; Tenembaum, S. Treatment of acute disseminated encephalomyelitis. *Curr. Treat. Options Neurol.* **2012**, *14*, 264–275. [CrossRef] [PubMed]
105. Jarius, S.; Wildemann, B. The history of neuromyelitis optica. *J. Neuroinflamm.* **2013**, *10*, 8. [CrossRef] [PubMed]
106. Lennon, P.V.A.; Wingerchuk, D.M.; Kryzer, T.J.; Pittock, S.J.; Lucchinetti, C.F.; Fujihara, K.; Nakashima, I.; Weinshenker, B.G. A serum autoantibody marker of neuromyelitis optica: Distinction from multiple sclerosis. *Lancet* **2004**, *364*, 2106–2112. [CrossRef]
107. Lennon, V.A.; Kryzer, T.J.; Pittock, S.J.; Verkman, A.S.; Hinson, S.R. IgG marker of optic-spinal multiple sclerosis binds to the aquaporin-4 water channel. *J. Exp. Med.* **2005**, *202*, 473–477. [CrossRef]
108. Wingerchuk, D.M.; Lennon, V.A.; Pittock, S.J.; Lucchinetti, C.F.; Weinshenker, B.G. Revised diagnostic criteria for neuromyelitis optica. *Neurology* **2006**, *66*, 1485–1489. [CrossRef]
109. Wingerchuk, D.M.; Lennon, V.A.; Lucchinetti, C.F.; Pittock, S.J.; Weinshenker, B.G. The spectrum of neuromyelitis optica. *Lancet Neurol.* **2007**, *6*, 805–815. [CrossRef]
110. Wingerchuk, D.M.; Banwell, B.; Bennett, J.L.; Cabre, P.; Carroll, W.; Chitnis, T.; de Seze, J.; Fujihara, K.; Greenberg, B.; Jacob, A.; et al. International consensus diagnostic criteria for neuromyelitis optica spectrum disorders. *Neurology* **2015**, *85*, 177–189. [CrossRef]
111. Saadoun, S.; Waters, P.; Bell, B.A.; Vincent, A.; Verkman, A.S.; Papadopoulos, M.C. Intra-cerebral injection of neuromyelitis optica immunoglobulin G and human complement produces neuromyelitis optica lesions in mice. *Brain* **2010**, *133*, 349–361. [CrossRef]
112. Ratelade, J.; Asavapanumas, N.; Ritchie, A.M.; Wemlinger, S.; Bennett, J.L.; Verkman, A.S. Involvement of antibody-dependent cell-mediated cytotoxicity in inflammatory demyelination in a mouse model of neuromyelitis optica. *Acta Neuropathol.* **2013**, *126*, 699–709. [CrossRef] [PubMed]
113. Bradl, M.; Misu, T.; Takahashi, T.; Watanabe, M.; Mader, S.; Reindl, M.; Adzemovic, M.; Bauer, J.; Berger, T.; Fujihara, K.; et al. Neuromyelitis optica: Pathogenicity of patient immunoglobulin in vivo. *Ann. Neurol.* **2009**, *66*, 630–643. [CrossRef] [PubMed]

114. Chang, V.T.W.; Chang, H.M. Review: Recent advances in the understanding of the pathophysiology of neuromyelitis optica spectrum disorder. *Neuropathol. Appl. Neurobiol.* **2020**, *46*, 199–218. [CrossRef] [PubMed]
115. Lucchinetti, C.F.; Mandler, R.N.; McGavern, D.; Bruck, W.; Gleich, G.; Ransohoff, R.M.; Trebst, C.; Weinshenker, B.; Wingerchuk, D.; Parisi, J.E.; et al. A role for humoral mechanisms in the pathogenesis of Devic's neuromyelitis optica. *Brain* **2002**, *125 Pt 7*, 1450–1461. [CrossRef]
116. Misu, T.; Fujihara, K.; Kakita, A.; Konno, H.; Nakamura, M.; Watanabe, S.; Takahashi, T.; Nakashima, I.; Takahashi, H.; Itoyama, Y. Loss of aquaporin 4 in lesions of neuromyelitis optica: Distinction from multiple sclerosis. *Brain* **2007**, *130*, 1224–1234. [CrossRef]
117. Pittock, S.J.; Lennon, V.A.; Krecke, K.; Wingerchuk, D.M.; Lucchinetti, C.F.; Weinshenker, B.G. Brain abnormalities in neuromyelitis optica. *Arch. Neurol.* **2006**, *63*, 390–396. [CrossRef]
118. Hinson, S.R.; Roemer, S.F.; Lucchinetti, C.F.; Fryer, J.P.; Kryzer, T.J.; Chamberlain, J.L.; Howe, C.L.; Pittock, S.J.; Lennon, V.A. Aquaporin-4-binding autoantibodies in patients with neuromyelitis optica impair glutamate transport by down- Regulating EAAT2. *J. Exp. Med.* **2008**, *205*, 2473–2481. [CrossRef]
119. Papadopoulos, M.; Verkman, A.S. Aquaporin 4 and neuromyelitis optica. *Lancet Neurol.* **2009**, *53*, 820–833. [CrossRef]
120. Rosenthal, J.F.; Hoffman, B.M.; Tyor, W.R. CNS inflammatory demyelinating disorders: MS, NMOSD and MOG antibody associated disease. *J. Investig. Med.* **2020**, *68*, 321–330. [CrossRef]
121. Jarius, S.; Ruprecht, K.; Wildemann, B.; Kuempfel, T.; Ringelstein, M.; Geis, C.; Kleiter, I.; Kleinschnitz, C.; Berthele, A.; Brettschneider, J.; et al. Contrasting disease patterns in seropositive and seronegative neuromyelitis optica: A multicentre study of 175 patients. *J. Neuroinflamm.* **2012**, *9*, 14. [CrossRef]
122. Ghezzi, A.; Bergamaschi, R.; Martinelli, V.; Trojano, M.; Tola, M.R.; Merelli, E.; Mancardi, L.; Gallo, P.; Filippi, M.; Zaffaroni, M.; et al. Clinical characteristics, course and prognosis of relapsing Devic's Neuromyelitis Optica. *J. Neurol.* **2004**, *251*, 47–52. [CrossRef] [PubMed]
123. Wingerchuk, D.M.; Hogancamp, W.F.; O'Brien, P.C.; Weinshenker, BG. The clinical course of neuromyelitis optica (Devic's syndrome). *Neurology* **1999**, *53*, 1107–1114. [CrossRef] [PubMed]
124. Yonezu, T.; Ito, S.; Mori, M.; Ogawa, Y.; Makino, T.; Uzawa, A.; Kuwabara, S. Bright spotty lesions on spinal magnetic resonance imaging differentiate neuromyelitis optica from multiple sclerosis. *Mult. Scler. J.* **2014**, *20*, 331–337. [CrossRef] [PubMed]
125. Flanagan, E.P.; Kaufmann, T.J.; Krecke, K.N.; Aksamit, A.J.; Pittock, S.J.; Keegan, B.M.; Giannini, C.; Weinshenker, B.G. Discriminating long myelitis of neuromyelitis optica from sarcoidosis. *Ann. Neurol.* **2016**, *79*, 437–447. [CrossRef] [PubMed]
126. Iorio, R.; Damato, V.; Mirabella, M.; Evoli, A.; Marti, A.; Plantone, D.; Frisullo, G.; Batocchi, A.P. Distinctive clinical and neuroimaging characteristics of longitudinally extensive transverse myelitis associated with aquaporin-4 autoantibodies. *J. Neurol.* **2013**, *260*, 2396–2402. [CrossRef]
127. Flanagan, E.P.; Weinshenker, B.G.; Krecke, K.N.; Lennon, V.A.; Lucchinetti, C.F.; McKeon, A.; Wingerchuk, D.M.; Shuster, E.A.; Jiao, Y.; Horta, E.S.; et al. Short myelitis lesions in aquaporin-4-IgG-positive neuromyelitis optica spectrum disorders. *JAMA Neurol.* **2015**, *72*, 81–87. [CrossRef]
128. Kim, S.H.; Huh, S.Y.; Kim, W.; Park, M.S.; Ahn, S.E.; Cho, J.Y.; Kim, B.J.; Kim, H.J. Clinical characteristics and outcome of multiple sclerosis in Korea: Does multiple sclerosis in Korea really differ from that in the Caucasian populations? *Mult. Scler. J.* **2013**, *19*, 1493–1498. [CrossRef]
129. Scott, T.F. Nosology of idiopathic transverse myelitis syndromes. *Acta Neurol. Scand.* **2007**, *115*, 371–376. [CrossRef]
130. Asgari, N.; Skejoe, H.P.B.; Lillevang, S.T.; Steenstrup, T.; Stenager, E.; Kyvik, K.O. Modifications of longitudinally extensive transverse myelitis and brainstem lesions in the course of neuromyelitis optica (NMO): A population-based, descriptive study. *BMC Neurol.* **2013**, *13*, 33. [CrossRef]
131. Hamid, S.H.M.; Elsone, L.; Mutch, K.; Solomon, T.; Jacob, A. The impact of 2015 neuromyelitis optica spectrum disorders criteria on diagnostic rates. *Mult. Scler. J.* **2017**, *23*, 228–233. [CrossRef]
132. Liu, Y.; Fu, Y.; Schoonheim, M.M.; Zhang, N.; Fan, M.; Su, L.; Shen, Y.; Yan, Y.; Yang, L.; Wang, Q.; et al. Structural MRI substrates of cognitive impairment in neuromyelitis optica. *Neurology* **2015**, *85*, 1491–1499. [CrossRef] [PubMed]

133. Ventura, R.E.; Kister, I.; Chung, S.; Babb, J.S.; Shepherd, T.M. Cervical spinal cord atrophy in NMOSD without a history of myelitis or MRI-visible lesions. *Neurol. Neuroimmunol. Neuroinflamm.* **2016**, *3*, e224. [CrossRef] [PubMed]
134. Hyun, J.W.; Jeong, I.H.; Joung, A.; Kim, S.H.; Kim, H.J. Evaluation of the 2015 diagnostic criteria for neuromyelitis optica spectrum disorder. *Neurology* **2016**, *86*, 1772–1779. [CrossRef] [PubMed]
135. Marignier, R.; Bernard-Valnet, R.; Giraudon, P.; Collongues, N.; Papeix, C.; Zéphir, H.; Cavillon, G.; Rogemond, V.; Casey, R.; Frangoulis, B.; et al. Aquaporin-4 antibody-negative neuromyelitis optica: Distinct assay sensitivity-dependent entity. *Neurology* **2013**, *80*, 2194–2200. [CrossRef]
136. Pittock, S.J.; Lennon, V.A.; Bakshi, N.; Shen, S.; McKeon, A.; Quach, H.; Briggs, F.B.S.; Bernstein, A.L.; Schaefer, C.A.; Barcellos, L.F. Seroprevalence of aquaporin-4-IgG in a northern California population representative cohort of multiple sclerosis. *JAMA Neurol.* **2014**, *71*, 1433–1436. [CrossRef]
137. Jarius, S.; Wildemann, B.; Paul, F. Neuromyelitis optica: Clinical features, immunopathogenesis and treatment. *Clin. Exp. Immunol.* **2014**, *176*, 149–164. [CrossRef]
138. van Pelt, E.D.; Wong, Y.Y.M.; Ketelslegers, I.A.; Hamann, D.; Hintzen, R.Q. Neuromyelitis optica spectrum disorders: Comparison of clinical and magnetic resonance imaging characteristics of AQP4-IgG versus MOG-IgG seropositive cases in the Netherlands. *Eur. J. Neurol.* **2016**, *23*, 580–587. [CrossRef]
139. Hamid, S.H.M.; Whittam, D.; Mutch, K.; Linaker, S.; Solomon, T.; Das, K.; Bhojak, M.; Jacob, A. What proportion of AQP4-IgG-negative NMO spectrum disorder patients are MOG-IgG positive? A cross sectional study of 132 patients. *J. Neurol.* **2017**, *264*, 2088–2094. [CrossRef]
140. Höftberger, R.; Sepulveda, M.; Armangue, T.; Blanco, Y.; Rostásy, K.; Cobo Calvo, A.; Olascoaga, J.; Ramió-Torrentà, L.; Reindl, M.; Benito-León, J.; et al. Antibodies to MOG and AQP4 in adults with neuromyelitis optica and suspected limited forms of the disease. *Mult. Scler. J.* **2015**, *21*, 866–874. [CrossRef]
141. Majed, M.; Fryer, J.P.; McKeon, A.; Lennon, V.A.; Pittock, S.J. Clinical utility of testing AQP4-IgG in CSF: Guidance for physicians. *Neurol. Neuroimmunol. NeuroInflamm.* **2016**, *3*, e231. [CrossRef]
142. Javed, A.; Balabanov, R.; Arnason, B.G.W.; Kelly, T.J.; Sweiss, N.J.; Pytel, P.; Walsh, R.; Blair, E.A.; Stemer, A.; Lazzaro, M.; et al. Minor salivary gland inflammation in Devic's disease and longitudinally extensive myelitis. *Mult. Scler. J.* **2008**, *14*, 809–814. [CrossRef] [PubMed]
143. Wandinger, K.P.; Stangel, M.; Witte, T.; Venables, P.; Charles, P.; Jarius, S.; Wildemann, B.; Probst, C.; Iking-Konert, C.; Schneider, M. Autoantibodies against aquaporin-4 in patients with neuropsychiatric systemic lupus erythematosus and primary Sjögren's syndrome. *Arthritis Rheumatol.* **2010**, *62*, 1198–1200. [CrossRef] [PubMed]
144. Jarius, S.; Paul, F.; Franciotta, D.; Ruprecht, K.; Ringelstein, M.; Bergamaschi, R.; Rommer, P.; Kleiter, I.; Stich, O.; Reuss, R.; et al. Cerebrospinal fluid findings in aquaporin-4 antibody positive neuromyelitis optica: Results from 211 lumbar punctures. *J. Neurol. Sci.* **2011**, *306*, 82–90. [CrossRef] [PubMed]
145. Weinshenker, B.G.; Wingerchuk, D.M. Neuromyelitis Spectrum Disorders. *Mayo Clin. Proc.* **2017**, *92*, 663–679. [CrossRef]
146. Kessler, R.A.; Mealy, M.A.; Levy, M. Treatment of Neuromyelitis Optica Spectrum Disorder: Acute, Preventive, and Symptomatic. *Curr. Treat. Options Neurol.* **2016**, *18*, 2. [CrossRef]
147. Trebst, C.; Jarius, S.; Berthele, A.; Paul, F.; Schippling, S.; Wildemann, B.; Borisow, N.; Kleiter, I.; Aktas, O.; Kümpfel, T.; et al. Update on the diagnosis and treatment of neuromyelitis optica: Recommendations of the Neuromyelitis Optica Study Group (NEMOS). *J. Neurol.* **2014**, *261*, 1–16. [CrossRef]
148. Palace, J.; Leite, I.; Jacob, A. A practical guide to the treatment of neuromyelitis optica. *Pract. Neurol.* **2012**, *12*, 209–214. [CrossRef]
149. Magaña, S.M.; Keegan, B.M.; Weinshenker, B.G.; Erickson, B.J.; Pittock, S.J.; Lennon, V.A.; Rodriguez, M.; Thomsen, K.; Weigand, S.; Mandrekar, J.; et al. Beneficial Plasma Exchange Response in CNS Inflammatory Demyelination. *Arch. Neurol.* **2012**, *68*, 870–878. [CrossRef]
150. Reeves, H.M.; Winters, J.L. The mechanisms of action of plasma exchange. *Br. J. Haematol.* **2014**, *164*, 342–351. [CrossRef]
151. Bonnan, M.; Valentino, R.; Debeugny, S.; Merle, H.; Fergé, J.L.; Mehdaoui, H.; Cabre, P. Short delay to initiate plasma exchange is the strongest predictor of outcome in severe attacks of NMO spectrum disorders. *J. Neurol. Neurosurg. Psychiatry* **2018**, *89*, 346–351. [CrossRef]

152. Lim, Y.M.; Pyun, S.Y.; Kang, B.H.; Kim, J.; Kim, K.K. Factors associated with the effectiveness of plasma exchange for the treatment of NMO-IgG-positive neuromyelitis optica spectrum disorders. *Mult. Scler. J.* **2013**, *19*, 1216–1218. [CrossRef] [PubMed]
153. Bonnan, M.; Valentino, R.; Olindo, S.; Mehdaoui, H.; Smadja, D.; Cabre, P. Plasma exchange in severe spinal attacks associated with neuromyelitis optica spectrum disorder. *Mult. Scler. J.* **2009**, *15*, 487–492. [CrossRef] [PubMed]
154. Watanabe, S.; Nakashima, I.; Misu, T.; Miyazawa, I.; Shiga, Y.; Fujihara, K.; Itoyama, Y. Therapeutic efficacy of plasma exchange in NMO-IgG-positive patients with neuromyelitis optica. *Mult. Scler. J.* **2007**, *13*, 128–132. [CrossRef] [PubMed]
155. Pittock, S.J.; Berthele, A.; Fujihara, K.; Kim, H.J.; Levy, M.; Palace, J.; Nakashima, I.; Terzi, M.; Totolyan, N.; Viswanathan, S.; et al. Eculizumab in aquaporin-4-positive neuromyelitis optica spectrum disorder. *N. Engl. J. Med.* **2019**, *381*, 614–625. [CrossRef]
156. Cree, B.A.C.; Bennett, J.L.; Kim, H.J.; Weinshenker, B.G.; Pittock, S.J.; Wingerchuk, D.M.; Fujihara, K.; Paul, F.; Cutter, G.R.; Marignier, R.; et al. Inebilizumab for the treatment of neuromyelitis optica spectrum disorder (N-MOmentum): A double-blind, randomised placebo-controlled phase 2/3 trial. *Lancet* **2019**, *394*, 1352–1363. [CrossRef]
157. Yamamura, T.; Kleiter, I.; Fujihara, K.; Palace, J.; Greenberg, B.; Zakrzewska-Pniewska, B.; Patti, F.; Tsai, C.P.; Saiz, A.; Yamazaki, H.; et al. Trial of satralizumab in neuromyelitis optica spectrum disorder. *N. Engl. J. Med.* **2019**, *381*, 2114–2124. [CrossRef]
158. Reindl, M.; Linington, C.; Brehm, U.; Egg, R.; Dilitz, E.; Deisenhammer, F.; Poewe, W.; Berger, T. Antibodies against the myelin oligodendrocyte glycoprotein and the myelin basic protein in multiple sclerosis and other neurological diseases: A comparative study. *Brain* **1999**, *122*, 2047–2056. [CrossRef]
159. Berger, T.; Rubner, P.; Schautzer, F.; Egg, R.; Ulmer, H.; Mayringer, I.; Dilitz, E.; Deisenhammer, F.; Reindl, M. Antimyelin antibodies as a predictor of clinically definite multiple sclerosis after a first demyelinating event. *N. Engl. J. Med.* **2003**, *349*, 139–145. [CrossRef]
160. Berger, T.; Reindl, M. Lack of association between antimyelin antibodies and progression to multiple sclerosis. *N. Engl. J. Med.* **2007**, *356*, 1888–1889.
161. Lampasona, V.; Franciotta, D.; Furlan, R.; Zanaboni, S.; Fazio, R.; Bonifacio, E.; Comi, G.; Martino, G. Similar low frequency of anti-MOG IgG and IgM in MS patients and healthy subjects. *Neurology* **2004**, *62*, 2092–2094. [CrossRef]
162. Lim, E.T.; Berger, T.; Reindl, M.; Dalton, C.M.; Fernando, K.; Keir, G.; Thompson, E.J.; Miller, D.H.; Giovannoni, G. Anti-myelin antibodies do not allow earlier diagnosis of multiple sclerosis. *Mult. Scler. J.* **2005**, *11*, 492–494. [CrossRef] [PubMed]
163. Hennes, E.M.; Baumann, M.; Schanda, K.; Anlar, B.; Bajer-Kornek, B.; Blaschek, A.; Brantner-Inthaler, S.; Diepold, K.; Eisenkölbl, A.; Gotwald, T.; et al. Prognostic relevance of MOG antibodies in children with an acquired demyelinating syndrome. *Neurology* **2017**, *89*, 900–908. [CrossRef] [PubMed]
164. Brilot, F.; Dale, R.C.; Selter, R.C.; Grummel, V.; Kalluri, S.R.; Aslam, M.; Busch, V.; Zhou, D.; Cepok, S.; Hemmer, B. Antibodies to native myelin oligodendrocyte glycoprotein in children with inflammatory demyelinating central nervous system disease. *Ann. Neurol.* **2009**, *66*, 833–842. [CrossRef] [PubMed]
165. Huppke, P.; Rostasy, K.; Karenfort, M.; Huppke, B.; Seidl, R.; Leiz, S.; Reindl, M.; Gärtner, J. Acute disseminated encephalomyelitis followed by recurrent or monophasic optic neuritis in pediatric patients. *Mult. Scler. J.* **2013**, *19*, 941–946. [CrossRef]
166. O'Connor, K.C.; McLaughlin, K.A.; De Jager, P.L.; Chitnis, T.; Bettelli, E.; Xu, C.; Robinson, W.H.; Cherry, S.V.; Bar-Or, A.; Banwell, B.; et al. Self-antigen tetramers discriminate between myelin autoantibodies to native or denatured protein. *Nat. Med.* **2007**, *13*, 211–217. [CrossRef]
167. Jarius, S.; Ruprecht, K.; Kleiter, I.; Borisow, N.; Asgari, N.; Pitarokoili, K.; Pache, F.; Stich, O.; Beume, L.A.; Hümmert, M.W.; et al. MOG-IgG in NMO and related disorders: A multicenter study of 50 patients. Part 1, Frequency, syndrome specificity, influence of disease activity, long-term course, association with AQP4-IgG, and origin. *J. Neuroinflamm.* **2016**, *13*, 279. [CrossRef]
168. Rostasy, K.; Mader, S.; Schanda, K.; Huppke, P.; Gärtner, J.; Kraus, V.; Karenfort, M.; Tibussek, D.; Blaschek, A.; Bajer-Kornek, B.; et al. Anti-myelin oligodendrocyte glycoprotein antibodies in pediatric patients with optic neuritis. *Arch. Neurol.* **2012**, *69*, 752–756. [CrossRef]

169. Mader, S.; Gredler, V.; Schanda, K.; Rostasy, K.; Dujmovic, I.; Pfaller, K.; Lutterotti, A.; Jarius, S.; Di Pauli, F.; Kuenz, B.; et al. Complement activating antibodies to myelin oligodendrocyte glycoprotein in neuromyelitis optica and related disorders. *J. Neuroinflamm.* **2011**, *8*, 184. [CrossRef]
170. Hyun, J.W.; Woodhall, M.R.; Kim, S.H.; Jeong, I.H.; Kong, B.; Kim, G.; Kim, Y.; Park, M.S.; Irani, S.R.; Waters, P.; et al. Longitudinal analysis of myelin oligodendrocyte glycoprotein antibodies in CNS inflammatory diseases. *J. Neurol. Neurosurg. Psychiatry* **2017**, *88*, 811–817. [CrossRef]
171. Ramanathan, S.; Mohammad, S.; Tantsis, E.; Nguyen, T.K.; Merheb, V.; Fung, V.S.C.; White, O.B.; Broadley, S.; Lechner-Scott, J.; Vucic, S.; et al. Clinical course, therapeutic responses and outcomes in relapsing MOG antibody-associated demyelination. *J. Neurol. Neurosurg. Psychiatry* **2018**, *89*, 127–137. [CrossRef]
172. Jarius, S.; Ruprecht, K.; Kleiter, I.; Borisow, N.; Asgari, N.; Pitarokoili, K.; Pache, F.; Stich, O.; Beume, L.A.; Hümmert, M.W.; et al. MOG-IgG in NMO and related disorders: A multicenter study of 50 patients. Part 2, Epidemiology, clinical presentation, radiological and laboratory features, treatment responses, and long-term outcome. *J. Neuroinflamm.* **2016**, *13*, 280. [CrossRef] [PubMed]
173. Sepúlveda, M.; Armangué, T.; Sola-Valls, N.; Arrambide, G.; Meca-Lallana, J.E.; Oreja-Guevara, C.; Mendibe, M.; Alvarez de Arcaya, A.; Aladro, Y.; Casanova, B.; et al. Neuromyelitis optica spectrum disorders: Comparison according to the phenotype and serostatus. *Neurol. Neuroimmunol. NeuroInflamm.* **2016**, *3*, e225. [CrossRef] [PubMed]
174. Jurynczyk, M.; Geraldes, R.; Probert, F.; Woodhall, M.R.; Waters, P.; Tackley, G.; DeLuca, G.; Chandratre, S.; Leite, M.I.; Vincent, A.; et al. Distinct brain imaging characteristics of autoantibody-mediated CNS conditions and multiple sclerosis. *Brain* **2017**, *140*, 617–627. [CrossRef] [PubMed]
175. Kim, H.J.; Paul, F.; Lana-Peixoto, M.A.; Tenembaum, S.; Asgari, N.; Palace, J.; Klawiter, E.C.; Sato, D.K.; de Seze, J.; Wuerfel, J.; et al. MRI characteristics of neuromyelitis optica spectrum disorder: An international update. *Neurology* **2015**, *84*, 1165–1173. [CrossRef]
176. Kim, S.M.; Woodhall, M.R.; Kim, J.S.; Kim, S.J.; Park, K.S.; Vincent, A.; Lee, K.W.; Waters, P. Antibodies to MOG in adults with inflammatory demyelinating disease of the CNS. *Neurol. Neuroimmunol. NeuroInflamm.* **2015**, *2*, e163. [CrossRef]
177. Jarius, S.; Kleiter, I.; Ruprecht, K.; Asgari, N.; Pitarokoili, K.; Borisow, N.; Hümmert, M.W.; Trebst, C.; Pache, F.; Winkelmann, A.; et al. MOG-IgG in NMO and related disorders: A multicenter study of 50 patients. Part 3, Brainstem involvement—Frequency, presentation and outcome. *J. Neuroinflamm.* **2016**, *13*, 281. [CrossRef]
178. Kitley, J.; Waters, P.; Woodhall, M.; Leite, M.I.; Murchison, A.; George, J.; Küker, W.; Chandratre, S.; Vincent, A.; Palace, J. Neuromyelitis optica spectrum disorders with aquaporin-4 and myelin-oligodendrocyte glycoprotein antibodies a comparative study. *JAMA Neurol.* **2014**, *71*, 276–283. [CrossRef]
179. Sato, D.K.; Callegaro, D.; Lana-Peixoto, M.A.; Waters, P.J.; de Haidar Jorge, F.M.; Takahashi, T.; Nakashima, I.; Apostolos-Pereira, S.L.; Talim, N.; Simm, R.F.; et al. Distinction between MOG antibody positive and AQP4 antibody-positive NMO spectrum disorders. *Neurology* **2014**, *82*, 474–481. [CrossRef]
180. Matthews, L.; Marasco, R.; Jenkinson, M.; Küker, W.; Luppe, S.; Leite, M.I.; Giorgio, A.; De Stefano, N.; Robertson, N.; Johansen-Berg, H.; et al. Distinction of seropositive NMO spectrum disorder and MS brain lesion distribution. *Neurology* **2013**, *80*, 1330–1337. [CrossRef]
181. Bensi, C.; Marrodan, M.; González, A.; Chertcoff, A.; Osa Sanz, E.; Chaves, H.; Schteinschnaider, A.; Correale, J.; Farez, M.F. Brain and spinal cord lesion criteria distinguishes AQP4-positive neuromyelitis optica and MOG-positive disease from multiple sclerosis. *Mult. Scler. Relat. Disord.* **2018**, *25*, 246–250. [CrossRef]
182. Cobo-Calvo, A.; Ruiz, A.; Maillart, E.; Audoin, B.; Zephir, H.; Bourre, B.; Ciron, J.; Collongues, N.; Brassat, D.; Cotton, F.; et al. Clinical spectrum and prognostic value of CNS MOG autoimmunity in adults: The MOGADOR study. *Neurology* **2018**, *90*, e1858–e1869. [CrossRef] [PubMed]
183. Chalmoukou, K.; Alexopoulos, H.; Akrivou, S.; Stathopoulos, P.; Reindl, M.; Dalakas, M.C. Anti-MOG antibodies are frequently associated with steroid-sensitive recurrent optic neuritis. *Neurol. Neuroimmunol. Neuroinflamm.* **2015**, *2*, e131. [CrossRef] [PubMed]
184. Kitley, J.; Woodhall, M.; Waters, P.; Leite, M.I.; Devenney, E.; Craig, J.; Palace, J.; Vincent, A. Myelin-oligodendrocyte glycoprotein antibodies in adults with a neuromyelitis optica phenotype. *Neurology* **2012**, *79*, 1273–1277. [CrossRef] [PubMed]

185. Kim, S.H.; Kim, W.; Li, X.F.; Jung, I.J.; Kim, H.J. Repeated treatment with rituximab based on the assessment of peripheral circulating memory B cells in patients with relapsing neuromyelitis optica over 2 years. *Arch. Neurol.* **2011**, *68*, 1412–1420. [CrossRef] [PubMed]
186. Montcuquet, A.; Collongues, N.; Papeix, C.; Zephir, H.; Audoin, B.; Laplaud, D.; Bourre, B.; Brochet, B.; Camdessanche, J.P.; Labauge, P.; et al. Effectiveness of mycophenolate mofetil as first-line therapy in AQP4-IgG, MOG-IgG, and seronegative neuromyelitis optica spectrum disorders. *Mult. Scler. J.* **2017**, *23*, 1377–1384. [CrossRef]
187. Flanagan, E.P.; Hinson, S.R.; Lennon, V.A.; Fang, B.; Aksamit, A.J.; Morris, A.P.; Basal, E.; Honorat, J.A.; Alfugham, N.N.; Linnoila, J.J.; et al. GFAP-IgG as Biomarker of Autoimmune Astrocytopathy: Analysis of 102 Patients. *Ann. Neurol.* **2017**, *81*, 298–309. [CrossRef]
188. Fang, B.; McKeon, A.; Hinson, S.R.; Kryzer, T.J.; Pittock, S.J.; Aksamit, A.J.; Lennon, V.A. Autoimmune glial fibrillary acidic protein astrocytopathy: A novel meningoencephalomyelitis. *JAMA Neurol.* **2016**, *73*, 1297–1307. [CrossRef]
189. Sasaki, K.; Bean, A.; Shah, S.; Schutten, E.; Huseby, P.G.; Peters, B.; Shen, Z.T.; Vanguri, V.; Liggitt, D.; Huseby, E.S. Relapsing–Remitting Central Nervous System Autoimmunity Mediated by GFAP-Specific CD8 T Cells. *J. Immunol.* **2014**, *192*, 3029–3042. [CrossRef]
190. Schweingruber, N.; Fischer, H.J.; Fischer, L.; van den Brandt, J.; Karabinskaya, A.; Labi, V.; Villunger, A.; Kretzschmar, B.; Huppke, P.; Simons, M.; et al. Chemokine-mediated redirection of T cells constitutes a critical mechanism of glucocorticoid therapy in autoimmune CNS responses. *Acta Neuropathol.* **2014**, *127*, 713–729. [CrossRef]
191. Sofroniew, M.V. Multiple roles for astrocytes as effectors of cytokines and inflammatory mediators. *Neuroscientist* **2014**, *20*, 160–172. [CrossRef]
192. Ramamoorthy, S.; Cidlowski, J.A. Corticosteroids: Mechanisms of Action in Health and Disease. *Rheum. Dis. Clin. N. Am.* **2016**, *42*, 15–31. [CrossRef] [PubMed]
193. Kunchok, A.; Zekeridou, A.; McKeon, A. Autoimmune glial fibrillary acidic protein astrocytopathy. *Curr. Opin. Neurol.* **2019**, *32*, 452–458. [CrossRef] [PubMed]
194. Iorio, R.; Damato, V.; Evoli, A.M.; Guessi, M.; Gaudino, S.; Di Lazzaro, V.; Spagni, G.; Sluijs, J.A.; Hol, E.M. Clinical and immunological characteristics of the spectrum of GFAP autoimmunity: A case series of 22 patients. *J. Neurol. Neurosurg. Psychiatry* **2018**, *89*, 138–146. [CrossRef] [PubMed]
195. Sechi, E.; Morris, P.P.; Mckeon, A.; Pittock, S.J.; Hinson, S.R.; Winshenker, B.G.; Aksamit, A.J.; Krecke, K.N.; Kaufmann, T.J.; Jolliffe, E.A.; et al. Glial fibrillary acidic protein IgG related myelitis: Characterisation and comparison with aquaporin-4-IgG myelitis. *J. Neurol. Neurosurg. Psychiatry* **2019**, *90*, 488–490. [CrossRef] [PubMed]
196. Shan, F.; Long, Y.; Qiu, W. Autoimmune Glial Fibrillary Acidic Protein Astrocytopathy: A Review of the Literature. *Front. Immunol.* **2018**, *9*, 2802. [CrossRef] [PubMed]

© 2020 by the authors. Licensee MDPI, Basel, Switzerland. This article is an open access article distributed under the terms and conditions of the Creative Commons Attribution (CC BY) license (http://creativecommons.org/licenses/by/4.0/).

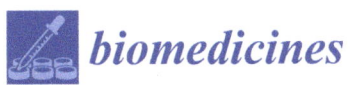

Review

Sphingosine-1-Phosphate: Its Pharmacological Regulation and the Treatment of Multiple Sclerosis: A Review Article

Stanley Cohan, Elisabeth Lucassen, Kyle Smoot, Justine Brink and Chiayi Chen *

Providence Multiple Sclerosis Center, Providence Brain and Spine Institute, Providence St, Vincent Medical Center, Portland, OR 97225, USA; Stanley.Cohan@providence.org (S.C.); elisabeth.lucassen@providence.org (E.L.); Kyle.smoot@providence.org (K.S.); Justine.Brink@providence.org (J.B.)
* Correspondence: Chiayi.Chen@providence.org; Tel.: +1-503-216-1012

Received: 27 May 2020; Accepted: 15 July 2020; Published: 18 July 2020

Abstract: Sphingosine-1-phosphate (S1P), via its G-protein-coupled receptors, is a signaling molecule with important regulatory properties on numerous, widely varied cell types. Five S1P receptors (S1PR1-5) have been identified, each with effects determined by their unique G-protein-driven downstream pathways. The discovery that lymphocyte egress from peripheral lymphoid organs is promoted by S1P via S1PR-1 stimulation led to the development of pharmacological agents which are S1PR antagonists. These agents promote lymphocyte sequestration and reduce lymphocyte-driven inflammatory damage of the central nervous system (CNS) in animal models, encouraging their examination of efficacy in the treatment of multiple sclerosis (MS). Preclinical research has also demonstrated direct protective effects of S1PR antagonists within the CNS, by modulation of S1PRs, particularly S1PR-1 and S1PR-5, and possibly S1PR-2, independent of effects upon lymphocytes. Three of these agents, fingolimod, siponimod and ozanimod have been approved, and ponesimod has been submitted for regulatory approval. In patients with MS, these agents reduce relapse risk, sustained disability progression, magnetic resonance imaging markers of disease activity, and whole brain and/or cortical and deep gray matter atrophy. Future opportunities in the development of more selective and intracellular S1PR-driven downstream pathway modulators may expand the breadth of agents to treat MS.

Keywords: multiple sclerosis; sphingosine-1-phosphate modulators

1. Introduction

Although it was long thought that sphingosine, largely generated from hydrolysis of ceramides within lysosomes [1,2], served primarily as a component of the structural sphingolipid family of molecules, it is now recognized for its importance as a component of sphingosine-1-phosphate (S1P), a crucial messenger molecule. S1P is generated by sphingosine kinase 1 or 2 (sk1, sk2), primarily in red blood cells, platelets and endothelial cells [3,4] (Figure 1). Their G-protein-coupled receptors are widely distributed in many organs and tissues, on cell surface plasma membranes, and on the endoplasmic reticulum and cell nuclei, but it is cytoplasmic membrane-bound receptor sites that have attracted the greatest attention [4]. Five S1P receptor (S1PR-1-5) subtypes have been identified [5,6] (Figure 2a). The translational intracellular pathways activated by S1P-receptor (S1PR) interaction are highly varied because of the multiplicity of receptor subtypes, the varied G-proteins to which they are coupled, the multiple downstream pathways linked to G proteins, and the wide variety cells which express S1PRs (Figure 2b; Table 1). Investigations into the physiological impact of S1P and its receptors, as well as its potential contribution to disease pathogenesis, have revealed important opportunities for therapeutic interventions. This is particularly the case in the treatment of multiple sclerosis (MS). In the past 10 years, three disease modifying therapies (DMT)s which modulate S1PRs, fingolimod (FGM), siponimod (SPM), and ozanimod (OZM), have been approved for treatment of MS, and a fourth agent, ponesimod (PNM) is under regulatory review.

The first part of this article describes the results of preclinical research, which has expanded the knowledge of the physiological roles of S1P and its receptors, and a discussion of the specific mechanisms of action of the S1PR modulators. This work did not only reveal important insights into S1PR-based DMT mechanisms of action, but also widened the perspective on future therapeutic opportunities for this class of molecules. The second part of this chapter summarizes the results of the pivotal clinical trials of FGM, SPM, OZM, and the phase II and phase III trials of PNM upon clinical efficacy, as well as the reported adverse events (AE) of these S1PR modulators.

Fingolimod (FGM) was the first S1PR modulator to be approved for the treatment of relapsing forms of MS (RMS). Preclinical and clinical studies demonstrated that its use results in the sequestration of lymphocytes, particularly central memory and naïve T and B cell lymphocytes in peripheral lymphoid organs [7–11]. Pathological studies also demonstrated reduced pro-inflammatory cells within the CNS following treatment with this class of agents, and it had been widely believed that the sequestration of these potentially pro-inflammatory cells within lymphoid organs accounted for their therapeutic efficacy in MS [7–10]. However, preclinical investigations, further detailed below, strongly suggest that these agents may also act directly within the CNS, where there is an abundance of S1PR expression, to ameliorate the impact of inflammatory disease.

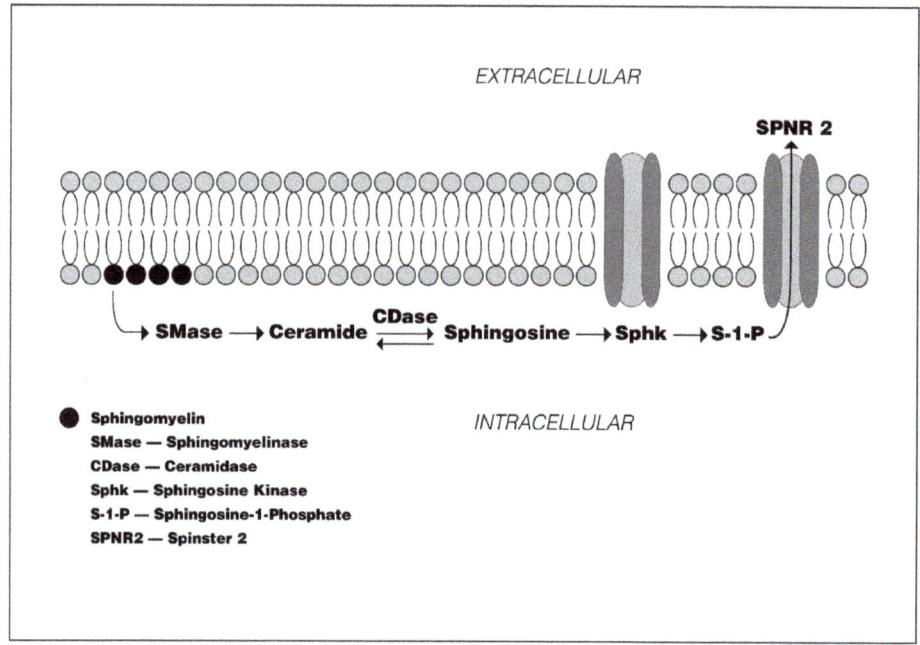

Figure 1. Metabolic Pathway to Sphingosine-1-phosphate Synthesis and Migration from the Intracellular to Extracellular Space via Sphingosine-1-phosphate Transmembrane Transporters.

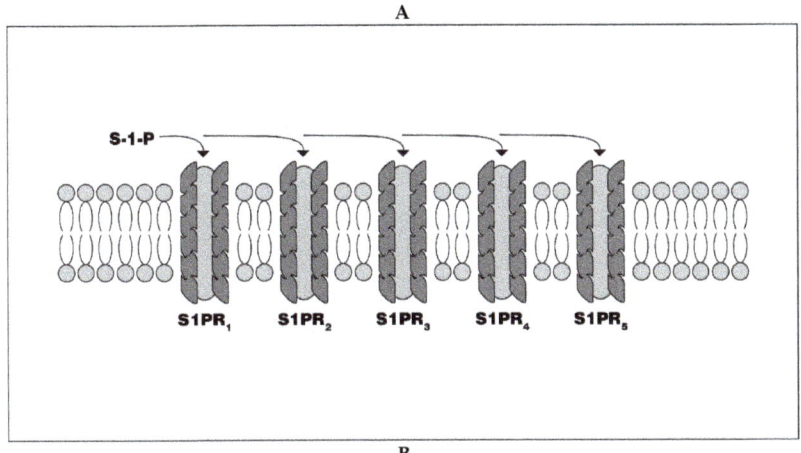

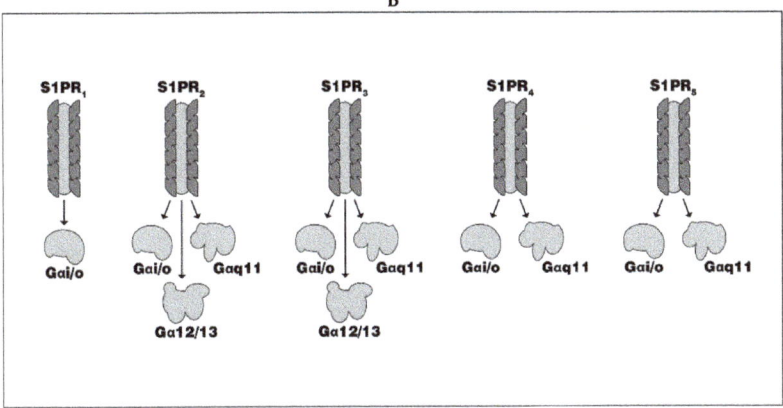

Figure 2. (**A**) Five G protein-coupled Sphingosine-1-phosphate receptors have been identified. (**B**) Each of the S1PRs is coupled to one or more G proteins, resulting in multiple different downstream messaging targets (See Table 1). S-1-P = Sphingosne-1-phosphate (S-1-P), S1PR = Sphingosine-1-phosphate Receptor.

Table 1. G protein-coupled Sphingosine-1-phosphate receptor subset modulation of downstream signaling pathways.

S1PR	G Protein	Downstream Signaling Pathways
S1PR 1–5	Gαi/o→	Akt→Ras→MAPK→Rac
S1PR 2–5	Gαq11→	DAG→PKC→Ca2+
S1PR 2 and 3	Gα12/13→	Rho→ROCK

S1PR = Sphingosine-1-phosphate Receptor, Akt = serine/threonine kinase (protein kinase B), Ras = small GTPase, MAPK = mitogen-activated protein kinase, Rac = member of Rho family of small GTPases, DAG = Diacyl Glycerol, PKC = protein kinase C, Rho = ras homolog gene family, ROCK = Rho kinase.

2. Preclinical Studies

As noted above, S1P is a major intracellular signaling molecule via its G-protein-coupled membrane bound receptors [12–15]. Because the S1PR subsets are coupled to different G-proteins, they can modulate multiple downstream intracellular pathways (Table 1).

Although S1P is critically essential for normal CNS development and maturation [3,4,16,17] and may regulate synaptic function [18], it may also be cytotoxic at elevated concentrations, such as when there is a genetic deficiency in its degradative enzymes, producing neuronal apoptosis [19–24]. S1P also regulates calcium signaling [25], and may promote presynaptic calcium overload and cell death [26].

It is now known that S1P, through its interaction with S1PR-1, expressed on the surface of CCR7+ naïve, central memory B, and T cell lymphocytes, regulates the trafficking of these cells from peripheral lymphoid organs [27–30]. The S1PR-1-expressing lymphocytes egress in response to the S1P gradient (Figure 3). This effect of S1P makes its metabolic and translational pathways attractive potential therapeutic targets for the treatment of cell-mediated immunologic disorders such as MS.

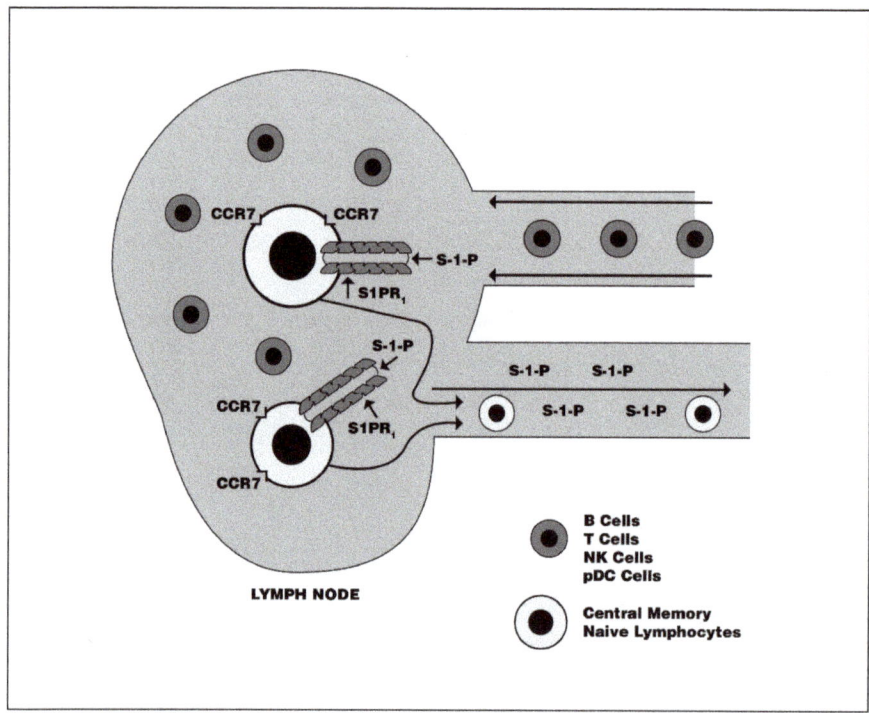

Figure 3. The effect of Sphingosine-1-phosphate on lymphocyte mobilization from peripheral lymphoid organs. Sphingosine-1-phosphate interaction with S1PR1-expressing lymphocytes over-rides CCR7-induced retention signaling, which results in mobilization and egress of naïve and central memory lymphocytes into circulation in response to the S-1-P gradient. Non-CCR7-expressing lymphocytes, such as effector memory cells, are not S-1-P dependent for their entry into the peripheral circulation. B Cells = B cell lymphocytes, T Cells = T cell lymphocyte, NK cells = natural killer cells, pDC Cells = plasmacytoid dendritic cell, S-1-P = Sphingosine-1-phosphate, S1PR1 = Sphingosine-1-Phosphate Receptor, CCR7 = Chemokine Receptor 7.

2.1. S1P Receptors

Fingolimod, approved for the treatment of relapsing forms of MS, is a non-selective S1PR modulator, which once phosphorylated (FGM-P) by sk2 [31], has affinity for S1PRs 1, 3, 4, and 5 [7,31]. The interaction of FGM-P with the S1PR-1 on the surface of CCR7+ lymphocytes results in the internalization and degradation of S1PR-1 [32,33] (Figure 4), promoting the sequestration of naïve, central memory T, and central memory B cell lymphocytes in peripheral lymphoid organs [34]. The circulation of central effector B and T cells, which do not express CCR7, are unaffected by FGM-P. When used in patients with relapsing forms of MS, FGM results in robust clinical and MRI evidence of efficacy, in parallel with marked reduction in circulating B and T cell numbers.

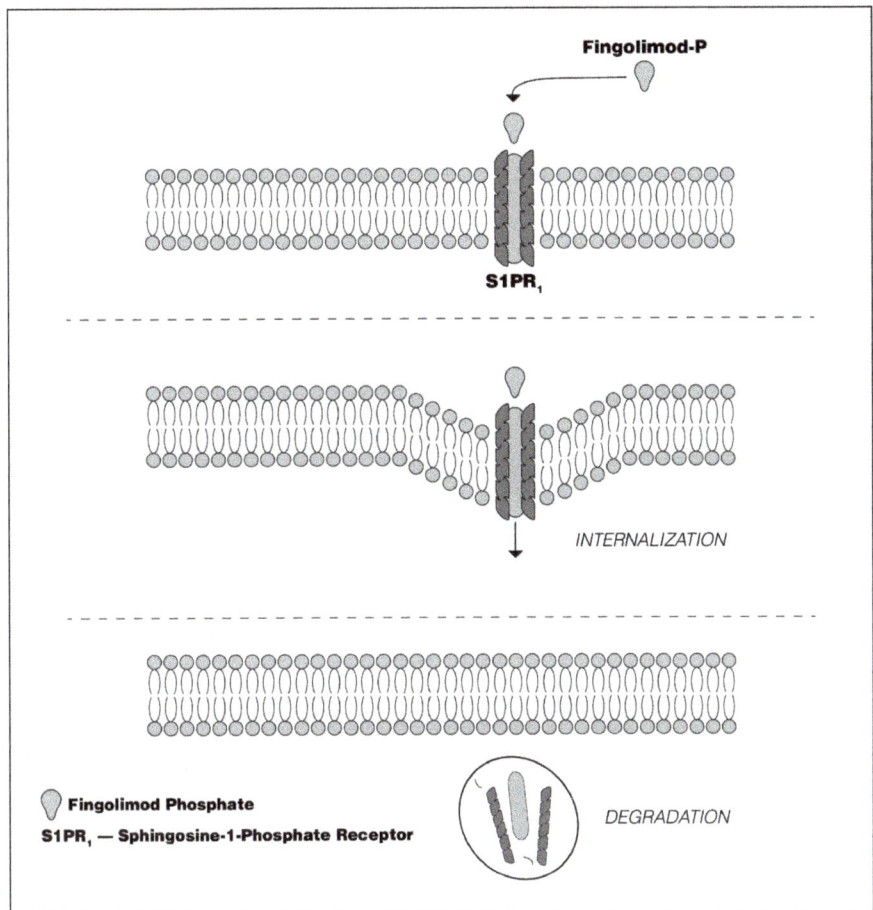

Figure 4. The effect of fingolimod-phosphate upon lymphocyte Sphinogosine-1-phosphate receptor-1. Although initially acting as an agonist, sustained exposure of sphingosine-1-phosphate receptor to fingolimod-phosphate results in receptor internalization and intracellular degradation. As a consequence of sphingosine-phosphate receptor-1 internalization, CCR7-expressing lymphocytes are no longer capable of responding to the sphingosine-1-phhosphate gradient. This results in naïve and central memory cell retention in peripheral lymphoid organs. $S1PR_1$ = Sphingosine-1-phosphate receptor-1.

It has been well-established that the CNS also expresses S1PRs, on neurons, astrocytes, microglia, and oligodendroglia (OLG) during development, maturation, and adult cell states [35–37]. Furthermore, FGM-P, and the newer S1PR modulators SPM, OZM, and PNM, readily cross the blood brain barrier (BBB), and are selectively accumulated within the CNS. Unlike FGM, these latter 3 agents do not require prior phosphorylation to be pharmacologically active. It is possible that some of the therapeutic benefits of S1PR modulators result directly from their effects upon CNS receptors, and in the discussion that follows, we present evidence that supports such a role for these agents. Furthermore, there is evidence to suggest that the therapeutic effects of these agents depends, at least in part, upon their interaction with CNS S1PRs [38].

The use of whole animal inflammatory CNS models, such as experimental allergic encephalitis (EAE), non-inflammatory models of CNS demyelination using in situ cuprizone or lyolecithin, in whole animal, brain tissue slice, and CNS cell culture models [39–42] have all provided important insights into fundamental S1P and S1PR physiology. They have also expanded knowledge of the mechanisms by which S1PR modulation regulates CNS development [4,17], and may protect the CNS during inflammatory insult [38]. What follows is a description of preclinical research which has provided important insights into the role of selective S1PR subtypes, the effects of their modulation/inhibition, and also the use of selective S1PR agonists and antagonists to further clarify the physiological roles of these receptors, and their impact on inflammatory CNS insults.

Although multiple S1PRs are expressed in the mammalian CNS, S1PR-1, 2 and 5 have attracted the most interest because of the pivotal roles they play in the development and myelinating function of OLGs, the regulation of astrocytes and microglia, and in maintaining the integrity of the BBB.

2.1.1. S1PR-1

During CNS inflammation, both S1PR-1 and S1PR-3 are up-regulated by astrocytes and are associated with astrocyte activation and increased production of glial acidic fibrillary protein (GFAP) [3]. The up-regulation of S1PR-1 is seen on activated GFAP-expressing astrocytes in or near active MS lesions [43–45]. During active inflammation there is also S1PR-1-dependent up-regulation of microglia (MGL) that is enhanced in the presence of S1P to further increase inflammation [46]. By contrast, in EAE produced in astrocyte S1PR-1 knockdown mice, there is an inhibition of astrocyte activation [38]. Furthermore, selective S1PR-1 blockade enhances maturation of OLGs [40]. Thus S1PR-1 blockade is a potentially important pharmacological target to reduce astrogliosis and promote remyelination in MS. Although S1PR3 up-regulation occurs in activated astrocytes, the role of S1PR-3 in producing significant cardiovascular effects, via its regulation of the KACh potassium channel [47–50], has diminished interest in it as a target for modulation in MS.

2.1.2. S1PR-2

S1PR-2 is expressed on oligodendroglial progenitor cells (OPC) and macrophages (MPG) [51,52]. In mice with EAE, S1PR-2 activation promotes breakdown of BBB, which is prevented by the use of selective endothelial cell S1PR-2 blocking agents [53], and in endothelial S1PR-2 knockout EAE mice. In these latter models there is also an inhibition of fibrinogen extravasation into the CNS, as well as the inhibition of MPG and MGL recruitment into CNS lesions [41]. To eliminate the potentially confounding effects of systemic inflammation in EAE, models employing in situ injection of lyolecithin-induced demyelination, have produced the same results: S1PR-2 knockout or pharmacologic S1PR-2 inhibition reduced MCP and MGL infiltration of the lesions [41]. S1PR-2 is also a negative regulator of oligodendroglial progenitor cell (OPC) maturation into OLGs. Following demyelination, the inhibition of S1PR-2 promoted maturation of OPCs, increased re-myelination and increased the number of mature myelinated axons [41]. In addition to being a receptor for S1P, S1PR-2 has a high affinity for NOGO A, which also inhibits remyelination [54], providing a second S1PR-2 pathway for the inhibition of re-myelination [55–57]. Consistent with these observations, the pharmacological inhibition of S1PR-2, or use of S1PR-2 knockout mice, results in improved EAE scores, reduced BBB leakage, less fibrinogen extravasation, reduced macrophage (MPG) and MGL recruitment, as well as increased OLG accumulation and re-myelination [53]. Although not a target of any current clinically employed S1PR modulators, S1PR-2 activation, because of its effects on BBB integrity, macrophage/MGL activation, and myelination, could be an important potential therapeutic target of future drug development.

2.1.3. S1P Neurotropism and S1PR-1/S1PR-2 Synergy

Sphingosine-1-P, by stimulating both S1PR-1 and S1PR-2, may induce gene expression encoding for the production of protective astrocyte neurotrophic factors, not achieved by S1PR-1 modulation alone [58]. Bi-receptor S1PR-1 and S1PR-2 stimulation [59] appears to be necessary to up-regulate neurotrophic mRNA expression, which only takes place in astrocytes [60,61]. To date there are no pharmacological agents of which we are aware that operate jointly or exclusively at both S1PR-1 and S1PR-2 under investigation as potential medications for MS, yet the importance of regulating astrocyte proliferation and astrogliosis would be reasons enough to examine agents that can synergistically modulate both receptor subsets.

2.1.4. S1PR-5

The S1PR-5 is mainly expressed on OLGs in white matter tracts, and on brain endothelial cells [51,62]. S1P5 receptor mRNA has been found primarily in the white matter of the CNS, but has not been detected in neurons, microglia, or astrocytes [63,64]. S1PR-5 is expressed throughout the development timeline of OLGs, from immature stages to the mature myelin-forming cell [62,65,66]. In mature OLGs, S1P5 receptors co-localize with myelin basic protein exclusively on myelinated axons and not on OLG cell bodies [64].

Although S1P5 appears to mediate S1P-induced survival of mature OLGs, it may also induce cell process retraction on immature OLGs [51,62], thus regulating a dual-signaling developmental pathway. It appears that activation of S1PR-5 may be important in the maturation and survival of OLGs by playing a role in their modulation, formation, and myelin repair [62].

As has been shown for S1PR-2, S1PR-5 influences BBB integrity and is highly expressed on human brain endothelial cells. Studies have demonstrated that S1PR-5 plays a key role in BBB maintenance and modulation of endothelial cell inflammatory state. S1PR-5 knockdown endothelial cells have reduced barrier integrity [67]. Activation of S1PR-5 reduces the expression of inflammatory cell adhesion molecules on their surface, and enhances the capacity of brain endothelial cells to prevent monocyte penetration. It has been suggested [67] that the role of S1PR-5 may include induction of specific BBB properties such as low paracellular permeability and increased expression of key brain endothelial proteins such as tight junction, ATP binding cassette and glucose transporter molecules. These results point out the potential importance of investigating pharmacological agents which have high affinity and selectivity to promote S1PR-5 preservation in maintaining BBB integrity and protecting OLG maturation and myelination.

2.2. Direct Pharmacological Actions of the S1PR Modulators in the CNS

Established and approved S1P agonists include fingolimod (FGM), siponimod (SPM), and ozanimod (OZM). Ponesimod (PNM) has recently been submitted for regulatory approval based upon Phase III clinical study outcomes. Because it has been available the longest, most data on modulation of S1P receptors by these agents come from studies utilizing FGM. At low doses, FGM has been shown to cause process extension of human OPCs via interaction with S1PR-1, but at high doses, causes process retraction via S1PR-3 and S1PR-5 [42]. Furthermore, short-term FGM treatment causes retraction and prevention of migration of OPCs via an S1PR-3 and S1PR-5-mediated pathway, whereas long-term exposure led to increased cell survival via an S1PR-1-driven pathway [42,51]. Fingolimod also enhances BBB integrity, probably by modulation of S1PR-5, reducing transendothelial migration of monocytes in vitro, the latter being an initial step in the formation of new MS lesions [67].

2.2.1. Fingolimod

As noted above, the therapeutic effects of FGM appear to result at least in part from control of lymphocyte trafficking via down-regulation of lymphocyte S1PR-1 (Figure 4) [68,69]. There is also growing evidence from preclinical studies, that some of FGM's therapeutic effects may be independent of lymphocyte sequestration in peripheral lymphoid organs [38,69]. FGM readily crosses the BBB, potentially enabling its subsequent modulation of S1PRs [35,69,70].

There is up-regulation of S1PR-1- and S1PR-3-expressing astrocytes [71] during active inflammation, and there is growing evidence that astrocytes expressing S1PR-1 may be a primary FGM therapeutic target in the CNS [72]. Consistent with this view has been the demonstration of diminished therapeutic benefit of FGM in EAE in the absence of S1PR-1 expression on astrocytes in genetic knock down mice [38].

Fingolimod, which causes the internalization and destruction of astrocytic S1PR-1 [38] also enhances remyelination in a number of different in vitro models and in EAE mice [40,45,73–75], prevents OLG death, reduces the number of reactive astrocytes and reduces the number of reactive MGL. These beneficial effects are mimicked by the selective S1PR-1 antagonist CYM5442, which also prevents the up-regulation of S1PR-1 on astrocytes [45]. As further evidence of the importance of the astrocyte S1PR-1 receptor, the S1PR-1 gene is primarily expressed in astrocytes, its coupled-G-protein-regulated pathway promotes astrocyte proliferation, and its selective blockade inhibits astrogliosis, potentially reducing OLG death and demyelination. These results are supporting evidence that at least some of the protective effects of FGM are mediated via S1PR-1 negative modulation in the CNS [45]. As further support, deletion of the astrocyte S1PR-1 gene reduces production of the pro-inflammatory cytokines IL-1β, IL-6 and IL-17, reduces demyelination, and eliminates any additive benefit of CNS protection by FGM treatment [38].

2.2.2. Siponimod

Siponimod is a selective modulator of S1PR-1 and S1PR-5 [76,77], and was originally synthesized to reduce cardiovascular effects by eliminating S1PR-3 affinity [78,79]. Its structure favors avid penetration of the BBB. It has a short T1/2 elimination, and lymphocyte counts may return to baseline within 48 h of the last dose (see Table 2) [78]. Recent studies in both human and rodent astrocytes have demonstrated that SPM modulates cellular pro-survival pathways [80–82], primarily via S1PR-1 [82]. SPM also demonstrates anti-inflammatory effects, reducing phosphatidyl choline, TNFα and IL-17-induced IL-6 production by via S1PR-1 modulation. In an in-situ injected curpizone mouse model, SPM treatment reduces myelin breakdown-associated proteins, decreases the number of damaged axons, decreases OLG loss, increases the number of myelinated axons, and reduces MPG and MGL infiltration [83]. In studies of EAE-induced excitotoxic synaptic degeneration, SPM treatment preserves gabaergic neurons in the striatum, and reduces microgliosis, even in the absence of pro-inflammatory lymphocyte affects. These results have been replicated in brain slices, further supporting a direct SPM affect upon the CNS. It has been hypothesized that SPM, via its actions on S1PR-1, reduces MGL activation, which in turn reduces pro-inflammatory lymphocyte recruitment into the CNS [83]. Lastly, since SPM is also a modulator of S1PR-5, preservation of OLGs and myelinated axons in demyelination models following its use is not unexpected. Although, to our knowledge, not yet reported, SPM may also preserve BBB function via S1PR-5 modulation.

Table 2. Pharmacokinetics and pharmacodynamics of the S1PR antagonists.

S1PR Antagonist	T$\frac{1}{2}$ Elimination	Time to Max Concentration	Median Decrease in Maximum Lymphocyte Count	Maximum Decrease in Steady State Lymphocyte Count	Median recovery Time to Normal Lymphocyte Count
fingolimod	6–9 days *	12–26 h	60% of baseline in 4–6 h	18–30% of baseline	1–2 months
siponimod	30 h	4 h	20–30% of baseline	20–30% of baseline	10 days, but up to 3–4 weeks for some patients
ozanimod CC112273 **	21 h 11 days	6–8 h	30% of baseline	45%	30 days ***
ponesimod	21–33 h	2.5–5 h	Not available	70%	4 days

* Increased by 50% in patients with moderate to severe heart disease, ** CC112273 the major ozanimod active metabolite, *** 90% recovery to baseline lymphocyte count with 3 months.

2.2.3. Ozanimod

Ozanimod has a high affinity for S1PR-1 and to a lesser extent for S1PR-5. It selectively crosses the BBB with brain to blood ratio of 10-16:1 [30] and its affinity for the S1PR-1 is comparable to FGM-P and SPM [30]. Like FGM-P and SPM, it induces rapid internalization and degradation of S1PR-1 in rodents and produces reduction in circulating B and T cell lymphocytes [30,84]. Compared to FGM and SPM, there is more rapid lymphocyte reconstitution after it is discontinued. The t1/2 elimination of its major active metabolites, cc112273 and cc1084037, is only 11 days (see Table 2) [85]. Of note, OZM treatment significantly improves EAE scores in mice, even in the presence of restored blood lymphocyte counts [30], supporting a direct CNS therapeutic role. We are unaware of extensive preclinical studies of OZM modulation of S1PR-5, its effects on OPCs, OLGs or myelination, or BBB integrity.

2.2.4. Ponesimod

Ponesimod is a selective S1PR-1 modulator [86,87], with a t1/2 elimination of 21-33 h [87], which like FGM, SPM and OZM, reduces circulating B and T cell lymphocytes by up to 70%, with return to baseline values within 4 days of cessation (see Table 2) [84,88–90], PNM readily crosses the BBB and reduces EAE scores in mice [84].

3. Clinical Trial Results

3.1. Fingolimod

Fingolimod was the first oral medication, approved in patients with relapsing forms of MS. The therapeutic efficacy of FGM for RMS was initially established in two pivotal, phase III, double-blind, randomized clinical trials of adults, comparing FGM to placebo (FREEDOMS) and comparing FGM to IFN-β-1a (TRANSFORMS). This was followed by the phase III extension studies FREEDOMS II and extended TRANSFORMS. The regulatory approval for use of FGM in the treatment of RRMS in children ages 10–17 years of age in 2018 [91] followed the results of the pivotal trial, PARADIGM [92].

3.1.1. FREEDOMS

FREEDOMS was a phase III double-blind, placebo-controlled trial with 1272 patients that demonstrated superior efficacy of FGM in RMS when compared to placebo [93]. Inclusion criteria included a diagnosis of RMS, Expanded Disability Status Scale (EDSS) score ≤5.5, and evidence of active disease over the previous 2 years. The median disease duration was 6.7 years, and median EDSS at baseline was 2.0. Patients were randomized in a 1:1:1 ratio to receive placebo, FGM 0.5 mg, or 1.25 mg once daily. The primary endpoint was annualized relapse rate (ARR) and the main secondary endpoint was time to three-month confirmed disability progression (CDP). Other secondary endpoints included: time to first relapse, change in EDSS score and the MS Functional Composite (MSFC) z-score at baseline compared to 24-months, conventional MRI measurements, drug tolerability, and safety. Because the 1.25 mg dose of FGM did not demonstrate therapeutic superiority to the 0.5 mg dose, it was the latter that received regulatory approval, and for that reason only the data for the 0.5 mg dose are presented.

The ARR was 0.18 for 0.5 mg FGM, and 0.40 for placebo-treated patients ($p < 0.0001$), a relative reduction of 54% in favor of FGM. Time to first relapse was significantly longer in FGM than in placebo-treated patients and more FGM patients remained relapse free over 24-months. Cumulative probability of three months of CDP was 17.7% for FGM and 24.1% for placebo (Hazard ratio 0.70). During the 24-month study period, EDSS score and MSFC z-scores remained stable in the FGM-treated group and minimally worsened in the placebo group. FGM treatment was associated with a significant relative decrease in the number of new or enlarging T2 lesions (74%), gadolinium-enhancing (Gd+) lesions (79%) and a relative reduction in brain volume loss (36%), all MRI comparisons being significant at 24 months ($p < 0.001$).

3.1.2. TRANSFORMS

TRANSFORMS was a Phase III clinical trial, enrolling 1292 patients, comparing efficacy of FGM to intramuscular IFNβ-1a in a 12-month, randomized, double-dummy, parallel group study in patients with active RMS over the previous 24 months [94]. The inclusion criteria included a diagnosis of RMS, EDSS ≤ 5.5. Patients were randomized 1:1:1 to oral FGM 0.5 mg or 1.25 mg once daily, or IFNβ-1a 30 μg IM once weekly, and we only report on the FGM 0.5 mg vs. IFNβ-1a results. The primary endpoint was ARR and major secondary endpoints included number of new or enlarging T2 MRI lesions at one year and 3-month CDP during the 12-month duration of the study. At 12 months, ARR was 0.16 for FGM, and 0.33 for IFNβ-1a patients ($p < 0.001$), a relative reduction in ARR of 52%. In the FGM arm time to first relapse was longer and more patients remained relapse free than the IFNβ-1a treated patients. FGM treatment was associated with a relative reduction in the mean number of new and enlarged T2 lesions (FGM 1.7 and IFNβ-1a 2.6; $p < 0.004$), a 54% relative reduction in Gd+ lesions ($p < 0.001$), a 31% relative reduction in percent brain volume loss from baseline ($p < 0.001$). In contrast, there was no significant difference observed between the treatment arms with respect to 3 month CDP.

3.1.3. FREEDOMS II

FREEDOMS II, a phase III trial to evaluate the efficacy and safety of FGM [95] was a 24-month, randomized, double-blind, placebo-controlled, evaluating the efficacy of FGM compared to placebo in 1083 patients. Inclusion criteria included: a diagnosis of RMS, evidence of active disease over the previous 24 months, and an EDSS ≤ 5.5. Patients were randomized in a 1:1:1 ratio to receive FGM 0.5 mg, or 1.25 mg, or placebo once daily but only the FGM 0.5 mg and placebo data are reported; patients randomized to the FGM 1.25 mg arm were switched to 0.5 mg a day at the recommendation of the data and safety committee. The primary endpoint of the trial was ARR. Secondary endpoints included the effect of FGM upon time to 3-month CDP, change in MSFC score, and effect on MRI measurements in comparison to placebo.

The ARR over 24 months was 0.21 for FGM and 0.40 for placebo ($p < 0.0001$), a relative reduction of 48%. The percent change in brain volume from baseline to 24 months, was 0.9% for FGM and 1.3% for placebo, a relative reduction of 31% ($p < 0.001$). The mean number of new and enlarged T2 lesions at 24 months was 2.3 for FGM, and 8.9 for placebo, a relative reduction of 74%; there was a 70% relative reduction in number of Gd+ lesions. There was no significant difference between FGM and placebo in 3- or 6-month CDP. The time to first confirmed relapse was longer, and more patients remained relapse-free in the FGM treated arm compared to placebo-treated patients at 24-months. MSFC scores were also improved at month 24 in the FGM versus the placebo-treated arm.

3.1.4. Extended TRANSFORMS

Extended TRANSFORMS reported long-term results (up to 4.5 years) for the core TRANSFORMS patients [96]. A total of 92% ($n = 1027$) of patients completing TRANSFORMS entered and 75.2% completed the extension phase. Patients randomized to FGM 0.5 mg or FGM 1.25 mg in the core study continued at the same dose in the extension study, whereas patients receiving IFNβ-1a were re-randomized 1:1 to either FGM 0.5 mg or FGM 1.25 mg daily. Following the sponsor's decision to discontinue FGM 1.25 mg in 2009, all patients subsequently received FGM 0.5 mg until completion of the extension phase. It is only the 0.5 mg FGM results vs. IFNβ-1a which are reported below.

The primary endpoint, ARR at 4.5 years, was significantly reduced in patients who initiated FGM treatment in TRANSFORMS compared to those patients switching from IFNβ-1a to FGM during Extended TRANSFORMS: (0.17 versus 0.27), a 35% relative reduction in risk of relapse ($p < 0.001$). Patients initially treated with IFNβ-1a who switched to FGM, experienced a subsequent 50% reduction in ARR, 0.4 to 0.2, by the end of the extension study. MRI outcomes in the extended TRANSFORMS revealed a 63% reduction in new or newly-enlarged T2 lesion count in the group switching from IFNβ-1a to FGM. The proportion of patients with no evidence of disease activity (NEDA: no relapses, no MRI worsening, and no sustained disability progression) increased by 50% in the first year after switching to FGM (43% to 66%). During the extension phase, there was no statistical difference in the number of patients in either group who remained without Gd+ lesions. The relative reduction in brain volume loss observed during the core study in patients continuously treated with FGM was maintained through the extension study, whereas the patients switched from IFNβ to FGM experienced a reduction in the rate of brain volume loss during the extension phase.

3.1.5. PARADIGM

PARADIGM [92] was a 24 month randomized double-blind, active-controlled, parallel group phase III study of 215 patients with RRMS between the ages of 10 and 17 years of age randomized to either daily oral FGM (107) 0.5 mg (0.25 mg for those weighing 40 kg or less), vs. IFNβ-1a 30 μg IM weekly. All patients had evidence of disease activity in the previous 2 years. The primary outcome, ARR, was 0.12 in FGM versus 0.67 in the IFNβ-1a treated patients, a relative decrease of 82% ($p < 0.001$). The mean percentage of relapse-free patients was 85.7 versus 38.8 favoring the FGM treatment arm. Secondary outcomes included the total number of new and enlarged T2 lesions, which was 4.39 in FGM versus 9.27 in IFNβ-1a treated patients, a 53% relative decrease ($p < 0.001$). The mean number of Gd+ lesions/scan was 0.44 in FGM versus 1.28 in IFNβ-1a treated patients. The mean rate in brain volume change was -0.48% in FGM versus −0.8% in IFNβ-1a treated patients.

3.2. Siponimod

As previously indicated, SPM is a selective S1P1R and S1P5R modulator that readily crosses the BBB [78]. Preclinical studies indicate that it may preserve neurons by preventing excitotoxic synaptic degeneration [83], enhancing cell survival pathways [80,82], and promoting remyelination in the CNS [83]. Given the results of these preclinical studies, and because of the need to develop DMTs that might slow disability worsening in patients with secondary progressive multiple sclerosis (SPMS), it was decided to evaluate SPM efficacy in this patient population.

EXPAND

EXPAND [97] was a double-blind, randomized phase III study of 1645 adults, age 18–60, with SPMS and an EDSS score of 3.0–6.5. Patients were assigned (2:1) to once daily oral SPM 2 mg or placebo for up to three years, or until the occurrence of a pre-specified number of CDP events. The primary endpoint was time to three-month CDP. At baseline, the mean time since first MS symptoms was 16.8 years and time since conversion to SPMS was 3.8 years. Sixty-four percent of patients ($n = 1055$) had not had a relapse in the previous two years; 56% ($n = 918$) needed walking assistance. Twenty-six percent (288/1096) of patients receiving SPM and 32% (173/545) receiving placebo had three-month CDP (hazard ratio 0.79, 95% CI 0.65–0.95), a relative risk reduction of 21% ($p = 0.013$). Of the secondary endpoints, there was no significant difference between SPM and placebo-treated patients in the time to three-month confirmed worsening of at least 20% in Timed 25 Foot Walk (T25FW). The increase in T2 lesion volume from baseline was significantly lower in SPM-treated versus placebo-treated patients, with a between group difference of -695.3 mm^3 (95% CI -877.3 to -513.3; $p < 0.0001$). Numerically more patients receiving SPM were free of Gd+ lesions (89% vs. 67%) and of new or enlarging T2 lesions (57% vs. 37%) than their placebo-treated counterparts. Siponimod was approved for the treatment of "active forms" of SPMS, defined as patients having had a relapse in the previous 2 years, because this was the only subgroup in which the primary end-point was achieved. Following completion of the core EXPAND trial, an open label extension was initiated which is expected to conclude in 2024.

3.3. Ozanimod

Ozanimod, a S1PR1 and S1PR5 modulator, that has been studied in two phase III clinical trials, RADIANCE Part B and SUNBEAM, the most recent agent in this class to receive regulatory approval. Each of these trials was a randomized, double-blind, double-dummy, parallel group, active-controlled study, evaluating the efficacy and safety of daily oral OZM 0.5 mg or 1 mg versus weekly IFNβ-1a 30 μg IM in patients with RRMS. Following its ingestion, OZM is partly transformed into 2 primary metabolites, CC112273 and CC1084037, which account for the bulk of OZM pharmacological effects, each with a t1/2 elimination of approximately 11 days, compared to 19–22 h for OZM itself [85].

3.3.1. RADIANCE Part B

RADIANCE Part B [98], a 24 month trial, included 1,313 patients with RRMS randomized to daily oral OZM 0.5 mg (n = 439), OZM 1 mg (n = 433) or weekly IFN β-1a 30 μg IM (n = 441). Inclusion criteria were ages 18–55 years, EDSS 0.0–5.0, diagnosis of RRMS, and evidence of active disease over the prior 24 months. Exclusion criteria included recent myocardial infarction, TIA, stroke, prolonged QTc interval, resting heart rate < 55 bpm, Type I diabetes, or uncontrolled Type II diabetes.

The primary endpoint in RADIANCE Part B was ARR at each OZM dose versus interferon β-1a over 24 months of treatment. Key secondary endpoints included number of new or enlarging T2 brain lesions, number of Gd+ brain lesions, and time to three-month CDP. Other secondary endpoints included relative rate of whole brain volume loss. Exploratory outcomes included relative changes in cortical grey matter and thalamic volumes over the 2 years of observation. Because of its superior efficacy, regulatory approval was only given the 1.0 mg dose. The 0.5 mg data are not presented. ARR at two years was 0.172 for OZM and 0.276 for IFN β-1a, a relative reduction of 38% favoring OZM ($p < 0.0001$). There was a 42% relative reduction in new and enlarging T2 lesions with OZM treatment compared to IFNβ-1a ($p < 0.001$). The relative reduction in number of Gd+ enhancing brain lesions at two years was 53% in OZM-treated patients ($p = 0.0006$) compared to patients treated with IFNβ-1a. There were no statistically significant differences between OZM and IFNβ-1a treatment in time to three-month CDP. Relative reduction in brain volume loss at 2 years was 27% less in OZM ($p < 0.0001$) than in IFNβ-1a treated patients. Relative cortical gray volume loss was reduced by 58% in patients treated with OZM ($p < 0.0001$) and relative thalamic volume loss at 2 years was reduced by 32% ($p < 0.0001$) in patients receiving OZM.

3.3.2. SUNBEAM

The SUNBEAM phase III study [99] included 1,346 patients with RRMS, randomized to daily oral OZM 0.5 mg (n = 451) or 1 mg (n = 447) versus weekly intramuscular 30 μg IFNβ-1a IM (n = 448). Inclusion criteria included ages 18–55 years, EDSS 0.0–5.0, diagnosis of RRMS, with the same remaining inclusion and exclusion criteria as RADIANCE Part B. Only the data for 1 mg OZM is presented.

The primary endpoint in SUNBEAM was ARR with OZM treatment versus IFNβ-1a over 12 months of observation. Key secondary endpoints included number of new or enlarging T2 brain lesions, number of Gd+ brain lesions at one year, and time to three-month CDP. Other secondary endpoints included whole brain volume loss. Exploratory endpoints included cortical grey matter and thalamic volume changes at one year. ARR at one year was 0.181 for OZM and 0.35 for IFNβ -1a treated patients, a relative risk reduction of 48% ($p < 0.0001$) favoring OZM treated patients. There was a 48% relative reduction in the number of new or enlarging T2 brain lesions favoring OZM-treated patients ($p < 0.001$) and total number of Gd+-brain lesions reduced by 63% in the OZM treatment arm ($p < 0.0001$) compared to IFNβ-1a. There was no statistically significant difference between OZM and IFNβ-1a for time to three-month CDP. There was a 33% relative reduction ($p < 0.0001$) in percentage whole brain volume decrease for OZM treated patients, as well as an 84% ($p < 0.0001$) relative reduction in cortical grey matter loss and a 39% ($p < 0.0001$) relative reduction in thalamic volume loss in OZM treated patients. It is of particular interest to learn the results of on-going studies which are focused on cognitive functioning and patient reported outcome status [100] in light of the demonstrated relative reduction in cortical gray matter and thalamic volume loss in OZM treated patients.

The regulatory approval for the higher OZM dose is a 92 mg capsule, as opposed to the 1.0 mg OZM hydrochloride tablets used in the clinical trials [85].

3.4. Ponesimod

Ponesimod (PNM), a selective S1PR-1 modulator without known effect on the remaining four S1PRs, has been studied in one phase III clinical trial.

OPTIMUM

OPTIMUM [101], was a 108 week multicenter, randomized, double-blind, parallel group, and active controlled study, evaluating the efficacy, safety, and tolerability of daily oral PNM 20 mg versus daily oral teriflunomide (TFM) 14 mg in adults with RRMS. OPTIMUM enrolled 1,133 patients, randomized to receive PNM ($n = 567$) or TFM ($n = 566$). Inclusion criteria included ages 18 to 55 years, EDSS 0.0-5.0, diagnosis of RRMS, and active disease in the 24 months prior to screening. The primary end-point was ARR over 108 weeks. Key secondary end-points included change from baseline to week 108 in fatigue-related symptoms, as measured by the symptoms domain of the FSIQ-RMS. Other secondary endpoints included the mean number of combined unique active lesions (CUAL) per year, defined as new Gd+1 lesions and any new or enlarging T2 lesions. In addition, time to 12-week and 24-week CDP was also determined.

There was a 30.5% relative reduction ($p = 0.0003$) in ARR in PNM treated patients (0.202 versus 0.290) compared to TFM treated patients. Ponesimod demonstrated superior improvement in fatigue scores at week 108 compared to TFM as measured by the FSIQ-RMS weekly symptom score (mean difference −3.57, $p = 0.0019$). There was a 56% relative reduction in CUALs per year (1.405 versus 3.164) in patients treated with PNM. No significant differences between PNM and TFM seen for 12-week or 24-week CDP.

4. Safety

4.1. Fingolimod

In FREEDOMS, 94% of patients receiving FGM compared to 93% of patients receiving placebo had an AE. The majority of these events were mild to moderate with 7.5% of patients on FGM stopping due to side effects compared to 7.7% on placebo. In TRANSFORMS, 86% of FGM 0.5 mg patients compared to 92% of patients on IFNβ-1a had an AE. However, 6% of patients on FGM versus 4% or patients on IFNβ-1a discontinued due to an AE [93,94].

In FREEDOMS, overall, incidence of infections was the same in all treatment groups; however, lower respiratory infections were more common in patients receiving FGM. There were two deaths in the 1.25 mg FGM group, one each of disseminated primary varicella zoster and herpes simplex encephalitis. The overall rate of herpes infections receiving FGM was 0.01 (10/854) and 0.01 (4/418) in placebo treated patients. As of this writing, there have been 36 confirmed cases of PML in greater than 746,700 patient years since FGM approval. In an analysis of 21 PML cases, age at treatment initiation was not a risk factor for the development of PML; however, longer duration of exposure to FGM increased the risk of developing PML [102]. As of February 2019, 46 cases of cryptococcal infections have been reported. (Novartis data on file), the majority of whom were treated for 2 or more years

Macular edema was slightly more common in patients on 0.5 mg of FGM compared to placebo, 0.5 verses 0.4%, and typically occurred within the first 3 to 4 months of therapy. Because patients with diabetes and uveitis are at higher risk of developing macular edema, they were excluded from the clinical trials. Given the risk of macular edema, a baseline eye exam is recommended within 6 months of starting and then 3 to 4 months after beginning FGM [91].

Fingolimod, on average, lowered the heart rate by eight beats per minute. Following the first dose, 0.6% of patients receiving FGM developed symptomatic bradycardia compared to 0.1% in the placebo group, with rare cases of second degree AV block reported. Nonetheless, patients are required to undergo an ECG prior to the first dose observation (FDO), and then at least a 6 h FDO, during which time hourly pulse and blood pressure are obtained, followed by an additional ECG at the end of monitoring. Medications which can cause bradycardia or prolong the QT interval, such as beta blockers. Selective serotonin and norepinephrine reuptake inhibitors are to be used with caution and may prompt, overnight or more prolonged ambulatory cardiac rhythm monitoring. Fingolimod is contraindicated in patients with recent myocardial infarction, unstable angina, stroke, transient ischemic attack, or heart failure within the last 6 months [91]. There was also an average 3 mm Hg increase in systolic blood pressure and 2 mm Hg increase in diastolic pressure in patients on FGM. Elevation in liver enzymes was more commonly seen in the patients receiving FGM, with elevations of three times the upper limit of normal (ULN) or greater were seen in 14% of patients treated with FGM and in 3% of patients on placebo, typically occurring within 6 to 9 months of starting FGM. Peripheral lymphocyte counts dropped by 73% on average in patients receiving FGM, and typically return to baseline values 1–2 after stopping FGM (Novartis data on file). To date, there has been no evidence that lower lymphocyte counts are predictive of increased infection risk [103].

Skin cancer, particularly basal cell carcinoma, may be more common in patients on FGM [91]. Post-marketing studies have also reported rare cases of cutaneous melanoma and squamous cell carcinoma [104,105].

In the pediatric population (PARADIGM), the incidence of AEs was 88.8% in FGM and 95.3% in IFNβ-1a treated patients. The most common side effects in the FGM treated patients were headache (31.8%), viral upper respiratory infections (21.5%), Upper respiratory infections (15.9%), leukopenia (14%), influenza (1.2%), cough (9%), and pyrexia (7.5%). Serious AEs occurred in the FGM treated cohort and 4.7 % of FGM treated patients discontinued the trial because of SAEs. These AEs included convulsions (5.6%), and 3.7% of patients had serious infections, including one case each of appendicitis, cellulitis, oral abscess, and viral pharyngitis. Single SAE cases also included agranulocytosis, arthralgia, auto-immune uveitis, gastrointestinal necrosis, vasculitis, second degree AV conduction block, and small bowel obstruction.

Fingolimod is not recommended during pregnancy and lactation, based upon its teratogenicity, increased fetal loss and its presence in the milk of lactating animals. Prescribing information currently recommends stopping FGM 3-months prior to planning conception; however this recommendation may require revision in light of recent reports of increased MS breakthrough activity, occurring in 10–25% of patients within 12 weeks of discontinuing FGM [106,107]. Patients with a higher annualized risk of relapse or higher EDSS prior to starting FGM may be at greater risk of rebound disease once stopping FGM [108].

4.2. Siponimod

The SPM safety profile is similar to that of FGM. In EXPAND [97], 89% of patients receiving SPM and 82% of patients receiving placebo had an AE. Non-serious adverse events leading to discontinuation in the study was 4% versus 3% respectively. Serious adverse events occurred in 18% of the SPM group compared to 15% in the placebo group.

Rate of infections were also similar in both groups, but upper and lower respiratory infections, as well as herpes zoster reactivation, were more common in the SPM treated group. The risk of herpes infection was 2.5% in SPM versus 0.7% in placebo treated patients. No cases of PML or cryptococcal infections were reported, although these opportunistic infections may emerge as larger populations are treated for longer durations, given the similar mechanism of action compared to FNM. The reduction in the peripheral lymphocyte count was between 20 to 30% which is less than that observed in patients treated with FGM [93,94], but whether this impacts the comparative rate of infection is yet to be determined.

Liver function abnormalities were observed in 10.7% of SPM treated patients and 3.7% in the placebo group.

Rate of macular edema was 1.8% in patients on SPM and 0.2% of patients treated with placebo. This is higher than 0.4% reported in the phase III clinical trials with FGM [93,94].

Seizures occurred in 1.7% of SPM treated patients and was 0.4% in the placebo group.

The reduction in heart rate was a mean of six beats per minute in the SPM treated group, with the maximum reduction occurring on average 4 h after the first dose. Bradycardia was reported as an AE in 6% of patients receiving SPM compared to 3% receiving placebo. Cases of Mobitz type II or higher degree atrio-ventricular (AV) block were not observed. As a result, first dose observation is not required except for patients with recent history of myocardial infarction, unstable angina, recent stroke, TIA or baseline heart rate of less than 55 beats per minute [109]. Clinicians may also recommend first dose observation for patients on medication which may lower heart rate, particularly those medication that slow AV conduction.

Elevation in liver enzymes was 10.1% in patients on SPM, versus 3.7% of patients on placebo. Overall, rate of malignancies was the same in each group.

Medications which inhibit the hepatic enzymes CYP2C9 and CYP3A4 can result in elevated concentration of SPM, and the opposite is true for hepatic enzyme inducers. Furthermore, in patients with the CYP2C9 genotype variants CYP2C9 1*/3* or 2*/3* should receive only 1.0 mg a day maintenance dosing and those with the 3*/3* genotype should not receive SPM at all due to their inhibition of SPM degradation in the liver [109].

4.3. Ozanimod

In RADIANCE and SUNBEAM, overall AEs and AEs leading to discontinuation were lower in both groups of patients taking OZM compared to interferon beta-1a. Nasopharyngitis, elevated liver enzymes, hypertension, and urinary tract infections were commonly seen in the OZM groups in both clinic trials. No serious opportunistic infections were reported, and the rate of herpes infections were the same across the three treatment groups.

There was one case of posterior reversible encephalopathy syndrome (PRES) in a patient receiving 1.0 mg OZM, occurring 10 months after starting the medication. Of note, post-approval cases have also been reported in patients treated with FGM [110,111]. Mean absolute lymphocyte count in patients on OZM 1.0 mg were reduced by approximately 45% by 3 months, and maintained at that level thereafter. The rate of macular edema was 0.3% in each OZM and the IFNβ-1a group. Maximum mean reduction in heart rate on day 1 was 0.6 bpm at 5 h in RADIANCE. Four patients treated with OZM had a heart rate less than 45, but had baseline heart rates of 55-64 bpm, and no symptoms were reported. In SUNBEAM, the maximum mean reduction was 1.8 bpm at 5 h, with no rate below 45 bpm reported. No second- or third-degree heart block was observed in either study. Given the minimal reduction in heart rate, FDO is not required for most patients.

As with the other S1PR-1 modulators, mild elevations in liver function enzymes were observed. In RADIANCE, 6.7% of patients on 1.0 mg of OZM had an ALT of 3 X ULN normal, as did 3.9% of patients on IFNβ-1a. In SUNBEAM, the rate was 4.3% for OZM and 2.2% for IFNβ-1a treated patients.

4.4. Contraindications and Cautions

The use of FGM, SPM, and OZM is contraindicated in patients with recent (within the past 6 months) myocardial infarction or stroke, unstable angina, class III/IV heart failure4.4, recent transient ischemic attack and in patients receiving class I and Class III anti-arrhythmics, patients with Mobitz type 2 s or third degree heart block, sino-atrial block, or sick sinus syndrome without a functioning pacemaker. In addition, specifically for OZM there is a contraindication for the concomitant use of monoamine oxidase inhibitors and in patients with untreated severe sleep apnea. The concomitant use of SSRIs, SNRIs and narcotics is not recommended for any of the S1PR modulators [85,91,109].

4.5. Ponesimod

The proportion of patients experiencing at least one treatment emergent AE (TEAE) in OPTIMUM was similar for both PNM and TFM, although discontinuation due to TEAE was higher in the PMN than the TFM group, 8.7% vs. 6.0% respectively. Premature discontinuations due to elevated liver enzymes and respiratory events were relatively higher in the PNM than TFM groups. The most common AEs of special interest were elevated liver function tests in the PNM group, (22.7% vs. 12.2%), hypertension (10.1% vs. 9.0%), and pulmonary events (8.0% vs. 2.7%). Most ALT increases ≥3X ULN were single transient asymptomatic events that spontaneously resolved on treatment or resulted in protocol mandated discontinuation. Eight seizures were reported in patients treated with PMN compared to one patient on TFM.

Skin malignancies occurred in five patients treated with PMN and in one patient in the TFM group. Four cases of bradycardia (0.7%) occurred in the PMN 20 mg group and an additional three patients experienced first degree atrioventricular block. None of the events were serious or led to treatment discontinuation.

5. Potential Therapeutic Opportunities

As is evident from the data presented, the S1PR modulators are an important addition to the list of DMTs for the treatment of MS. In addition to their oral route of administration, an important addition to patient quality of life, with a higher likelihood of compliance and persistence, they offer significant improvement in clinical efficacy at acceptable levels of risk in studies in which they have been compared to "platform" injectable or oral therapies. Important questions and research opportunities remain. Will agents with more potent S1PR-5 modulation improve remyelination, as a result of improved maturation of OPCs and enhanced myelin formation by OLGs? Will their use reduce inflammatory impact of MS by the enhancement of BBB integrity? Will selective S1PR-2 inhibition stimulate remyelination by blocking the NOGO/LOGO membrane complex, and will simultaneous S1PR-1 and S1PR-2 provide greater synergistic regulation of astrocytes than either agent alone? Since S1PR-3 is up-regulated on astrocytes during CNS inflammation [112] can CNS selective S1PR-3 modulators be developed which do not also increase cardiovascular side effects? Lastly, as more is learned about the intracellular pathways activated or inhibited by S1P and its receptors, the development of pharmacological agents which can manipulate these pathways, and the development of agents that can interact with intracellular S1PRs, offer highly specific, potentially fruitful therapeutic opportunities for MS and numerous other diseases, including rheumatoid arthritis [113–115], systemic lupus [116,117], polymyotisis [118], ulcerative colitis [119], psoriasis [120], colon cancer [121–123], breast cancer [124–126], lung cancer [127,128] and atherosclerosis [129,130].

Author Contributions: Conceptualization, S.C., E.L., K.S., and J.B.; writing—original draft preparation, S.C., E.L., K.S., J.B., and C.C.; writing—review and editing, S.C. and C.C. All authors have read and agreed to the published version of the manuscript.

Funding: The authors received no funding for writing this review article.

Acknowledgments: The authors acknowledge and thank Jessica Garten for producing Figures 1–4.

Conflicts of Interest: S.C. has served on advisory boards or steering committees for AbbVie, Biogen, Novartis, Sanofi Genzyme, and Pear Therapeutics; has received research support from AbbVie, Adamas, Biogen, Novartis, Sanofi Genzyme, MedDay, and Roche Genentech; has received speaker honoraria from Biogen, Novartis, Sanofi Genzyme, and Roche Genentech. EL has served on the advisory board for Genentech and Celgene/Bristol Myers Squibb, and received speaking honoraria from Biogen, Genentech, EMD Serono, Genzyme, and Novartis, and research support from Biogen, Novartis, and Celgene/Bristol Myers Squibb. K.S. has received research support from AbbVie, Biogen, Genentech, EMD Serono, MedDay, and IMS Health and consulting fees from Acorda, Biogen, EMD Serono, Genzyme, Genentech, Novartis, and Teva. J.B. has received speaker honoraria from Teva and served on an advisory board for Biogen. C.C. declares no conflict of interest.

References

1. Spiegel, S.; Milstien, S. Sphingosine-1-phosphate: An enigmatic signalling lipid. *Nat. Rev. Mol. Cell Boil.* **2003**, *4*, 397–407. [CrossRef] [PubMed]
2. Merrill, A.H. Sphingolipid and Glycosphingolipid Metabolic Pathways in the Era of Sphingolipidomics. *Chem. Rev.* **2011**, *111*, 6387–6422. [CrossRef] [PubMed]
3. Grassi, S.; Mauri, L.; Prioni, S.; Cabitta, L.; Sonnino, S.; Prinetti, A.; Giussani, P. Sphingosine 1-Phosphate Receptors and Metabolic Enzymes as Druggable Targets for Brain Diseases. *Front. Pharmacol.* **2019**, *10*, 807. [CrossRef] [PubMed]
4. Proia, R.L.; Hla, T. Emerging biology of sphingosine-1-phosphate: Its role in pathogenesis and therapy. *J. Clin. Investig.* **2015**, *125*, 1379–1387. [CrossRef]

5. Brunkhorst, R.; Vutukuri, R.; Pfeilschifter, W. Fingolimod for the treatment of neurological diseases-state of play and future perspectives. *Front. Cell. Neurosci.* **2014**, *8*. [CrossRef]
6. Blaho, V.A.; Hla, T. An update on the biology of sphingosine 1-phosphate receptors. *J. Lipid Res.* **2014**, *55*, 1596–1608. [CrossRef]
7. Brinkmann, V.; Davis, M.D.; Heise, C.E.; Albert, R.; Cottens, S.; Hof, R.; Bruns, C.; Prieschl, E.; Baumruker, T.; Hiestand, P.; et al. The Immune Modulator FTY720 Targets Sphingosine 1-Phosphate Receptors. *J. Boil. Chem.* **2002**, *277*, 21453–21457. [CrossRef]
8. Webb, M.; Tham, C.-S.; Lin, F.-F.; Lariosa-Willingham, K.; Yu, N.; Hale, J.; Mandala, S.; Chun, J.; Rao, T.S. Sphingosine 1-phosphate receptor agonists attenuate relapsing–remitting experimental autoimmune encephalitis in SJL mice. *J. Neuroimmunol.* **2004**, *153*, 108–121. [CrossRef]
9. Matloubian, M.; Lo, C.G.; Cinamon, G.; Lesneski, M.J.; Xu, Y.; Brinkmann, V.; Allende, M.L.; Proia, R.L.; Cyster, J.G. Lymphocyte egress from thymus and peripheral lymphoid organs is dependent on S1P receptor 1. *Nature* **2004**, *427*, 355–360. [CrossRef]
10. Pappu, R.; Schwab, S.R.; Cornelissen, I.; Pereira, J.P.; Regard, J.B.; Xu, Y.; Camerer, E.; Zheng, Y.-W.; Huang, Y.; Cyster, J.G.; et al. Promotion of Lymphocyte Egress into Blood and Lymph by Distinct Sources of Sphingosine-1-Phosphate. *Science* **2007**, *316*, 295–298. [CrossRef]
11. Cyster, J.G.; Schwab, S.R. Sphingosine-1-Phosphate and Lymphocyte Egress from Lymphoid Organs. *Annu. Rev. Immunol.* **2012**, *30*, 69–94. [CrossRef] [PubMed]
12. Harrison, S.M.; Reavill, C.; Brown, G.; Brown, J.T.; Cluderay, J.E.; Crook, B.; Davies, C.H.; Dawson, L.A.; Grau, E.; Heidbreder, C.; et al. LPA1 receptor-deficient mice have phenotypic changes observed in psychiatric disease. *Mol. Cell Neurosci.* **2003**, *24*, 1170–1179. [CrossRef] [PubMed]
13. Chun, J.; Brinkmann, V. Faculty Opinions recommendation of A mechanistically novel, first oral therapy for multiple sclerosis: The development of fingolimod (FTY720, Gilenya). *Fac. Opin. Post-Pub. Peer Rev. Biomed. Lit.* **2014**, *12*, 213–228. [CrossRef]
14. Choi, J.W.; Chun, J. Lysophospholipids and their receptors in the central nervous system. *Biochim. Biophys. Acta (BBA)-Mol. Cell Boil. Lipids* **2013**, *1831*, 20–32. [CrossRef]
15. Giussani, P.C.; Tringali, C.A.; Riboni, L.; Viani, P.; Venerando, B. Sphingolipids: Key Regulators of Apoptosis and Pivotal Players in Cancer Drug Resistance. *Int. J. Mol. Sci.* **2014**, *15*, 4356–4392. [CrossRef] [PubMed]
16. Bassi, R.; Anelli, V.V.; Giussani, P.C.; Tettamanti, G.; Viani, P.; Riboni, L. Sphingosine-1-phosphate is released by cerebellar astrocytes in response to bFGF and induces astrocyte proliferation through Gi-protein-coupled receptors. *Glia* **2006**, *53*, 621–630. [CrossRef]
17. Mizugishi, K.; Yamashita, T.; Olivera, A.; Miller, G.F.; Spiegel, S.; Proia, R.L. Essential Role for Sphingosine Kinases in Neural and Vascular Development. *Mol. Cell. Boil.* **2005**, *25*, 11113–11121. [CrossRef]
18. Riganti, L.; Antonucci, F.; Gabrielli, M.; Prada, I.; Giussani, P.C.; Viani, P.; Valtorta, F.; Menna, E.; Matteoli, M.; Verderio, C. Sphingosine-1-Phosphate (S1P) Impacts Presynaptic Functions by Regulating Synapsin I Localization in the Presynaptic Compartment. *J. Neurosci.* **2016**, *36*, 4624–4634. [CrossRef]
19. Moore, A.N.; Kampfl, A.W.; Zhao, X.; Hayes, R.L.; Dash, P.K. Sphingosine-1-phosphate induces apoptosis of cultured hippocampal neurons that requires protein phosphatases and activator protein-1 complexes. *Neuroscience* **1999**, *94*, 405–415. [CrossRef]
20. Hagen, N.; Van Veldhoven, P.P.; Proia, R.L.; Park, H.; Merrill, A.H.; Van Echten-Deckert, G. Subcellular Origin of Sphingosine 1-Phosphate Is Essential for Its Toxic Effect in Lyase-deficient Neurons. *J. Boil. Chem.* **2009**, *284*, 11346–11353. [CrossRef]
21. Hagen, N.; Hans, M.; Hartmann, D.; Swandulla, D.; Van Echten-Deckert, G. Sphingosine-1-phosphate links glycosphingolipid metabolism to neurodegeneration via a calpain-mediated mechanism. *Cell Death Differ.* **2011**, *18*, 1356–1365. [CrossRef] [PubMed]
22. Mitroi, D.N.; Karunakaran, I.; Gräler, M.; Saba, J.D.; Ehninger, D.; Ledesma, M.D.; Van Echten-Deckert, G. SGPL1 (sphingosine phosphate lyase 1) modulates neuronal autophagy via phosphatidylethanolamine production. *Autophagy* **2017**, *13*, 885–899. [CrossRef]
23. Karunakaran, I.; Alam, S.; Jayagopi, S.; Frohberger, S.J.; Hansen, J.N.; Kuehlwein, J.; Hölbling, B.V.; Schumak, B.; Hübner, M.P.; Gräler, M.H.; et al. Neural sphingosine 1-phosphate accumulation activates microglia and links impaired autophagy and inflammation. *Glia* **2019**, *67*, 1859–1872. [CrossRef] [PubMed]
24. Choi, Y.-J.; Saba, J.D. Sphingosine phosphate lyase insufficiency syndrome (SPLIS): A novel inborn error of sphingolipid metabolism. *Adv. Boil. Regul.* **2019**, *71*, 128–140. [CrossRef] [PubMed]

25. Giussani, P.C.; Ferraretto, A.; Gravaghi, C.; Bassi, R.; Tettamanti, G.; Riboni, L.; Viani, P. Sphingosine-1-Phosphate and Calcium Signaling in Cerebellar Astrocytes and Differentiated Granule Cells. *Neurochem. Res.* **2006**, *32*, 27–37. [CrossRef] [PubMed]
26. Mitroi, D.N.; Deutschmann, A.U.; Raucamp, M.; Karunakaran, I.; Glebov, K.; Hans, M.; Walter, J.; Saba, J.; Gräler, M.; Ehninger, D.; et al. Sphingosine 1-phosphate lyase ablation disrupts presynaptic architecture and function via an ubiquitin- proteasome mediated mechanism. *Sci. Rep.* **2016**, *6*, 37064. [CrossRef] [PubMed]
27. Brinkmann, V.; Cyster, J.G.; Hla, T. FTY720: Sphingosine 1-Phosphate Receptor-1 in the Control of Lymphocyte Egress and Endothelial Barrier Function. *Arab. Archaeol. Epigr.* **2004**, *4*, 1019–1025. [CrossRef]
28. Chiba, K. FTY720, a new class of immunomodulator, inhibits lymphocyte egress from secondary lymphoid tissues and thymus by agonistic activity at sphingosine 1-phosphate receptors. *Pharmacol. Ther.* **2005**, *108*, 308–319. [CrossRef]
29. Thangada, S.; Khanna, K.M.; Blaho, V.A.; Oo, M.L.; Im, D.-S.; Guo, C.; Lefrancois, L.; Hla, T. Cell-surface residence of sphingosine 1-phosphate receptor 1 on lymphocytes determines lymphocyte egress kinetics. *J. Exp. Med.* **2010**, *207*, 1475–1483. [CrossRef]
30. Scott, F.L.; Clemons, B.; Brooks, J.; Brahmachary, E.; Powell, R.; Dedman, H.; Desale, H.G.A.; Timony, G.; Martinborough, E.; Rosen, H.; et al. Ozanimod (RPC1063) is a potent sphingosine-1-phosphate receptor-1 (S1P1) and receptor-5 (S1P5) agonist with autoimmune disease-modifying activity. *Br. J. Pharmacol.* **2016**, *173*, 1778–1792. [CrossRef]
31. Mandala, S. Alteration of Lymphocyte Trafficking by Sphingosine-1-Phosphate Receptor Agonists. *Science* **2002**, *296*, 346–349. [CrossRef] [PubMed]
32. Oo, M.L.; Thangada, S.; Wu, M.T.; Liu, C.H.; Macdonald, T.L.; Lynch, K.R.; Lin, C.Y.; Hla, T. Immunosuppressive and anti-angiogenic sphingosine 1-phosphate receptor-1 agonists induce ubiquitinylation and proteasomal degradation of the receptor. *J. Biol. Chem.* **2007**, *282*, 9082–9089. [CrossRef]
33. Gräler, M.H.; Goetzl, E.J. The immunosuppressant FTY720 down-regulates sphingosine 1-phosphate G protein-coupled receptors. *FASEB J.* **2004**, *18*, 551–553. [CrossRef]
34. Mullershausen, F.; Zecri, F.; Çetin, C.; Billich, A.; Guerini, D.; Seuwen, K. Persistent signaling induced by FTY720-phosphate is mediated by internalized S1P1 receptors. *Nat. Methods* **2009**, *5*, 428–434. [CrossRef] [PubMed]
35. Groves, A.; Kihara, Y.; Chun, J. Fingolimod: Direct CNS effects of sphingosine 1-phosphate (S1P) receptor modulation and implications in multiple sclerosis therapy. *J. Neurol. Sci.* **2013**, *328*, 9–18. [CrossRef] [PubMed]
36. Subei, A.M.; Cohen, J.A. Sphingosine 1-phosphate receptor modulators in multiple sclerosis. *CNS Drugs* **2015**, *29*, 565–575. [CrossRef] [PubMed]
37. Mao-Draayer, Y.; Sarazin, J.; Fox, D.; Schiopu, E. The sphingosine-1-phosphate receptor: A novel therapeutic target for multiple sclerosis and other autoimmune diseases. *Clin. Immunol.* **2016**, *175*, 10–15. [CrossRef]
38. Choi, J.W.; Gardell, S.E.; Herr, D.R.; Rivera, R.; Lee, C.-W.; Noguchi, K.; Teo, S.T.; Yung, Y.C.; Lu, M.; Kennedy, G.; et al. FTY720 (fingolimod) efficacy in an animal model of multiple sclerosis requires astrocyte sphingosine 1-phosphate receptor 1 (S1P1) modulation. *Proc. Natl. Acad. Sci. USA* **2010**, *108*, 751–756. [CrossRef]
39. Kim, H.J.; Miron, V.E.; Dukala, D.; Proia, R.L.; Ludwin, S.K.; Traka, M.; Antel, J.P.; Soliven, B. Neurobiological effects of sphingosine 1-phosphate receptor modulation in the cuprizone model. *FASEB J.* **2011**, *25*, 1509–1518. [CrossRef]
40. Nystad, A.E.; Lereim, R.R.; Wergeland, S.; Oveland, E.; Myhr, K.-M.; Bø, L.; Torkildsen, Ø. Fingolimod downregulates brain sphingosine-1-phosphate receptor 1 levels but does not promote remyelination or neuroprotection in the cuprizone model. *J. Neuroimmunol.* **2020**, *339*, 577091. [CrossRef]
41. Seyedsadr, M.S.; Weinmann, O.; Amorim, A.; Ineichen, B.V.; Egger, M.; Mirnajafi-Zadeh, J.; Becher, B.; Javan, M.; Schwab, M.E. Inactivation of sphingosine-1-phosphate receptor 2 (S1PR2) decreases demyelination and enhances remyelination in animal models of multiple sclerosis. *Neurobiol. Dis.* **2019**, *124*, 189–201. [CrossRef]
42. Miron, V.E.; Jung, C.-G.; Kim, H.J.; Kennedy, T.E.; Soliven, B.; Antel, J.P. FTY720 modulates human oligodendrocyte progenitor process extension and survival. *Ann. Neurol.* **2008**, *63*, 61–71. [CrossRef]

43. Brana, C.; Frossard, M.J.; Gobert, R.P.; Martinier, N.; Boschert, U.; Seabrook, T.J. Immunohistochemical detection of sphingosine-1-phosphate receptor 1 and 5 in human multiple sclerosis lesions. *Neuropathol. Appl. Neurobiol.* **2014**, *40*, 564–578. [CrossRef]
44. Van Doorn, R.; Van Horssen, J.; Verzijl, D.; Witte, M.; Ronken, E.; Hof, B.V.H.; Lakeman, K.; Dijkstra, C.D.; Van Der Valk, P.; Reijerkerk, A.; et al. Sphingosine 1-phosphate receptor 1 and 3 are upregulated in multiple sclerosis lesions. *Glia* **2010**, *58*, 1465–1476. [CrossRef] [PubMed]
45. Kim, S.; Bielawski, J.; Yang, H.; Kong, Y.; Zhou, B.; Li, J. Functional antagonism of sphingosine-1-phosphate receptor 1 prevents cuprizone-induced demyelination. *Glia* **2017**, *66*, 654–669. [CrossRef] [PubMed]
46. Assi, E.; Cazzato, D.; De Palma, C.; Perrotta, C.; Clementi, E.; Cervia, D. Sphingolipids and Brain Resident Macrophages in Neuroinflammation: An Emerging Aspect of Nervous System Pathology. *Clin. Dev. Immunol.* **2013**, *2013*, 1–8. [CrossRef]
47. Koyrakh, L.; Roman, M.I.; Brinkmann, V.; Wickman, K. The Heart Rate Decrease Caused by Acute FTY720 Administration Is Mediated by the G Protein-Gated Potassium Channel I KACh. *Arab. Archaeol. Epigr.* **2005**, *5*, 529–536. [CrossRef] [PubMed]
48. Bünemann, M.; Brandts, B.; Zu Heringdorf, D.M.; Van Koppen, C.J.; Jakobs, K.H.; Pott, L. Activation of muscarinic K+ current in guinea-pig atrial myocytes by sphingosine-1-phosphate. *J. Physiol.* **1995**, *489*, 701–707. [CrossRef] [PubMed]
49. Sanna, M.G.; Liao, J.; Jo, E.; Alfonso, C.; Ahn, M.-Y.; Peterson, M.S.; Webb, B.; Lefebvre, S.; Chun, J.; Gray, N.; et al. Sphingosine 1-Phosphate (S1P) Receptor Subtypes S1P1and S1P3, Respectively, Regulate Lymphocyte Recirculation and Heart Rate. *J. Boil. Chem.* **2004**, *279*, 13839–13848. [CrossRef] [PubMed]
50. Li, N.; Zhang, F. Implication of sphingosin-1-phosphate in cardiovascular regulation. *Front. Biosci.* **2016**, *21*, 1296–1313. [CrossRef] [PubMed]
51. Novgorodov, A.S.; El-Alwani, M.; Bielawski, J.; Obeid, L.M.; Gudz, T.I. Activation of sphingosine-1-phosphate receptor S1P5 inhibits oligodendrocyte progenitor migration. *FASEB J.* **2007**, *21*, 1503–1514. [CrossRef] [PubMed]
52. Adada, M.; Canals, D.; Hannun, Y.A.; Obeid, L.M. Sphingosine-1-phosphate receptor 2. *FEBS J.* **2013**, *280*, 6354–6366. [CrossRef] [PubMed]
53. Cruz-Orengo, L.; Daniels, B.P.; Dorsey, D.; Basak, S.A.; Grajales-Reyes, J.G.; McCandless, E.E.; Piccio, L.; Schmidt, R.E.; Cross, A.H.; Crosby, S.D.; et al. Enhanced sphingosine-1-phosphate receptor 2 expression underlies female CNS autoimmunity susceptibility. *J. Clin. Investig.* **2014**, *124*, 2571–2584. [CrossRef]
54. Kempf, A.; Tews, B.; Arzt, M.; Weinmann, O.; Obermair, F.J.; Pernet, V.; Zagrebelsky, M.; Delekate, A.; Iobbi, C.; Zemmar, A.; et al. The Sphingolipid Receptor S1PR2 Is a Receptor for Nogo-A Repressing Synaptic Plasticity. *PLoS Boil.* **2014**, *12*, e1001763. [CrossRef] [PubMed]
55. Chong, S.Y.C.; Rosenberg, S.S.; Fancy, S.P.J.; Zhao, C.; Shen, Y.-A.A.; Hahn, A.T.; McGee, A.W.; Xu, X.; Zheng, B.; Zhang, L.I.; et al. Neurite outgrowth inhibitor Nogo-A establishes spatial segregation and extent of oligodendrocyte myelination. *Proc. Natl. Acad. Sci. USA* **2011**, *109*, 1299–1304. [CrossRef]
56. Ishii, M.; Kikuta, J.; Shimazu, Y.; Meier-Schellersheim, M.; Germain, R.N. Chemorepulsion by blood S1P regulates osteoclast precursor mobilization and bone remodeling in vivo. *J. Exp. Med.* **2010**, *207*, 2793–2798. [CrossRef]
57. Thurnherr, T.; Benninger, Y.; Wu, X.; Chrostek, A.; Krause, S.M.; Nave, K.-A.; Franklin, R.; Brakebusch, C.; Suter, U.; Relvas, J.B. Cdc42 and Rac1 Signaling Are Both Required for and Act Synergistically in the Correct Formation of Myelin Sheaths in the CNS. *J. Neurosci.* **2006**, *26*, 10110–10119. [CrossRef]
58. Hoffmann, F.S.; Hofereiter, J.; Rübsamen, H.; Melms, J.; Schwarz, S.; Faber, H.; Weber, P.; Pütz, B.; Loleit, V.; Weber, F.; et al. Fingolimod induces neuroprotective factors in human astrocytes. *J. Neuroinflamm.* **2015**, *12*, 184. [CrossRef] [PubMed]
59. Tran, C.; Heng, B.; Teo, J.D.; Humphrey, S.J.; Qi, Y.; Couttas, T.A.; Stefen, H.; Brettle, M.; Fath, T.; Guillemin, G.J.; et al. Sphingosine 1-phosphate but not Fingolimod protects neurons against excitotoxic cell death by inducing neurotrophic gene expression in astrocytes. *J. Neurochem.* **2019**, *153*, 173–188. [CrossRef]
60. Zhang, Y.; Chen, K.; Sloan, S.A.; Bennett, M.L.; Scholze, A.R.; O'Keeffe, S.; Phatnani, H.P.; Guarnieri, P.; Caneda, C.; Ruderisch, N.; et al. An RNA-Sequencing Transcriptome and Splicing Database of Glia, Neurons, and Vascular Cells of the Cerebral Cortex. *J. Neurosci.* **2014**, *34*, 11929–11947. [CrossRef] [PubMed]

61. Zhang, Y.; Sloan, S.A.; Clarke, L.E.; Caneda, C.; Plaza, C.A.; Blumenthal, P.D.; Vogel, H.; Steinberg, G.K.; Edwards, M.S.B.; Li, G.; et al. Purification and Characterization of Progenitor and Mature Human Astrocytes Reveals Transcriptional and Functional Differences with Mouse. *Neuron* **2016**, *89*, 37–53. [CrossRef] [PubMed]
62. Jaillard, C.; Harrison, S.; Stankoff, B.; Aigrot, M.S.; Calver, A.R.; Duddy, G.; Walsh, F.S.; Pangalos, M.N.; Arimura, N.; Kaibuchi, K.; et al. Edg8/S1P5: An oligodendroglial receptor with dual function on process retraction and cell survival. *J. Neurosci.* **2005**, *25*, 1459–1469. [CrossRef] [PubMed]
63. Allard, J.; Barron, S.; Diaz, J.; Lubetzki, C.; Zalc, B.; Schwartz, J.C.; Sokoloff, P. A rat G protein-coupled receptor selectively expressed in myelin-forming cells. *J. Neurosci.* **1998**, *10*, 1045–1053. [CrossRef] [PubMed]
64. Im, N.-S.; Clemens, J.; Macdonald, T.L.; Lynch, K.R. Characterization of the Human and Mouse Sphingosine 1-Phosphate Receptor, S1P5(Edg-8): Structure–Activity Relationship of Sphingosine1-Phosphate Receptors. *Biochemistry* **2001**, *40*, 14053–14060. [CrossRef]
65. Terai, K.; Soga, T.; Takahashi, M.; Kamohara, M.; Ohno, K.; Yatsugi, S.; Okada, M.; Yamaguchi, T. Edg-8 receptors are preferentially expressed in oligodendrocyte lineage cells of the rat CNS. *Neuroscice* **2003**, *116*, 1053–1062. [CrossRef]
66. Yu, N.; Lariosa-Willingham, K.D.; Lin, F.-F.; Webb, M.; Rao, T.S. Characterization of lysophosphatidic acid and sphingosine-1-phosphate-mediated signal transduction in rat cortical oligodendrocytes. *Glia* **2003**, *45*, 17–27. [CrossRef]
67. Van Doorn, R.; Pinheiro, M.A.L.; Kooij, G.; Lakeman, K.; Hof, B.V.H.; Van Der Pol, S.M.A.; Geerts, D.; Van Horssen, J.; Van Der Valk, P.; Van Der Kam, E.; et al. Sphingosine 1-phosphate receptor 5 mediates the immune quiescence of the human brain endothelial barrier. *J. Neuroinflamm.* **2012**, *9*, 133. [CrossRef] [PubMed]
68. Brinkmann, V.; Pinschewer, D.; Chiba, K.; Feng, L. FTY720: A novel transplantation drug that modulates lymphocyte traffic rather than activation. *Trends Pharmacol. Sci.* **2000**, *21*, 49–52. [CrossRef]
69. Chun, J.; Hartung, H.-P. Mechanism of Action of Oral Fingolimod (FTY720) in Multiple Sclerosis. *Clin. Neuropharmacol.* **2010**, *33*, 91–101. [CrossRef] [PubMed]
70. Brinkmann, V. Sphingosine 1-phosphate receptors in health and disease: Mechanistic insights from gene deletion studies and reverse pharmacology. *Pharmacol. Ther.* **2007**, *115*, 84–105. [CrossRef] [PubMed]
71. Farez, M.F.; Correale, J.; Information, P.E.K.F.C. Sphingosine 1-phosphate signaling in astrocytes: Implications for progressive multiple sclerosis. *J. Neurol. Sci.* **2016**, *361*, 60–65. [CrossRef] [PubMed]
72. Rothhammer, V.; Kenison, J.E.; Tjon, E.; Takenaka, M.C.; De Lima, K.A.; Borucki, D.M.; Chao, C.-C.; Wilz, A.; Blain, M.; Healy, L.; et al. Sphingosine 1-phosphate receptor modulation suppresses pathogenic astrocyte activation and chronic progressive CNS inflammation. *Proc. Natl. Acad. Sci. USA* **2017**, *114*, 2012–2017. [CrossRef]
73. Miron, V.E.; Ludwin, S.K.; Darlington, P.J.; Jarjour, A.A.; Soliven, B.; Kennedy, T.E.; Antel, J.P. Fingolimod (FTY720) Enhances Remyelination Following Demyelination of Organotypic Cerebellar Slices. *Am. J. Pathol.* **2010**, *176*, 2682–2694. [CrossRef] [PubMed]
74. Yazdi, A.; Baharvand, H.; Javan, M. Enhanced remyelination following lysolecithin-induced demyelination in mice under treatment with fingolimod (FTY720). *Neuroscience* **2015**, *311*, 34–44. [CrossRef] [PubMed]
75. Zhang, J.; Zhang, Z.; Li, Y.; Ding, X.; Shang, X.; Lü, M.; Elias, S.B.; Chopp, M. Fingolimod treatment promotes proliferation and differentiation of oligodendrocyte progenitor cells in mice with experimental autoimmune encephalomyelitis. *Neurobiol. Dis.* **2015**, *76*, 57–66. [CrossRef] [PubMed]
76. Fryer, R.M.; Muthukumarana, A.; Harrison, P.C.; Nodop, M.S.; Chen, R.R.; Harrington, K.E.; Dinallo, R.M.; Horan, J.C.; Patnaude, L.; Modis, L.K.; et al. The clinically-tested S1P receptor agonists, FTY720 and BAF312, demonstrate subtype-specific bradycardia (S1P(1)) and hypertension (S1P(3)) in rat. *PLoS ONE* **2012**, *7*, e52985. [CrossRef]
77. Gergely, P.; Nuesslein-Hildesheim, B.; Guerini, D.; Brinkmann, V.; Traebert, M.; Bruns, C.; Pan, S.; Gray, N.; Hinterding, K.; Cooke, N.; et al. The selective sphingosine 1-phosphate receptor modulator BAF312 redirects lymphocyte distribution and has species-specific effects on heart rate. *Br. J. Pharmacol.* **2012**, *167*, 1035–1047. [CrossRef]
78. Pan, S.; Gray, N.S.; Gao, W.; Mi, Y.; Fan, Y.; Wang, X.; Tuntland, T.; Che, J.; Lefebvre, S.; Chen, Y.; et al. Discovery of BAF312 (Siponimod), a Potent and Selective S1P Receptor Modulator. *ACS Med. Chem. Lett.* **2013**, *4*, 333–337. [CrossRef]

79. Forrest, M.; Sun, S.-Y.; Hajdu, R.; Bergstrom, J.; Card, D.; Doherty, G.; Hale, J.; Keohane, C.; Meyers, C.; Milligan, J.; et al. Immune Cell Regulation and Cardiovascular Effects of Sphingosine 1-Phosphate Receptor Agonists in Rodents Are Mediated via Distinct Receptor Subtypes. *J. Pharmacol. Exp. Ther.* **2004**, *309*, 758–768. [CrossRef]
80. Coelho, R.P.; Payne, S.G.; Bittman, R.; Spiegel, S.; Sato-Bigbee, C. The Immunomodulator FTY720 Has a Direct Cytoprotective Effect in Oligodendrocyte Progenitors. *J. Pharmacol. Exp. Ther.* **2007**, *323*, 626–635. [CrossRef]
81. Jung, C.G.; Kim, H.J.; Miron, V.E.; Cook, S.; Kennedy, T.E.; Foster, C.A.; Antel, J.P.; Soliven, B. Functional consequences of S1P receptor modulation in rat oligodendroglial lineage cells. *Glia* **2007**, *55*, 1656–1667. [CrossRef] [PubMed]
82. O'Sullivan, C.; Schubart, A.; Mir, A.K.; Dev, K.K. The dual S1PR1/S1PR5 drug BAF312 (Siponimod) attenuates demyelination in organotypic slice cultures. *J. Neuroinflamm.* **2016**, *13*, 31.
83. Gentile, A.; Musella, A.; Bullitta, S.; Fresegna, D.; De Vito, F.; Fantozzi, R.; Piras, E.; Gargano, F.; Borsellino, G.; Battistini, L.; et al. Siponimod (BAF312) prevents synaptic neurodegeneration in experimental multiple sclerosis. *J. Neuroinflamm.* **2016**, *13*, 207. [CrossRef]
84. Cohen, J.A.; Comi, G.; Arnold, D.L. Efficacy and safety of ozanimod in multiple sclerosis: Dose-blinded extension of a randomized phase II study. *Mult. Scler.* **2019**, *25*, 1255–1262. [CrossRef]
85. ZEPOSIA (Ozanimod) (Package Insert). Celgene Corporation: Summit, NJ, USA. 2020. Available online: https://www.accessdata.fda.gov/drugsatfda_docs/label/2020/209899s000lbl.pdf (accessed on 18 July 2020).
86. Bolli, M.H.; Abele, S.; Binkert, C.; Bravo, R.; Buchmann, S.; Bur, D.; Gatfield, J.; Hess, P.; Kohl, C.; Mangold, C.; et al. 2-Imino-thiazolidin-4-one Derivatives as Potent, Orally Active S1P1Receptor Agonists. *J. Med. Chem.* **2010**, *53*, 4198–4211. [CrossRef] [PubMed]
87. D'Ambrosio, D.; Freedman, M.S.; Prinz, J. Ponesimod, a selective S1P1 receptor modulator: A potential treatment for multiple sclerosis and other immune-mediated diseases. *Ther. Adv. Chronic Dis.* **2016**, *7*, 18–33. [CrossRef]
88. You, S.; Piali, L.; Kuhn, C.; Steiner, B.; Sauvaget, V.; Valette, F.; Clozel, M.; Bach, J.-F.; Chatenoud, L. Therapeutic Use of a Selective S1P1 Receptor Modulator Ponesimod in Autoimmune Diabetes. *PLoS ONE* **2013**, *8*, e77296. [CrossRef]
89. Piali, L.; Froidevaux, S.; Hess, P.; Nayler, O.; Bolli, M.H.; Schlosser, E.; Kohl, C.; Steiner, B.; Clozel, M. The Selective Sphingosine 1-Phosphate Receptor 1 Agonist Ponesimod Protects against Lymphocyte-Mediated Tissue Inflammation. *J. Pharmacol. Exp. Ther.* **2011**, *337*, 547–556. [CrossRef]
90. Brossard, P.; Derendorf, H.; Xu, J.; Maatouk, H.; Halabi, A.; Dingemanse, J. Pharmacokinetics and pharmacodynamics of ponesimod, a selective S1P1 receptor modulator, in the first-in-human study. *Br. J. Clin. Pharmacol.* **2013**, *76*, 888–896. [CrossRef]
91. GILENYA (Fingolimod) (Package Insert). Novartis Pharmaceuticals Coporation: East Hanover, NJ, USA. 2019. Available online: https://www.novartis.us/sites/www.novartis.us/files/gilenya.pdf (accessed on 18 July 2020).
92. Chitnis, T.; Arnold, U.L.; Banwell, B.; Brück, W.; Ghezzi, A.; Giovannoni, G.; Greenberg, B.M.; Krupp, L.; Rostásy, K.; Tardieu, M.; et al. Trial of Fingolimod versus Interferon Beta-1a in Pediatric Multiple Sclerosis. *N. Engl. J. Med.* **2018**, *379*, 1017–1027. [CrossRef]
93. Kappos, L.; Radue, E.-W.; O'Connor, P.; Polman, C.; Hohlfeld, R.; Calabresi, P.; Selmaj, K.; Agoropoulou, C.; Leyk, M.; Zhang-Auberson, L.; et al. A Placebo-Controlled Trial of Oral Fingolimod in Relapsing Multiple Sclerosis. *N. Engl. J. Med.* **2010**, *362*, 387–401. [CrossRef] [PubMed]
94. Cohen, J.; Barkhof, F.; Comi, G.; Hartung, H.-P.; Khatri, B.O.; Montalban, X.; Pelletier, J.; Capra, R.; Gallo, P.; Izquierdo, G.; et al. Oral Fingolimod or Intramuscular Interferon for Relapsing Multiple Sclerosis. *N. Engl. J. Med.* **2010**, *362*, 402–415. [CrossRef] [PubMed]
95. Kappos, L.; Li, D.K.B.; Stuve, O.; Hartung, H.-P.; Freedman, M.S.; Hemmer, B.; Rieckmann, P.; Montalban, X.; Ziemssen, F.; Hunter, B.; et al. Safety and Efficacy of Siponimod (BAF312) in Patients with Relapsing-Remitting Multiple Sclerosis. *JAMA Neurol.* **2016**, *73*, 1089–1098. [CrossRef] [PubMed]
96. Cohen, J.; Khatri, B.; Barkhof, F.; Comi, G.; Hartung, H.-P.; Montalban, X.; Pelletier, J.; Stites, T.; Ritter, S.; Von Rosenstiel, P.; et al. Long-term (up to 4.5 years) treatment with fingolimod in multiple sclerosis: Results from the extension of the randomised TRANSFORMS study. *J. Neurol. Neurosurg. Psychiatry* **2015**, *87*, 468–475. [CrossRef]

97. Kappos, L.; Bar-Or, A.; Cree, B.A.C.; Fox, R.J.; Giovannoni, G.; Gold, R.; Vermersch, P.; Arnold, D.L.; Arnould, S.; Scherz, T.; et al. Siponimod versus placebo in secondary progressive multiple sclerosis (EXPAND): A double-blind, randomised, phase 3 study. *Lancet* **2018**, *391*, 1263–1273. [CrossRef]
98. Cohen, J.; Comi, G.; Selmaj, K.W.; Bar-Or, A.; Arnold, D.L.; Steinman, L.; Hartung, H.-P.; Montalban, X.; Havrdová, E.K.; Cree, B.A.C.; et al. Safety and efficacy of ozanimod versus interferon beta-1a in relapsing multiple sclerosis (RADIANCE): A multicentre, randomised, 24-month, phase 3 trial. *Lancet Neurol.* **2019**, *18*, 1021–1033. [CrossRef]
99. Comi, G.; Kappos, L.; Selmaj, K.W.; Bar-Or, A.; Arnold, D.L.; Steinman, L.; Hartung, H.-P.; Montalban, X.; Havrdová, E.K.; Cree, B.A.C.; et al. Safety and efficacy of ozanimod versus interferon beta-1a in relapsing multiple sclerosis (SUNBEAM): A multicentre, randomised, minimum 12-month, phase 3 trial. *Lancet Neurol.* **2019**, *18*, 1009–1020. [CrossRef]
100. Deluca, J.; Huang, D.; Cohen, J.A.; Cree, B.A.C.; Chen, Y.; Campanolo, D.; Sheffield, J.K.; Comi, G.; Kappos, L. *Ozanimod-Treated Patients Exhibited Improvements in Cognitive Processing Speed in the Phase 3 SUNBEAM Trial of Relapsing Multiple Sclerosis (RMS)*; ECTRIMS: Berlin, Germany, 2018.
101. Kappos, L.; Burcklen, M.; Freedman, M.S.; Fox, R.; Havrdová, E.K.; Hennessy, B.; Hohlfeld, R.; Lublin, F.; Montalban, X.; Pozzilli, C.; et al. *Efficacy and Safety of Ponesimod Compared to Teriflunomide in Patients with Relapsing Multiple Sclerosis: Results of the Randomized, Active-Controlled, Double-Blind, Parallel-Group Phase 3 OPTIMUM Study*; ECTRIMS: Stockholm, Sweden, 2019.
102. Ontaneda, D.; Moore, A.; Bakshi, R.; Zajicheck, A.; Kattan, M.; Fox, R. *Risk Estimates of Progressive Multifocal Leukoencephalopathy Related to Fingolimod*; ECTRIMS: Berlin, Germany, 2018.
103. Boffa, G.; Bruschi, N.; Cellerino, M.; Lapucci, C.; Novi, G.; Sbragia, E.; Capello, E.; Uccelli, A.; Inglese, M. Fingolimod and Dimethyl-Fumarate-Derived Lymphopenia is not Associated with Short-Term Treatment Response and Risk of Infections in a Real-Life MS Population. *CNS Drugs* **2020**, *34*, 425–432. [CrossRef]
104. Conzett, K.B.; Kolm, I.; Jelčić, I.; Kamarachev, J.; Dummer, R.; Braun, R.; French, L.; Linnebank, M.; Hofbauer, G.F.L. Melanoma Occurring During Treatment with Fingolimod for Multiple Sclerosis: A Case Report. *Arch. Dermatol.* **2011**, *147*, 991–992. [CrossRef]
105. Robinson, C.L.; Guo, M. Fingolimod (Gilenya) and melanoma. *BMJ Case Rep.* **2016**, *2016*. [CrossRef]
106. Hatcher, S.E.; Waubant, E.; Nourbakhsh, B.; Crabtree-Hartman, E.; Graves, J.S. Rebound Syndrome in Patients with Multiple Sclerosis After Cessation of Fingolimod Treatment. *JAMA Neurol.* **2016**, *73*, 790. [CrossRef]
107. Frau, J.; Sormani, M.P.; Signori, A.; Realmuto, S.; Baroncini, D.; Annovazzi, P.; Signoriello, E.; Maniscalco, G.T.; La Gioia, S.; Cordioli, C.; et al. Clinical activity after fingolimod cessation: Disease reactivation or rebound? *Eur. J. Neurol.* **2018**, *25*, 1270–1275. [CrossRef] [PubMed]
108. Uygunoğlu, U.; Tütüncü, M.; Altintas, A.; Saip, S.; Siva, A. Factors Predictive of Severe Multiple Sclerosis Disease Reactivation After Fingolimod Cessation. *Neurology* **2018**, *23*, 12–16. [CrossRef]
109. Bobes, N.S. Package inserts. *N. Engl. J. Med.* **1968**, *278*, 282.
110. Linda, H.; von Heijne, A. A case of posterior reversible encephalopathy syndrome associated with gilenya((R)) (fingolimod) treatment for multiple sclerosis. *Front. Neurol.* **2015**, *6*, 39. [CrossRef] [PubMed]
111. Downey, C.; Robertson, D.; Casady, L.; Maldonado, J. A Rare Complication of Fingolimod: Case Report of Posterior Reversible Encephalopathy Syndrome. *Neurology* **2019**, *92*, 2–16.
112. Fischer, A.; Prüfer, K.; Good, J.M.; Halbwax, M.; Wiebe, V.; Andre, C.; Atencia, R.; Mugisha, L.; Ptak, S.E.; Pääbo, S. Bonobos Fall within the Genomic Variation of Chimpanzees. *PLoS ONE* **2011**, *6*, e21605. [CrossRef] [PubMed]
113. Zhao, C.; Fernandes, M.J.; Turgeon, M.; Tancrède, S.; Di Battista, J.; Poubelle, P.E.; Bourgoin, S.G. Specific and overlapping sphingosine-1-phosphate receptor functions in human synoviocytes: Impact of TNF-α. *J. Lipid Res.* **2008**, *49*, 2323–2337. [CrossRef] [PubMed]
114. Tsunemi, S.; Iwasaki, T.; Kitano, S.; Imado, T.; Miyazawa, K.; Sano, H. Effects of the novel immunosuppressant FTY720 in a murine rheumatoid arthritis model. *Clin. Immunol.* **2010**, *136*, 197–204. [CrossRef]
115. Militsakh, O.; Day, T.; Hornig, J.; Lentsch, E.; Skoner, J.; Gillespie, M.B.; Sharma, A.; Neville, B.; Rumboldt, Z.; James, R.; et al. Sphingosine-1-Phosphate. *Encyclopedia Cancer* **2011**, *38*, 3485. [CrossRef]
116. Clark, D.N.; Markham, J.L.; Sloan, C.S.; Poole, B. Cytokine inhibition as a strategy for treating systemic lupus erythematosus. *Clin. Immunol.* **2013**, *148*, 335–343. [CrossRef]
117. Gottschalk, T.; Tsantikos, E.; Hibbs, M.L. Pathogenic Inflammation and Its Therapeutic Targeting in Systemic Lupus Erythematosus. *Front. Immunol.* **2015**, *6*, 1. [CrossRef] [PubMed]

118. Danko, K.; Vencovsky, J.; Lundberg, I.; Amato, A.; Oddis, C.; Malnar, M.; Moher, A.; Colin, L. *The Selective Sphingosine-1-Phosphate Receptor 1/5 Modulator Siponimod (BAF312) Shows Beneficial Effects in Patients with Active, Treatment Refractory Polymyositis and Dermatomyositis: A Phase IIa Proof-of-Concept, Double-Blind, Randomized Trial*; American College of Rheumatology: Boston, MA, USA, 2014.
119. Sandborn, W.J.; Feagan, B.G.; Mutneja, H.; Arora, S.; Vij, A. Ozanimod Treatment for Ulcerative Colitis. *N. Engl. J. Med.* **2016**, *375*, e17. [CrossRef] [PubMed]
120. Vaclavkova, A.; Chimenti, S.; Arenberger, P.; Hollo, P.; Sator, P.G.; Burcklen, M.; Stefani, M.; D'Ambrosio, D. Oral ponesimod in patients with chronic plaque psoriasis: A randomised, double-blind, placebo-controlled phase 2 trial. *Lancet* **2014**, *384*, 2036–2045. [CrossRef]
121. Oskouian, B.; Sooriyakumaran, P.; Borowsky, A.D.; Crans, A.; Dillard-Telm, L.; Tam, Y.Y.; Bandhuvula, P.; Saba, J.D. Sphingosine-1-phosphate lyase potentiates apoptosis via p53- and p38-dependent pathways and is down-regulated in colon cancer. *Proc. Nat. Acad. Sci. USA* **2006**, *103*, 17384–17389. [CrossRef] [PubMed]
122. Degagne, E.; Pandurangan, A.; Bandhuvula, P.; Kumar, A.; Eltanawy, A.; Zhang, M.; Yoshinaga, Y.; Nefedov, M.; de Jong, P.J.; Fong, L.G.; et al. Sphingosine-1-phosphate lyase downregulation promotes colon carcinogenesis through STAT3-activated microRNAs. *J. Clin. Investig.* **2014**, *124*, 5368–5384. [CrossRef]
123. Bao, Y.; Guo, Y.; Zhang, C.; Fan, F.; Yang, W. Sphingosine Kinase 1 and Sphingosine-1-Phosphate Signaling in Colorectal Cancer. *Int. J. Mol. Sci.* **2017**, *18*, 2109. [CrossRef]
124. Wang, S.; Liang, Y.; Chang, W.; Hu, B.; Zhang, Y. Triple Negative Breast Cancer Depends on Sphingosine Kinase 1 (SphK1)/Sphingosine-1-Phosphate (S1P)/Sphingosine 1-Phosphate Receptor 3 (S1PR3)/Notch Signaling for Metastasis. *Med. Sci. Monit.* **2018**, *24*, 1912–1923. [CrossRef]
125. Watson, C.; Long, J.S.; Orange, C.; Tannahill, C.L.; Mallon, E.; McGlynn, L.M.; Pyne, S.; Pyne, N.J.; Edwards, J. High expression of sphingosine 1-phosphate receptors, S1P1 and S1P3, sphingosine kinase 1, and extracellular signal-regulated kinase-1/2 is associated with development of tamoxifen resistance in estrogen receptor-positive breast cancer patients. *Am. J. Pathol.* **2010**, *177*, 2205–2215. [CrossRef]
126. Ohotski, J.; Long, J.S.; Orange, C.; Elsberger, B.; Mallon, E.; Doughty, J.; Pyne, S.; Pyne, N.J.; Edwards, J. Expression of sphingosine 1-phosphate receptor 4 and sphingosine kinase 1 is associated with outcome in oestrogen receptor-negative breast cancer. *Br. J. Cancer* **2012**, *106*, 1453–1459. [CrossRef]
127. Zhao, J.; Liu, J.; Lee, J.F.; Zhang, W.; Kandouz, M.; VanHecke, G.C.; Chen, S.; Ahn, Y.H.; Lonardo, F.; Lee, M.J. TGF-beta/SMAD3 Pathway Stimulates Sphingosine-1 Phosphate Receptor 3 Expression: Implication of sphingosine-1 phosphate receptor 3 in lung adenocarcinoma progression. *J. Biol. Chem.* **2016**, *291*, 27343–27353. [CrossRef] [PubMed]
128. Hsu, A.; Zhang, W.; Lee, J.F.; An, J.; Ekambaram, P.; Liu, J.; Honn, K.V.; Klinge, C.M.; Lee, M.J. Sphingosine-1-phosphate receptor-3 signaling up-regulates epidermal growth factor receptor and enhances epidermal growth factor receptor-mediated carcinogenic activities in cultured lung adenocarcinoma cells. *Int. J. Oncol.* **2012**, *40*, 1619–1626. [PubMed]
129. Kurano, M.; Yatomi, Y. Sphingosine 1-Phosphate and Atherosclerosis. *J. Atheroscler. Thromb.* **2018**, *25*, 16–26. [CrossRef] [PubMed]
130. Skoura, A.; Michaud, J.; Im, D.S.; Thangada, S.; Xiong, Y.; Smith, J.D.; Hla, T. Sphingosine-1-phosphate receptor-2 function in myeloid cells regulates vascular inflammation and atherosclerosis. *Arterioscler. Thromb. Vasc. Biol.* **2011**, *31*, 81–85. [CrossRef] [PubMed]

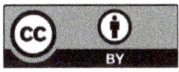

© 2020 by the authors. Licensee MDPI, Basel, Switzerland. This article is an open access article distributed under the terms and conditions of the Creative Commons Attribution (CC BY) license (http://creativecommons.org/licenses/by/4.0/).

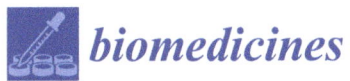

Article

Longitudinal Serum Neurofilament Levels of Multiple Sclerosis Patients Before and After Treatment with First-Line Immunomodulatory Therapies

André Huss [1], Makbule Senel [1], Ahmed Abdelhak [1,2,3], Benjamin Mayer [4], Jan Kassubek [1], Albert C. Ludolph [1], Markus Otto [1] and Hayrettin Tumani [1,5,*]

1. Department of Neurology, University Hospital of Ulm, Oberer Eselsberg 45, 89081 Ulm, Germany; andre.huss@uni-ulm.de (A.H.); makbule.senel@uni-ulm.de (M.S.); ahmed.abdelhak@ucsf.edu (A.A.); jan.kassubek@uni-ulm.de (J.K.); Albert.Ludolph@rku.de (A.C.L.); markus.otto@uni-ulm.de (M.O.)
2. Department of Neurology and Stroke, University Hospital of Tübingen, Hoppe-Seyler-Alle 3, 72076 Tübingen, Germany
3. Hertie institute of clinical of clinical brain research, University of Tübingen, Hoppe-Seyler-Alle 3, 72076 Tübingen, Germany
4. Institute of Epidemiology and Medical Biometry, Ulm University, Schwabstraße 13, 89075 Ulm, Germany; benjamin.mayer@uni-ulm.de
5. Speciality Clinic of Neurology Dietenbronn, Dietenbronn 7, 88477 Schwendi, Germany
* Correspondence: hayrettin.tumani@uni-ulm.de

Received: 9 July 2020; Accepted: 25 August 2020; Published: 28 August 2020

Abstract: Serum neurofilament light chain (NfL) has been shown to correlate with neuroaxonal damage in multiple sclerosis (MS) and various other neurological diseases. While serum NfL is now regularly reported in clinical approval studies, there is a lack of longitudinal data from patients treated with established basic immunotherapies outside of study conditions. In total, 34 patients with early relapsing-remitting MS (RRMS) were included. The follow-up period was 24 months with regular follow-up visits after 3, 6, 9, 12 and 18 months. Therapy with glatiramer acetate was initiated in 20 patients and with interferon-beta in 12 patients. The disease course was monitored by the events of relapses, Expanded Disability Status Scale (EDSS) score and MRI parameters. Overall, serum NfL levels were higher at time points with a current relapse event than at time points without relapse (12.8 pg/mL vs. 9.7 pg/mL, $p = 0.011$). At follow-up, relapse-free patients showed significantly reduced serum NfL levels starting from 9 months compared to baseline ($p < 0.05$) and reduced levels after 12 months compared to baseline ($p = 0.013$) in patients without EDSS progression for 12 months. In this explorative observational study, our data suggest that the longitudinal measurement of serum NfL may be useful in addition to MRI to monitor disease activity and therapy response.

Keywords: multiple sclerosis; serum neurofilament; immunomodulatory therapies; therapy-response marker

---

1. Introduction

Multiple sclerosis (MS) is a chronic inflammatory disease of the central nervous system (CNS) characterized by demyelination and axonal loss [1]. The current concept of MS pathology is based on infiltrating immune B- and T-cells via the blood–brain barrier, local antibody production and activation of glial cells [2,3]. These processes are thought to lead to primary demyelination followed by neurodegeneration [2]. In recent years, several neurochemical markers have been established for the characterization of pathological molecular processes. One of the most extensively investigated markers for neuroaxonal loss is neurofilament light chain (NfL) [4–6]. NfL is one of four neurofilament subunits and the most abundant one, making it a popular target for neurological diseases [7]. Here, NfL showed superior sensitivity for MS than the phosphorylated subunit of neurofilament [8].

Initially investigated using standard immunoassays, NfL in the cerebrospinal fluid (CSF) from MS patients was found to correlate with disease course and activity [9,10]. In the early phase of the disease, it has a prognostic value [5,11,12] and can be used as a treatment response marker [13]. However, NfL is not specific for MS, is rather a general marker for neurodegenerative processes [14,15] and changes with the normal aging brain [16], which needs to be considered when looking at NfL changes over time.

As detection methods were developed over the years, highly sensitive immunoassays became available and allowed the analysis of brain-derived proteins, not only in the CSF, but in serum as well [17]. Beyond showing a good correlation with CSF values, serum NfL has already thoroughly been investigated in MS [18], i.e., it has been shown to correlate with clinical and radiological disease activity (relapses, new/enlarged T2 lesions and gadolinium-enhancing lesions in magnetic resonance imaging (MRI)) [19–22]. The most important advantage of serum analyses is the possibility of serial sampling and consecutive analysis of biomarkers. Thus, NfL is regularly used in clinical trials to monitor therapy efficacy, and it is on the footsteps of being used as a secondary outcome parameter in clinical trials [23].

In most studies, group effects of treatments on neurofilaments are investigated, which already indicate the applicability of serum NfL as a therapy response marker [22,24] and as a prognostic marker for long-term clinical outcomes in MS [25]. However, longitudinal data of intraindividual NfL levels over disease course under immunomodulatory therapies in well-characterized MS patients are widely missing and only described rarely [26,27].

In this study, we analyzed consecutive samples of MS patients in the early phase of the disease, before and after the initiation of disease-modifying treatment with either glatiramer acetate or interferon-beta over a follow-up period of 24 months. Serum NfL levels at each visit were correlated to clinical outcome parameters (relapse and Expanded Disability Status Scale (EDSS)), serum cytokine profile, cognitive functions and MRI parameters of disease activity and progression.

The aim of this study was (a) to show the effect of immunomodulatory therapies on serum NfL levels in MS patients over disease course, (b) to evaluate the relationship between NfL and MRI parameters reflecting disease progression, such as T2 lesion load, (c) to evaluate possible correlation with cognitive functions and (d) to compare serum NfL levels with the serum cytokine profile.

2. Experimental Section

2.1. Patients

In total, 34 patients who attended the Department of Neurology at the University Hospital Ulm between 2002 and 2004 before initiation of disease-modifying treatment (DMT) were included in the study. Initially, the MS diagnosis was made on the diagnostic criteria valid at time of study inclusion (McDonald 2001), but were adjusted for the most recent updates of the McDonald criteria (McDonald 2017). After study inclusion, 20 patients started treatment with glatiramer acetate, 12 patients were treated with interferon-beta (Avonex, Betaferon and Rebif) and 2 patients rejected DMT. All patients were then followed-up for 24 months with visits every 3 months in the first year and every 6 months in the second year. At all visits, clinical assessments including relapse evaluation, EDSS, Paced Auditory Serial Addition Test (PASAT), and serum sampling were performed. Relapses were defined as focal neurological disturbance lasting more than 24 h, without an alternate explanation. Furthermore, 17 patients received magnetic resonance imaging (MRI) scans at baseline, 12 months and 24 months. Detailed patients' characteristics are shown in Table 1 and the study schedule is shown in Table 2. Relapses were treated with high-dose corticosteroids (50–1000 mg) over 3–5 days after exclusion of contraindications. Age did not differ between patients with and without at least one relapse during follow-up and did not correlate with serum NfL levels at baseline.

Table 1. Patients' characteristics.

Characteristics	Median Values with IQR, $n = 34$
Age	33 (29–40)
EDSS baseline	1.5 (1.0–2.0)
Serum NfL baseline (pg/mL)	10.2 (8.4–14.7)
Relapse within 12 months (n)	14
Relapse within 24 months (n)	16
Treatment after baseline	
Glatiramer acetate	20
Interferon-beta	12
No disease-modifying therapy	2

EDSS = Expanded Disability Status Scale; NfL = Neurofilament light chain; IQR = Interquartile range.

Table 2. Study schedule and number of available data.

	Baseline	3 Months	6 Months	9 Months	12 Months	18 Months	24 Months
Clinical assessment	34	32	32	32	33	34	34
EDSS	31	30	27	30	32	32	32
Serum NfL	34	29	29	32	33	31	24
MRI (T2 lesion load)	17				17		17
Serum cytokine profile	29	29	29	29	29	29	29
PASAT	32	32	31	30	32	30	31

EDSS, Expanded Disability Status Scale; PASAT, Paced Auditory Serial Addition Test; NfL, neurofilament light chain; MRI, magnetic resonance imaging.

2.2. NfL Measurements

Serum samples were stored in the local biobank according to recommended biobanking protocols at −80 °C [28]. Serum NfL was measured using the Simoa technology (Quanterix Corporation, Lexington, MA, USA). Samples were diluted, as recommended by the manufacturer, and concentrations were calculated using the corresponding standard curve.

2.3. Cytokines Measurements

Cytokine profiles including IFN-γ, osteopontin (OPN), IL-2, IL-4 and IL-10 were determined in serum at study onset and at every visit during follow-up using the electrochemiluminescence detection multiplex technology of Meso Scale Discovery (MSD, Gaithersburg, MD, USA) according to the manufacturer's instructions as previously reported [29].

2.4. MRI Scans

MRI scans of the brain and spinal cord were performed on a 1.5 Tesla clinical MRI scanner (Symphony Siemens, Erlangen, Germany) and the total number of hyperintense lesions in T2-weighted scans at the different time points were visually quantified by an experienced rater.

2.5. Cognitive Functions

Cognitive functions were assessed at every time point by the Paced Auditory Serial Addition Test (PASAT). Here, information processing speed and flexibility, as well as calculation ability are tested, which also means that this is not a global measure of cognitive dysfunction, but rather targets specific cognitive executive functions frequently affected in MS.

2.6. Statistical Methods

All statistical tests were performed using the GraphPad Prism 8 software (GraphPad Software Inc., La Jolla, CA, USA). Shapiro–Wilk test was used to examine the distribution of the data. Mann–Whitney U test was used to compare medians in skewed distributed parameters for unpaired samples and Wilcoxon matched-pairs signed-rank test for paired samples. Correlation analyses were performed with Spearman's rank correlation and corrected for multiple testing by the Bonferroni method. A p-value ≤ 0.05 was considered as statistically significant.

2.7. Ethical Statement

The study was reviewed by the appropriate ethics committee of the University of Ulm (approval number 79/2001, approval date 14.11.2001) and was performed in accordance with the ethical standards of the current version of the Declaration of Helsinki. Written informed consent was obtained from all patients participating in this study.

3. Results

3.1. Serum NfL at Time Points With and Without Active Relapse

We categorized serum NfL levels of all time points accordingly whether an active relapse was present or not. Additionally, the change of serum NfL values at a time point with an active relapse in comparison with the previous time point was determined. Here, the absolute change of serum NfL values (pg/mL) and the percentage change was calculated (tx-tx-1). Significantly higher serum NfL levels were observed for time points with an active relapse compared with time points with no relapse (Figure 1A, $p < 0.05$). This was also true for the percentage change (Figure 1C, $p < 0.05$), but not for the absolute change of serum NfL (Figure 1B, $p = 0.15$).

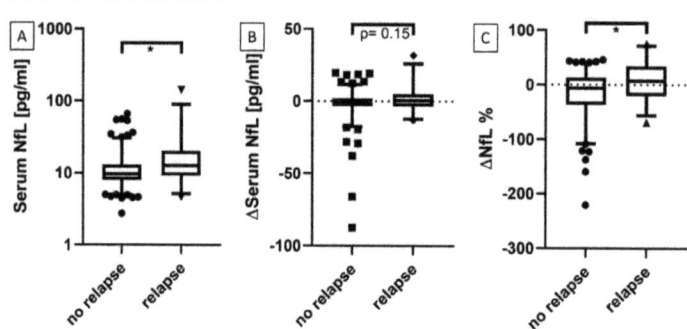

Figure 1. Serum NfL and time points with or without an active relapse. (**A**) Comparison of serum NfL levels during time points with and without an active relapse. (**B**) Comparison of the change of serum NfL between a time point with an active relapse and the previous time point. (**C**) Comparison of the percentage change of serum NfL between a time point with an active relapse and the previous time point. * $p < 0.05$.

3.2. Serum NfL Levels During Follow-Up Period of 24 Months

3.2.1. Patients with Relapses vs. No Relapse

In patients with a relapse-free disease course of 12 months and 24 months, serum NfL decreased significantly between baseline and time points 12 months and 18 months and time points 9, 12, 18 and

24 months, respectively (Figure 2A,B, blue triangles facing down, $p < 0.05$). There were no significant differences for baseline and follow-up visits of serum NfL levels in patients with at least one relapse within 12 or 24 months (Figure 2A,B). Furthermore, serum NfL levels in patients with a relapse within 12 months were significantly higher than in patients without a relapse within 12 months at time points 9 and 12 months (Figure 2A, $p < 0.05$).

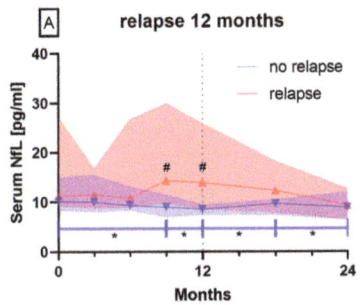 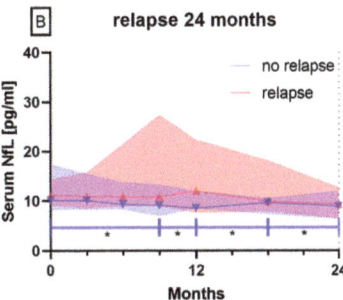

Figure 2. Serum NfL levels over 12 and 24 months in patients with (red triangle facing up) and without relapse (blue triangle facing down) for (**A**) 12 or (**B**) 24 months. Symbols show median values, colored range indicates 95% confidence interval (CI), * $p < 0.05$ for intragroup differences, # $p < 0.05$ for intergroup differences.

3.2.2. Patients with EDSS Progression vs. Stable or Improved EDSS

In patients showing EDSS progression within 12 months and patients with a stable or improved EDSS for 24 months, no differences concerning their NfL levels were observed. However, in patients with a stable or improving EDSS within 12 months, serum NfL levels decreased significantly between baseline and time points 12 and 18 months (Figure 3A, $p < 0.05$). Considering 24 months of observation, patients with EDSS progression showed serum NfL levels that differed significantly from baseline serum NfL levels after 3 and 18 months (Figure 3B, $p < 0.05$).

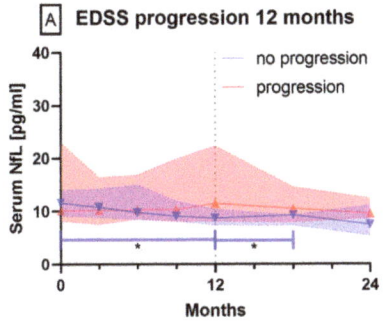 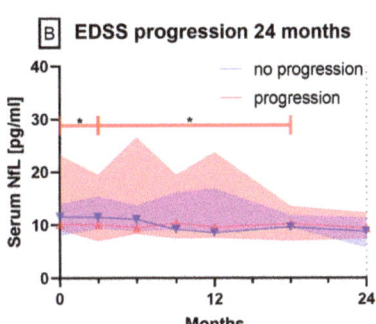

Figure 3. Serum NfL levels over 12 and 24 months in patients with (red triangle up) and without EDSS progression (blue triangle down) within (**A**) 12 or (**B**) 24 months. Symbols show median values, colored range indicates 95% CI, * $p < 0.05$.

3.3. Correlation of Serum NfL with

3.3.1. Age

There was no significant correlation of serum NfL and age in our cohort ($r < 0.3, p > 0.05$). However, age effects on serum NfL have been described [9,16]. As we mainly compared longitudinal sNfL values from the same individual over a limited period (24 months), no correction for age was made.

3.3.2. Serum Cytokine Profile in All Patients

We performed correlation analyses for serum NfL and serum IFN-γ, OPN, IL-2, IL-4 and IL-10 and for all time points. There was no significant correlation between serum NfL and the cytokine profile (r < 0.3, p > 0.05).

3.4. PASAT

To see whether serum NfL is associated with cognitive decline in MS patients, we performed a correlation analysis of serum NfL and PASAT at all time points (Figure 4). After correcting for multiple testing, a significant correlation between PASAT at month 24 and serum NfL at time points 3 and 18 remained (Spearman r = 0.64 and 0.57 and adjusted p-value = 0.005 and 0.029, respectively).

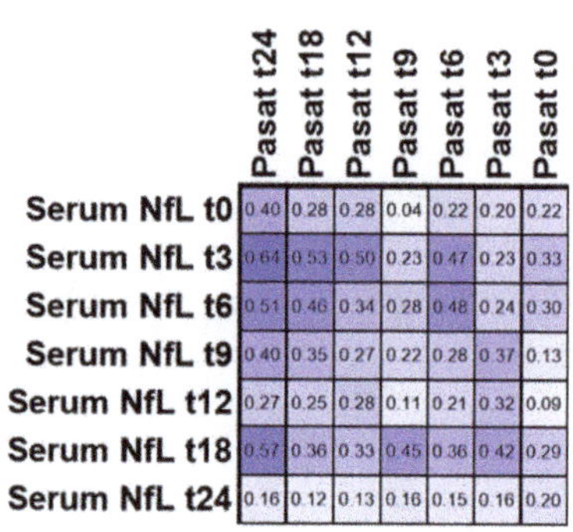

	Pasat t24	Pasat t18	Pasat t12	Pasat t9	Pasat t6	Pasat t3	Pasat t0
Serum NfL t0	0.40	0.28	0.28	0.04	0.22	0.20	0.22
Serum NfL t3	0.64	0.53	0.50	0.23	0.47	0.23	0.33
Serum NfL t6	0.51	0.46	0.34	0.28	0.48	0.24	0.30
Serum NfL t9	0.40	0.35	0.27	0.22	0.28	0.37	0.13
Serum NfL t12	0.27	0.25	0.28	0.11	0.21	0.32	0.09
Serum NfL t18	0.57	0.36	0.33	0.45	0.36	0.42	0.29
Serum NfL t24	0.16	0.12	0.13	0.16	0.15	0.16	0.20

Figure 4. Correlation matrix of Spearman correlation analysis for serum NfL and PASAT. Numbers in the cells are showing the respective Spearman correlation coefficient.

3.5. EDSS in Patients with Active Disease within 24 Months

To see whether serum NfL is associated with the disability in MS patients, we performed a correlation analysis of serum NfL and EDSS at all time points (Figure 5).

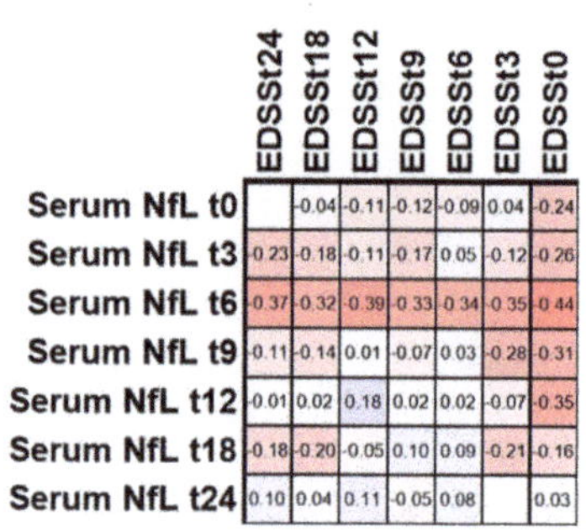

	EDSSt24	EDSSt18	EDSSt12	EDSSt9	EDSSt6	EDSSt3	EDSSt0
Serum NfL t0		-0.04	-0.11	-0.12	-0.09	0.04	-0.24
Serum NfL t3	-0.23	-0.18	-0.11	-0.17	0.05	-0.12	-0.26
Serum NfL t6	-0.37	-0.32	-0.39	-0.33	-0.34	-0.35	-0.44
Serum NfL t9	-0.11	-0.14	0.01	-0.07	0.03	-0.28	-0.31
Serum NfL t12	-0.01	0.02	0.18	0.02	0.02	-0.07	-0.35
Serum NfL t18	-0.18	-0.20	-0.05	0.10	0.09	-0.21	-0.16
Serum NfL t24	0.10	0.04	0.11	-0.05	0.08		0.03

Figure 5. Correlation matrix of Spearman correlation analysis for serum NfL and EDSS. Numbers in the cells are showing the respective Spearman correlation coefficient.

We did not observe significant correlations for serum NfL and EDSS at any time point in the group with active disease (at least one relapse) within 24 months.

3.6. Individual Serum NfL Courses in Patients Treated with Glatiramer Acetate

The serum NfL courses of all patients treated with glatiramer acetate with available MRI scans (T2 lesions) are illustrated. Additionally, for every available time point, the EDSS and occurred relapses are shown (Figure 6).

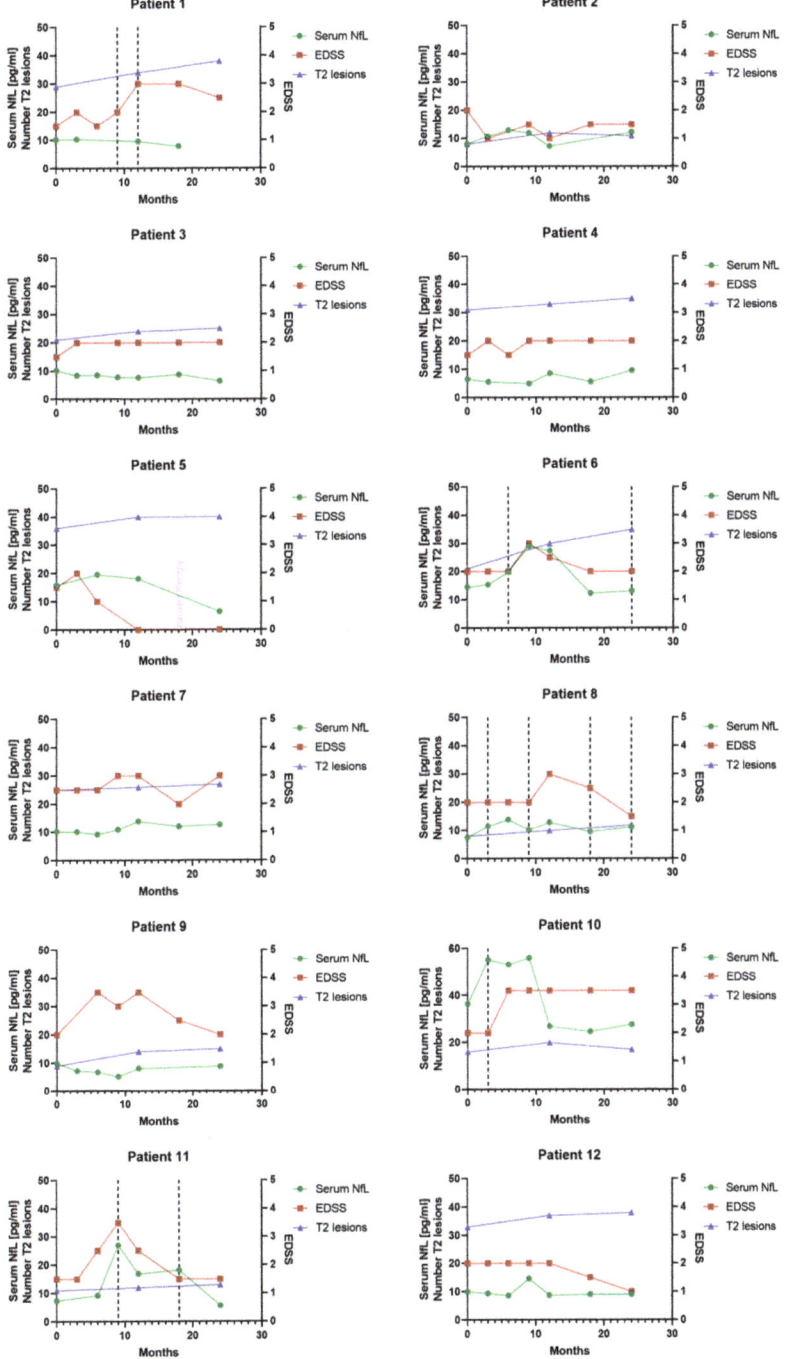

Figure 6. *Cont.*

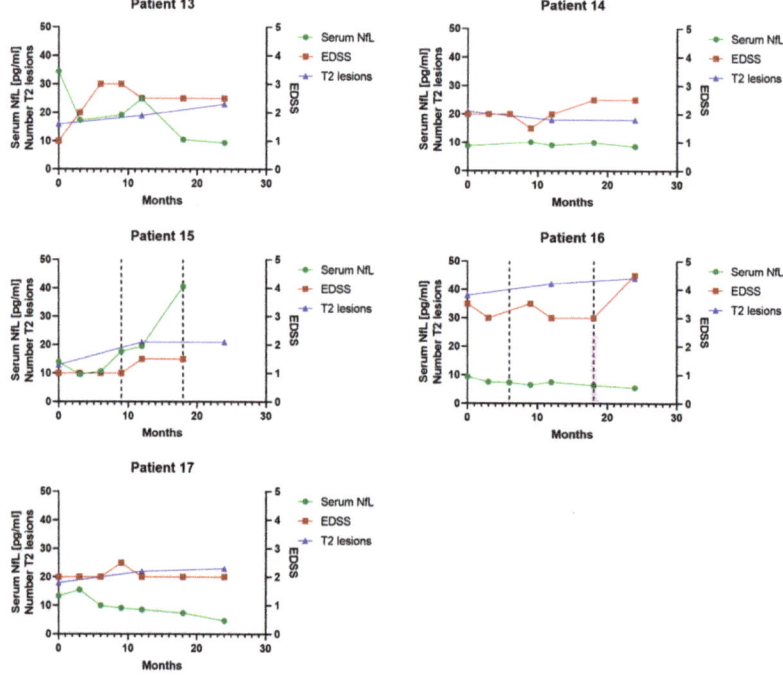

Figure 6. Illustration of individual serum NfL courses over 24 months in patients with initiation of disease-modifying treatment with glatiramer acetate after baseline. Green circles, red squares and blue triangles show serum NfL values (left y-axis), EDSS (right y-axis) and the number of T2 lesions (left y-axis), respectively. Vertical dashed lines show events of clinical activity in the form of a relapse at this time point.

4. Discussion

Neurodegeneration and axonal loss are major hallmarks of MS [2]. NfL has been extensively investigated as a biomarker for those molecular processes [6,9,11]. Initially NfL was exclusively analyzed in CSF, but with improved analytical sensitivity, serum analyses became possible as well [17]. Serum NfL shows a good correlation with CSF level and thereby offers a window to monitor axonal loss in MS patients consecutively [18,22]. Therefore, numerous studies including serum NfL in MS are available and it is used frequently in clinical trials [9,11,23,30]. However, longitudinal serum NfL assessments are scarce [26,27], especially in individual MS patients before and after initiation of first-line therapies. For this purpose, we aimed at characterizing the influence of those therapies on serum NfL levels.

Our data suggested that serum NfL may be suitable as a marker for therapy responsiveness based on the following findings: (a) sNfL levels stayed at a consistent low level or even dropped significantly in relapse-free patients over time and (b) sNfL levels after 9 and 12 months were significantly lower in patients without relapse within 12 months compared with patients suffering from a relapse during this time period.

However, we want to point out that most MS patients in the early phase of the disease, which is the case for most of our patients, show serum NfL levels that are within a normal age-adjusted range [16].

Furthermore, our data showed that serum NfL levels were associated with relapses as they were higher in time points with a present relapse compared with non-relapse time points.

The individual serum NfL courses showed that effects that were seen on a group basis did not always hold for every individual. Although serum NfL levels increased during the event of a relapse and decreased after high-dose corticosteroid therapy in most patients, there were exceptions (e.g., patient 16). More consistently, in our cohort, we observed that serum NfL levels stayed at a constant low level in therapy-responsive patients, which might be helpful in therapy monitoring of patients treated with first-line therapies. Our data suggested that this effect can be seen after 9 months. Whereas a sampling interval of 3 or even 6 months seems appropriate in patients without disease activity, other studies of highly active and more severely affected patients suggest a sampling interval and serum NfL testing every month [26]. We did not observe a positive correlation between serum NfL and EDSS for all time points, which is not surprising as this was also not seen in other studies [31] or only described in larger cohorts and with patients more severely affected by the disease and accordingly with higher EDSS [22,32]. The same was true for the correlation of serum NfL and PASAT as cognitive functions are only mildly affected in the early phase of the disease [33]. Even though, in a previous study, we observed an association of a more active disease course with higher levels of pro-inflammatory cytokines and lower levels of anti-inflammatory cytokines in a subpopulation of our study cohort [29], there was no correlation of serum NfL with any of the observed cytokines in the present study.

We also want to discuss the shortcomings of this study. As this was a retrospective analysis of serum NfL in a prospectively collected cohort, pre-analytical effects on serum NfL outcomes must be considered as samples were stored for more than 10 years. However, the observed values were in the same range as those of comparable patients [30,34,35] and of particular interest as no other therapies were available at this time and thereby we were able to monitor long-term outcomes of serum NfL in this specific study population. We can also not completely rule out spontaneous processes or regression that influences serum NfL (sNfL) levels, as we did not include untreated, stable MS patients. As this was an explorative study, these findings need to be confirmed in independent studies and it is desirable to have more detailed MRI data (e.g., number of gadolinium-enhanced lesions, atrophy, etc.) and complete data sets for every patient in those future studies because, for example, T1-hypointense lesions explain the severity of clinical disability better than T2-hyperintense white matter lesions and gadolinium-enhancing lesions correlate better with active disease status. Missing correlation with EDSS was similar to previous findings [31]. However, we were also unable to detect any correlations with the analyzed cytokines. This might be due to the small sample size or that inflammatory processes were either not present in patients or not displayed in the serum of those patients.

Monitoring of subclinical disease activity using MRI is an established procedure in the care of MS patients. Due to the method's invasiveness, this is not possible for CSF examination, although CSF parameters are appropriate to reflect intrathecal inflammatory processes. Serum NfL appears to be a promising marker for monitoring subclinical disease activity, as demonstrated in this cohort with longitudinal data collection under the same therapy over 24 months. However, this effect may not be seen in every patient as shown in our single-patient illustrations. In a heterogeneous disease like MS, a single biomarker is not sufficient to completely monitor and evaluate therapy efficacy. For this reason, all available information, clinical and paraclinical, should be gathered and taken into account for clinical decision making.

In summary, our study presents the first results on the effect of first-line therapies on serum NfL levels in mildly affected MS patients over 24 months. Here, serum NfL seems especially helpful in detecting therapy-responsive patients, but we also want to address the need for identifying factors that might influence serum NfL values. Among others, this includes processes involved in the transport of NfL from the CSF into serum as well as NfL clearance. The more we know about non-disease-related mechanisms that affect serum NfL, the better we can model serum NfL courses and identify real changes that are caused by pathological processes.

Author Contributions: Conceptualization, H.T.; data curation, A.H.; analysis, A.H. and B.M.; funding acquisition, H.T.; investigation, A.H.; methodology, J.K. and M.O.; project administration, A.C.L. and H.T.; resources, M.O.;

supervision, A.C.L. and H.T.; validation, M.S. and A.A.; visualization, A.H.; writing—original draft, A.H.; writing—review and editing, M.S., A.A., J.K., A.C.L., M.O. and H.T. All authors have read and agreed to the published version of the manuscript.

Funding: This study was supported in part by the German Federal Ministry of Education and Research (KKNMS), the German Research Foundation/DFG (SFB1279) and the foundation of the state Baden-Württemberg.

Acknowledgments: We kindly thank all patients for their participation in this study and all members of our local biobank, CSF and research lab for their excellent work. We would like to thank Paula Klassen for the linguistic and grammatical revision of the manuscript.

Conflicts of Interest: A.H. has nothing to disclose. M.S. has received consulting and/or speaker honoraria from Alexion, Bayer, Biogen, Merck, Roche and Sanofi Genzyme. She has received travel support from Celgene and Teva. She has received research funding from the Hertha-Nathorff-Program. A.A. received research funding from DMSG and travel grants from Biogen, all not related to the current study. B.M. has nothing to disclose. J.K. has nothing to disclose. A.C.L. has nothing to disclose. M.O. has nothing to disclose. H.T. reports funding for research projects, lectures and travel from Bayer, Biogen, Genzyme, Fresenius, Merck, Mylan, Novartis, Roche, Siemens Health Diagnostics and Teva, and received research support from Hertie-Stiftung, DMSG, BMBF and University of Ulm.

References

1. Compston, A.; Coles, A. Multiple sclerosis. *Lancet* **2002**, *359*, 1221–1231. [CrossRef]
2. Compston, A.; Coles, A. Multiple Sclerosis. *Lancet* **2008**, *372*, 1502–1517. [CrossRef]
3. Kamm, C.P.; Uitdehaag, B.M.; Polman, C.H. Multiple sclerosis: Current knowledge and future outlook. *Eur. Neurol.* **2014**, *72*, 132–141. [CrossRef] [PubMed]
4. Petzold, A.; Keir, G.; Green, A.J.E.; Giovannoni, G.; Thompson, E.J. A specific ELISA for measuring neurofilament heavy chain phosphoforms. *J. Immunol. Methods* **2003**, *278*, 179–190. [CrossRef]
5. Teunissen, C.E.; Khalil, M. Neurofilaments as biomarkers in multiple sclerosis. *Mult. Scler. J.* **2012**, *18*, 552–556. [CrossRef] [PubMed]
6. Yuan, A.; Rao, M.; Veeranna; Nixon, R.A. Neurofilaments and neurofilament proteins in health and disease. *Cold Spring Harb. Perspect. Biol.* **2017**, *9*, a018309. [CrossRef]
7. Gaetani, L.; Blennow, K.; Calabresi, P.; Di Filippo, M.; Parnetti, L.; Zetterberg, H. Neurofilament light chain as a biomarker in neurological disorders. *J. Neurol. Neurosurg. Psychiatry* **2019**, *90*, 870–881. [CrossRef]
8. Kuhle, J.; Plattner, K.; Bestwick, J.P.; Lindberg, R.L.; Ramagopalan, S.V.; Norgren, N.; Nissim, A.; Malaspina, A.; Leppert, D.; Giovannoni, G.; et al. A comparative study of CSF neurofilament light and heavy chain protein in MS. *Mult. Scler. J.* **2013**, *19*, 1597–1603. [CrossRef]
9. Khalil, M.; Teunissen, C.E.; Otto, M.; Piehl, F.; Sormani, M.P.; Gattringer, T.; Barro, C.; Kappos, L.; Comabella, M.; Fazekas, F.; et al. Neurofilaments as biomarkers in neurological disorders. *Nat. Rev. Neurol.* **2018**, *14*, 577–589. [CrossRef]
10. Khalil, M.; Salzer, J. CSF neurofilament light. *Neurology* **2016**, *87*, 1068–1069. [CrossRef]
11. Brettschneider, J.; Petzold, A.; Junker, A.; Tumani, H. Axonal damage markers in the cerebrospinal fluid of patients with clinically isolated syndrome improve predicting conversion to definite multiple sclerosis. *Mult. Scler. J.* **2006**, *12*, 143–148. [CrossRef] [PubMed]
12. Arrambide, G.; Espejo, C.; Eixarch, H.; Villar, L.M.; Alvarez-Cermeño, J.C.; Picón, C.; Kuhle, J.; Disanto, G.; Kappos, L.; Sastre-Garriga, J.; et al. Neurofilament light chain level is a weak risk factor for the development of MS. *Neurology* **2016**, *87*, 1076–1084. [CrossRef] [PubMed]
13. Gunnarsson, M.; Malmeström, C.; Axelsson, M.; Sundström, P.; Dahle, C.; Vrethem, M.; Olsson, T.P.; Piehl, F.; Norgren, N.; Rosengren, L.E.; et al. Axonal damage in relapsing multiple sclerosis is markedly reduced by natalizumab. *Ann. Neurol.* **2010**, *69*, 83–89. [CrossRef]
14. Bridel, C.; Van Wieringen, W.N.; Zetterberg, H.; Tijms, B.M.; Teunissen, C.E.; Alvarez-Cermeño, J.C.; Andreasson, U.; Axelsson, M.; Bäckström, D.C.; Bartos, A.; et al. Diagnostic value of cerebrospinal fluid neurofilament light protein in neurology. *JAMA Neurol.* **2019**, *76*, 1035–1048. [CrossRef] [PubMed]
15. Delaby, C.; Alcolea, D.; Carmona-Iragui, M.; Illán-Gala, I.; Morenas-Rodríguez, E.; Barroeta, I.; Altuna, M.; Estellés, T.; Santos-Santos, M.; Turon-Sans, J.; et al. Differential levels of Neurofilament Light protein in cerebrospinal fluid in patients with a wide range of neurodegenerative disorders. *Sci. Rep.* **2020**, *10*, 1–8. [CrossRef] [PubMed]

16. Khalil, M.; Pirpamer, L.; Hofer, E.; Voortman, M.M.; Barro, C.; Leppert, D.; Benkert, P.; Ropele, S.; Enzinger, C.; Fazekas, F.; et al. Serum neurofilament light levels in normal aging and their association with morphologic brain changes. *Nat. Commun.* **2020**, *11*, 812. [CrossRef]
17. Rissin, D.M.; Kan, C.W.; Campbell, T.G.; Howes, S.C.; Fournier, D.R.; Song, L.; Piech, T.; Patel, P.P.; Chang, L.; Rivnak, A.J.; et al. Single-molecule enzyme-linked immunosorbent assay detects serum proteins at subfemtomolar concentrations. *Nat. Biotechnol.* **2010**, *28*, 595–599. [CrossRef]
18. Kuhle, J.; Barro, C.; Andreasson, U.; Derfuss, T.; Lindberg, R.; Sandelius, Å.; Liman, V.; Norgren, N.; Blennow, K.; Zetterberg, H. Comparison of three analytical platforms for quantification of the neurofilament light chain in blood samples: ELISA, electrochemiluminescence immunoassay and Simoa. *Clin. Chem. Lab. Med.* **2016**, *54*, 1655–1661. [CrossRef]
19. Kuhle, J.; Barro, C.; Disanto, G.; Mathias, A.; Soneson, C.; Bonnier, G.; Yaldizli, Ö.; Regeniter, A.; Derfuss, T.; Canales, M.; et al. Serum neurofilament light chain in early relapsing remitting MS is increased and correlates with CSF levels and with MRI measures of disease severity. *Mult. Scler. J.* **2016**, *22*, 1550–1559. [CrossRef]
20. Kuhle, J.; Nourbakhsh, B.; Grant, D.; Morant, S.; Barro, C.; Yaldizli, Ö.; Pelletier, D.; Giovannoni, G.; Waubant, E.; Gnanapavan, S. Serum neurofilament is associated with progression of brain atrophy and disability in early MS. *Neurology* **2017**, *88*, 826–831. [CrossRef]
21. Siller, N.; Kuhle, J.; Muthuraman, M.; Barro, C.; Uphaus, T.; Groppa, S.; Kappos, L.; Zipp, F.; Bittner, S. Serum neurofilament light chain is a biomarker of acute and chronic neuronal damage in early multiple sclerosis. *Mult. Scler. J.* **2018**, *25*, 678–686. [CrossRef] [PubMed]
22. Disanto, G.; Barro, C.; Benkert, P.; Naegelin, Y.; Schädelin, S.; Giardiello, A.; Zecca, C.; Blennow, K.; Zetterberg, H.; Leppert, D.; et al. Serum Neurofilament light: A biomarker of neuronal damage in multiple sclerosis. *Ann. Neurol.* **2017**, *81*, 857–870. [CrossRef]
23. Sormani, M.P.; Haering, D.A.; Kropshofer, H.; Leppert, D.; Kundu, U.; Barro, C.; Kappos, L.; Tomic, D.; Kuhle, J. Blood neurofilament light as a potential endpoint in Phase 2 studies in MS. *Ann. Clin. Transl. Neurol.* **2019**, *6*, 1081–1089. [CrossRef]
24. Sejbæk, T.; Nielsen, H.H.; Penner, N.; Plavina, T.; Mendoza, J.P.; Martin, N.A.; Elkjaer, M.L.; Ravnborg, M.H.; Illes, Z. Dimethyl fumarate decreases neurofilament light chain in CSF and blood of treatment naïve relapsing MS patients. *J. Neurol. Neurosurg. Psychiatry* **2019**, *90*, 1324–1330. [CrossRef]
25. Thebault, S.; Abdoli, M.; Fereshtehnejad, S.-M.; Tessier, D.; Tabard-Cossa, V.; Freedman, M.S. Serum neurofilament light chain predicts long term clinical outcomes in multiple sclerosis. *Sci. Rep.* **2020**, *10*, 10381. [CrossRef] [PubMed]
26. Akgün, K.; Kretschmann, N.; Haase, R.; Proschmann, U.; Kitzler, H.H.; Reichmann, H.; Ziemssen, T. Profiling individual clinical responses by high-frequency serum neurofilament assessment in MS. *Neurol. Neuroimmunol. Neuroinflamm.* **2019**, *6*, e555. [CrossRef] [PubMed]
27. Hyun, J.-W.; Kim, Y.; Kim, G.; Kim, S.-H.; Kim, H.J. Longitudinal analysis of serum neurofilament light chain: A potential therapeutic monitoring biomarker for multiple sclerosis. *Mult. Scler. J.* **2019**, *26*, 659–667. [CrossRef]
28. Teunissen, C.E.; Petzold, A.; Bennett, J.L.; Berven, F.S.; Brundin, L.; Comabella, M.; Franciotta, D.; Frederiksen, J.L.; Fleming, J.O.; Furlan, R.; et al. A consensus protocol for the standardization of cerebrospinal fluid collection and biobanking. *Neurology* **2009**, *73*, 1914–1922. [CrossRef]
29. Tumani, H.; Kassubek, J.; Hijazi, M.; Lehmensiek, V.; Unrath, A.; Süssmuth, S.; Lauda, F.; Kapfer, T.; Fang, L.; Senel, M.; et al. Patterns of TH1/TH2 cytokines predict clinical response in multiple sclerosis patients treated with glatiramer acetate. *Eur. Neurol.* **2011**, *65*, 164–169. [CrossRef]
30. Novakova, L.; Zetterberg, H.; Sundström, P.; Axelsson, M.; Khademi, M.; Gunnarsson, M.; Malmeström, C.; Svenningsson, A.; Olsson, T.; Piehl, F.; et al. Monitoring disease activity in multiple sclerosis using serum neurofilament light protein. *Neurology* **2017**, *89*, 2230–2237. [CrossRef]
31. Abdelhak, A.; Huss, A.; Kassubek, J.; Tumani, H.; Otto, M. Serum GFAP as a biomarker for disease severity in multiple sclerosis. *Sci. Rep.* **2018**, *8*, 14798. [CrossRef]
32. Högel, H.; Rissanen, E.; Barro, C.; Matilainen, M.; Nylund, M.; Kuhle, J.; Airas, L. Serum glial fibrillary acidic protein correlates with multiple sclerosis disease severity. *Mult. Scler. J.* **2018**, *26*, 210–219. [CrossRef] [PubMed]

33. Johnen, A.; Bürkner, P.-C.; Landmeyer, N.C.; Ambrosius, B.; Calabrese, P.; Motte, J.; Hessler, N.; Antony, G.; König, I.R.; Klotz, L.; et al. Can we predict cognitive decline after initial diagnosis of multiple sclerosis? Results from the German National early MS cohort (KKNMS). *J. Neurol.* **2018**, *266*, 386–397. [CrossRef] [PubMed]
34. Håkansson, I.; Tisell, A.; Cassel, P.; Blennow, K.; Zetterberg, H.; Lundberg, P.; Dahle, C.; Vrethem, M.; Ernerudh, J. Neurofilament levels, disease activity and brain volume during follow-up in multiple sclerosis. *J. Neuroinflamm.* **2018**, *15*, 209. [CrossRef] [PubMed]
35. Bittner, S.; Steffen, F.; Uphaus, T.; Muthuraman, M.; Fleischer, V.; Salmen, A.; Luessi, F.; Berthele, A.; Klotz, L.; Meuth, S.G.; et al. Clinical implications of serum neurofilament in newly diagnosed MS patients: A longitudinal multicentre cohort study. *EBioMedicine* **2020**, *56*, 102807. [CrossRef]

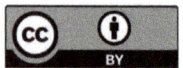

© 2020 by the authors. Licensee MDPI, Basel, Switzerland. This article is an open access article distributed under the terms and conditions of the Creative Commons Attribution (CC BY) license (http://creativecommons.org/licenses/by/4.0/).

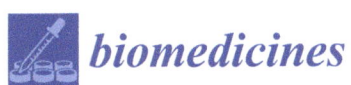

Article

Whole-Transcriptome Analysis in Peripheral Blood Mononuclear Cells from Patients with Lipid-Specific Oligoclonal IgM Band Characterization Reveals Two Circular RNAs and Two Linear RNAs as Biomarkers of Highly Active Disease

Leire Iparraguirre [1], Danel Olaverri [1,2], Telmo Blasco [1,2], Lucía Sepúlveda [1,3], Tamara Castillo-Triviño [4], Mercedes Espiño [5], Lucienne Costa-Frossard [5], Álvaro Prada [6], Luisa María Villar [3,5], David Otaegui [1,3] and Maider Muñoz-Culla [1,3,*]

1. Multiple Sclerosis Group, Neurosciences Area, Biodonostia Health Research Institute, 20014 San Sebastian, Spain; leire.iparraguirre@biodonostia.org (L.I.); a904612@alumni.unav.es (D.O.); tblasco@tecnun.es (T.B.); lucia.sepulveda@biodonostia.org (L.S.); david.otaegui@biodonostia.org (D.O.)
2. Department of Biomedical Engineering and Sciences, Tecnun-Universidad de Navarra, Manuel de Lardizábal 15, 20018 San Sebastián, Spain
3. Spanish Network of Multiple Sclerosis, 08028 Barcelona, Spain; luisamaria.villar@salud.madrid.org
4. Multiple Sclerosis Group, Neurosciences Area, Biodonostia Health Research Institute, Neurology Department, Basque Health Service, 20014 San Sebastian, Spain; TAMARA.CASTILLOTRIVINO@osakidetza.eus
5. Departments of Immunology and Neurology, Multiple Sclerosis Unit, Hospital Ramon y Cajal, (IRYCIS), 28034 Madrid, Spain; mercedes.espino@salud.madrid.org (M.E.); lucienne.costa@salud.madrid.org (L.C.-F.)
6. Multiple Sclerosis Group, Neurosciences Area, Biodonostia Health Research Institute, Immunology Department, Basque Health Service, 20014 San Sebastian, Spain; ALVAROJOSE.PRADAINURRATEGUI@osakidetza.eus
* Correspondence: maider.munoz@biodonostia.org

Received: 26 October 2020; Accepted: 23 November 2020; Published: 26 November 2020

Abstract: The presence of anti-myelin lipid-specific oligoclonal IgM bands (LS-OCMBs) has been defined as an accurate predictor of an aggressive evolution of multiple sclerosis. However, the detection of this biomarker is performed in cerebrospinal fluid, a quite invasive liquid biopsy. In the present study we aimed at studying the expression profile of miRNA, snoRNA, circRNA and linearRNA in peripheral blood mononuclear cells (PBMCs) from patients with lipid-specific oligoclonal IgM band characterization. We included a total of 89 MS patients, 47 with negative LS-OCMB status and 42 with positive status. Microarray (miRNA and snoRNA) and RNA-seq (circular and linear RNAs) were used to perform the profiling study in the discovery cohort and candidates were validated by RT-qPCR in the whole cohort. The biomarker potential of the candidates was evaluated by ROC curve analysis. RNA-seq and RT-qPCR validation revealed that two circular (hsa_circ_0000478 and hsa_circ_0116639) and two linear RNAs (*IRF5* and *MTRNR2L8*) are downregulated in PBMCs from patients with positive LS-OCMBs. Finally, those RNAs show a performance of a 70% accuracy in some of the combinations. The expression of hsa_circ_0000478, hsa_circ_0116639, *IRF5* and *MTRNR2L8* might serve as minimally invasive biomarkers of highly active disease.

Keywords: multiple sclerosis; biomarkers; transcriptome; microRNAs; circular RNAs; oligoclonal bands

1. Introduction

Multiple sclerosis (MS) is a chronic, inflammatory, neurodegenerative and demyelinating disease of the central nervous system (CNS). It is considered an autoimmune disease, in which peripheral autoreactive lymphocytes enter the CNS and develop an immune response, leading to demyelinating lesions, both in white and grey matter [1]. It is estimated that about 2–3 million people have MS and it typically affects young adults, with an onset between 20 and 40 years of age. Moreover, MS is three times more prevalent in women than men and there is evidence that this ratio has increased in the last 70 years [1], a phenomenon shared with several other autoimmune diseases.

Both the disease course and clinical phenotype of MS are highly variable among patients and also with time in the same individual. For this reason, biomarkers can aid in the diagnosis, the differentiation of MS phenotypes and also in the monitoring of disease progression [2,3].

Disease activity biomarkers can be associated with the different pathophysiological processes of the disease and they could ideally help to distinguish between patients with an aggressive course and those with a more benign form [2]. In this context, the presence restricted to cerebrospinal fluid (CSF) of anti-myelin lipid-specific oligoclonal IgM bands (LS-OCMBs) has been defined as an accurate predictor of an aggressive evolution [4]. However, for this test, cerebrospinal fluid sample is needed, a quite invasive liquid biopsy. Therefore, a great effort has been done towards the discovery of minimally invasive biomarkers such as blood biomarkers [5].

In this context, gene expression profiling studies have been widely used for new biomarker discovery, but also to elucidate the molecular mechanisms underlying the pathogenic processes occurring in the disease [6,7]. In addition to the classical protein-coding transcriptome, non-coding transcriptome has gained great interest in the last decades, and several authors, including our group, have demonstrated that it has a role in MS pathogenesis [8–10]. MicroRNAs are the best studied class of small non-coding RNAs, although others such as small nucleolar RNAs have also been related to MS [11,12]. MiRNAs are single-strand small non-coding RNAs that regulate gene expression at a post-transcriptional level, binding to their target mRNAs, and they participate in almost all known biological processes [13]. More recently, circular RNAs (circRNAs) have emerged as new players in the RNA field, with an important role in the post-transcriptional regulatory mechanisms. They have been found to participate in several processes such as tumor, metabolism and immune-related pathways and consequently, they have also been linked to various diseases such as neurological and autoimmune diseases including a few studies in MS [14–18]. Both miRNA and circRNA have been proposed as promising source of biomarkers in a wide variety of sample types, such as blood, serum, saliva, urine and CSF [19–21].

In light of these evidences, and due to the increasing need for a solid, reproducible and accessible biomarker for MS, we hypothesized that a whole-transcriptome study of peripheral blood mononuclear cells (PBMCs) from patients with LS-OCMBs characterization could reveal new biomarkers that correlate with this stablished CSF marker. Such a biomarker could be used more easily to monitor patients on an ongoing basis, since blood sampling is less invasive, with less adverse effects, than doing a lumbar puncture.

With this in mind, in the present study we analyzed the expression of small non-coding RNA, circRNA and linear RNAs in peripheral blood mononuclear cells (PBMCs), from 89 patients with positive ($n = 42$) and negative ($n = 47$) LS-OCMBs characterization, and found two circular RNAs and two linear RNAs, with differential expression between the two groups, that could serve as future blood biomarkers of highly active disease.

2. Experimental Section

2.1. Patients, Sample Collection and RNA Isolation

MS patients were recruited in the Hospital Ramon y Cajal after giving informed consent. Blood samples were obtained and PBMCs were isolated following a standard Ficol gradient separation protocol and frozen in liquid nitrogen until used. Total RNA was isolated using the miRNeasy mini kit (Qiagen, Hilden, Germany) following the manufacturer's instructions. RNA concentration was measured using the NanoDrop ND-1000 spectrophotometer (ThermoFisher Scientific, Waltham, Massachusetts, MA, USA), and the que quality of the samples included in microarray and RNA-seq experiments was assessed using the Agilent 2100 Bioanalyzer (Agilent Technologies, Santa Clara, CA, USA), obtaining a RNA integrity number higher than 6 in all the samples. CSF was obtained to analyze the status of LS-OCMBs as previously described [4,22].

The main clinical and demographical characteristics of patients are summarized in Table 1. A complete list of samples and the experiment in which each of them was included is available in Table S1. The study was approved by the hospital's ethics committee (MMC-UEM-2018-01, October 2018). The profiling cohort includes only female samples, aiming at reducing the source of variability and considering that MS is three times more prevalent in females than men in this disease [1].

Table 1. Summary of patients' clinical and demographical data.

	Microarrays			RNAseq					
	LS-OCMB status	Sex	Age	LS-OCMB status	Sex	Age			
Profiling cohort	P = 5	F = 5 M = 0	35 (23–58)	P = 4	F = 4 M = 0	38 (23–58)			
	N = 6	F = 6 M = 0	34.5 (27–53)	N = 4	F = 4 M = 0	35 (27–44)			
	miRNA validation *			circRNA validation *			linear RNA validation		
	LS-OCMB status	Sex	Age	LS-OCMB status	Sex	Age	LS-OCMB status	Sex	Age
Validation cohort	P = 42	F = 24 M = 18	34 (17–58)	P = 42	F = 24 M = 18	34 (17–58)	P = 30	F = 18 M = 12	33.4 (17–51)
	N = 47	F = 39 M = 8	37 (20–53)	N = 46	F = 38 M = 8	37 (20–53)	N = 30	F = 24 M = 6	36.9 (20–49)

* Including patients in profiling cohort. Age—mean (range). LS-OCMB—lipid-specific oligoclonal IgM bands. P—positive. N—negative. F—females. M—males. There are 7 subjects (1 positive and 6 negative) in validation cohorts for which we do not have age data.

2.2. Microarray Analysis

Total RNA (200 ng) was labeled using the FlashTag HSR Biotin labelling kit (Genisphere LLC, Hatfield, Pennsylvania, PA, USA) and hybridized to the GeneChip miRNA 4.0 Array (Affymetrix, Santa Clara, CA, USA), which covers 2578, 2025 and 1996 human mature miRNAs, pre-miRNAs and snoRNAs, respectively. Labeled RNA was hybridized to the array, washed and stained in a GeneChip Fluidics Station 450 and scanned in a GeneChip Scanner 7G (Affymetrix, Santa Clara, CA, USA).

Microarray data analysis was carried out in Transcriptome Analysis Console 4.0 software (Affymetrix, Santa Clara, CA, USA), applying the RMA + DABG algorithm only to human probesets for normalization, detection and summarization purposes. We performed a classical differential expression analysis between patients with positive and negative LS-OCMBs, considering as differentially expressed those probesets showing a p-value lower than 0.01 and an absolute fold-change (FC) value higher or equal to 1.5.

2.3. RNAseq

Library preparation and Next Generation Sequencing was performed at CD Genomics (Shirley, New York, NY, USA). The concentration and quality of the RNA samples was again measured using Agilent 2100 Bioanalyzer before library preparation. After normalization, rRNA was depleted from the total RNA sample using the Ribo-Zero rRNA removal kit and followed by purification and fragmentation steps. To construct the sequencing libraries, a strand-specific cDNA synthesis was performed, the 3′ ends were adenylated and adaptors were ligated. The resulting libraries were subjected to a quality control and normalization process. Paired-end sequencing was performed with Illumina HiSeq X Ten PE150 (Illumina, San Diego, CA, USA).

The data presented in this study (raw data of microarray and RNA-seq experiments) are openly available in Gene Expression Omnibus (GEO) under the series reference GSE159036.

2.4. CircRNA Detection and Quantification in RNA-Seq Data

First, quality of the sequencing was checked and, then, reads were mapped to the human genome (hg19, downloaded from UCSC Genome Browser [23]) using STAR version 2.5.4b (https://code.google.com/archive/p/rna-star/) [24] or BWA version 0.7.17-1 (http://maq.sourceforge.net) [25]. Subsequently, circRNA prediction was performed by CIRCexplorer2 version 2.3.3 (https://circexplorer2.readthedocs.io/en/latest/) [26] and CIRI2 version 2.0.5 (https://sourceforge.net/projects/ciri/) [27] adhering to the recommendation by the authors. Moreover, only circRNAs supported by both algorithms were considered as bona fide circRNAs and used in subsequent analyses, a method that has been described in the literature by other authors [28]. CircRNA expression was based on back-spliced junctions-spanning reads according to CIRI2 quantification. After filtering out circRNAs with low expression (sum of reads < 10), differential expression analysis was performed using DESeq2 version 1.28.1 (http://www.bioconductor.org/packages/release/bioc/html/DESeq2.html) [29] package for R (version 3.6.3) (https://www.r-project.org/) in R-studio (Version 1.0.136) (https://rstudio.com/), considering as differentially expressed those circRNA showing a *p*-value < 0.05 and a fold-change higher than 2. To select a group of candidates for validation purposes, two additional filters were applied: (1) BaseMean value higher than five (BM > 5) and (2) the transcripts having a read count value of zero in any of the samples were removed. Finally, we selected ten candidate circRNAs having the highest absolute fold-change value.

2.5. Linear RNA Detection and Quantification in RNA-Seq Data

After sequencing and quality control, the Kallisto version 0.44.0 (http://pachterlab.github.io/kallisto/) [30] algorithm was used for transcript pseudoalignment, identification and quantification. Differential expression analysis was performed using DESeq2 package. Before running the DESeq2 algorithm, we applied a filter of a minimum number of reads (sum of number of reads higher than or equal to 10) to remove low expression transcripts. For subsequent analysis, due to the large number of transcripts detected and our small sample size, we added a filter to keep only the most robust transcripts regarding their read count. Therefore, we created a detection filter, as follows: (1) Transcripts detected in both groups—transcripts having at least two reads in $\frac{3}{4}$ of samples from each group. (2) Transcripts detected only in one of the groups—transcripts having at least two reads in $\frac{3}{4}$ of samples in the negative group but only in 1 sample from the positive group (detected only in negative group), and transcripts having at least two reads in $\frac{3}{4}$ of positive group but only in 1 from negative group (detected only in positive group). Transcripts selected with this detection filter were considered as consistent linear RNAs. Finally, differentially expressed transcripts were considered those showing a *p*-value < 0.05 and an absolute fold-change value higher than two. For validation purposes, we selected ten candidate linear RNAs having the highest absolute fold-change value and having an assigned gene name.

All these profiling experiments and data analysis steps, tools and filters are summarized in Figure 1.

2.6. cDNA Synthesis and Quantitative PCR

For the validation of candidate microRNAs, total RNA (10 ng) was reverse transcribed into cDNA using TaqMan™ Advanced miRNA cDNA synthesis kit (Applied Biosystems™, Foster City, CA, USA). To quantify miRNA expression, we used TaqMan Advanced miRNA assays and TaqMan Fast Advanced Master Mix (Applied Biosystems™, Foster City, CA, USA), following the manufacturer's protocol. Assay for hsa-miR-191-5p was used as a reference miRNA for normalization purposes.

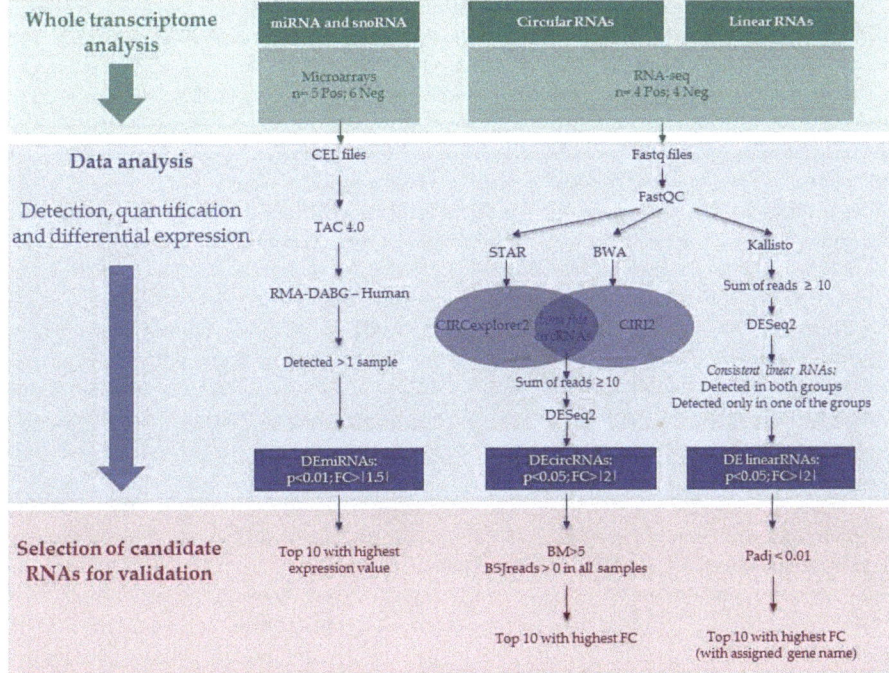

Figure 1. Summary of the study indicating profiling experiments, data analysis tools, filters and candidate selection criteria. Pos—positive. Neg—negative. DE—differentially expressed. FC—fold-change. BM—BaseMean. BSJ—backspliced junction. Padj—adjusted *p*-value. BWA—Burrows-Wheeler Aligner.

For the validation of candidate circRNA, total RNA (500 ng) was reverse transcribed into cDNA with random primers using the High Capacity cDNA Reverse Transcription Kit (Applied Biosystems, Foster City, CA, USA), following the kit protocol. PCR reaction was set up using 10 ng of cDNA as the template and using Power SYBRGreen Master Mix (Applied Biosystems™ Foster City, CA, USA) with the following thermal cycling program: A temperature of 50 °C for 2 min, 95 °C for 10 min, 40 cycles of 95 °C for 15 s and 60 °C for 1 min, followed by a dissociation curve analysis. Divergent primers were used so that the amplicon spans the backspliced junction (BSJ), as described previously [18]. EEF1A1 and B2M were used as the reference genes, using the mean value of both genes for normalization purposes. The presence of a single-peak in the melting curve indicated the specificity of the amplification.

For the validation of candidate linear RNAs, total RNA (500 ng) was reverse transcribed into cDNA with oligo-dT and random primers using the miScript II RT (Qiagen, Hilden, Germany) kit with the HiFlex buffer, as indicated in manufacturer's protocol. PCR reaction was set up using 10 ng of cDNA as template and using miSscript SYBRGreen PCR kit (Qiagen, Hilden, Germany) with the following thermal cycling program: A temperature of 95 °C for 15 min, 40 cycles of 94 °C for 15 s, 55 °C for 30 s and 70 °C for 30 s, followed by a dissociation curve analysis. The amplification of each linear RNA was carried out with QuantiTect primer Assays (Qiagen, Hilden, Germany) (Table S2) and B2M was used as a reference gene for normalization. The presence of a single-peak in the melting curve indicated the specificity of the amplification.

All retrotranscription reactions were run in a Veriti Thermal Cycler (Applied Biosytems, Foster City, CA, USA) and quantitative PCR reactions were performed in a CFX384 Touch Real-Time PCR Detection System (Bio-Rad laboratories, Inc., Hercules, CA, USA).

Prior to run all the validation experiments, a technical validation of the circRNA amplification was carried out. The RT-qPCR amplification products were subsequently purified with the ExoSAP-IT™ PCR Product Cleanup Reagent (Applied Biosystems, Foster City, CA, USA) following the manufacturer's instructions and Sanger sequenced (ABIprism 3130) (Applied Biosystems, Foster City, CA, USA) in order to check for the presence of the BSJ. In addition, the PCR products were also subjected to electrophoresis on agarose gel to confirm the presence of a single amplification product.

The Raw Cq values and melting curves were analyzed in CFX Maestro 1.0 (Bio-Rad laboratories, Inc., Hercules, CA, USA). Expression levels represented as fold-change (FC) were calculated using the $2^{\char`\^}DDCq$ method. Statistical analysis was done by R in RStudio on DCq data. Distribution of data was tested with Shapiro–Wilk test and the difference of the distribution was assessed by Student t-test or non-parametric Wilcoxon Rank sum test. In each circRNA and linear RNA dataset, outlier samples were removed before the statistical analysis, identifying those values using boxplot.stat function in R.

2.7. Gene Overrepresentation Test

In order to describe the function of differentially expressed transcripts, the PANTHER overrepresentation test was applied (released 7 November 2019, Panther [31]), based on the Complete Biological Process from Gene Ontology database (released 9 December 2019). As a reference background, we used the list of genes giving rise to detected transcripts defined above. Fisher test was carried out and false discovery rate (FDR) correction was applied to raw p-values, taking as a significant threshold FDR values below 0.05.

2.8. ROC Curve Analysis

Based on DCq values obtained by RT-qPCR, we performed a receiver operating characteristic curve (ROC curve) analysis in R environment in RStudio. Three different datasets were used: (1) circRNA validation data, (2) linear RNA validation data and (3) samples in both datasets to test different combination of transcripts. This last dataset was smaller given that we needed to include only samples without any missing value (Table S1). The combination of different transcripts was computed with ROC function of "Epi" package.

3. Results

3.1. microRNA Expression Profile

Microarray analysis was able to detect 2827 probesets in at least one sample out of the total 6659 human probesets (42.45%) (Figure 2A). Among detected probesets, 33 showed a differential expression between positive and negative patients for LS-OCMBs, and more importantly, the top 10 probesets that show the highest expression are able to group patients according to their LS-OCMBs status (Figure 2B). Among these 10 probesets, we can find five mature miRNA, two pre-miRNA and two small nucleolar RNAs. For validation purposes, we selected the four mature miRNA for which TaqMan Advanced miRNA Assays were available (hsa-miR-6800-5p, hsa-miR-6821-5p, hsa-miR-4485 and hsa-miR-4741). However, RT-qPCR validation results did not confirm the alteration of these four miRNAs (Figure 2C).

3.2. circRNA Expression Profile

RNA-seq analysis pipeline of circular transcriptome detected 27,630 bona fide circRNAs and 5431 circRNAs (19.6%) with sum of reads ≥ 10 (Figure 3A). Differential expression analysis revealed that 124 circRNAs are altered ($p < 0.05$; FC > |2|) between the two groups, 72 of them being upregulated, while 52 are downregulated.

We selected ten candidate circRNAs to confirm their differential expression by RT-qPCR in a larger cohort. First, the technical test for primer amplification confirmed a single and specific circRNA amplification for nine out of the 10 circRNA candidates. circMETRNL was the one that did not show a good amplification and a single band in agarose gel, so we discarded it in subsequent validation experiments. Additionally, Sanger sequencing of the PCR product confirmed that the amplicons span the BSJ (Figure S1). As it can be observed in Figure 3C, the lower expression of hsa_circ_0000478 and hsa_circ_0116639 was confirmed by qPCR in PBMCs from patients with positive LS-OCMBs (FC = −1.5 and FC = −1.65, respectively; $p < 0.01$).

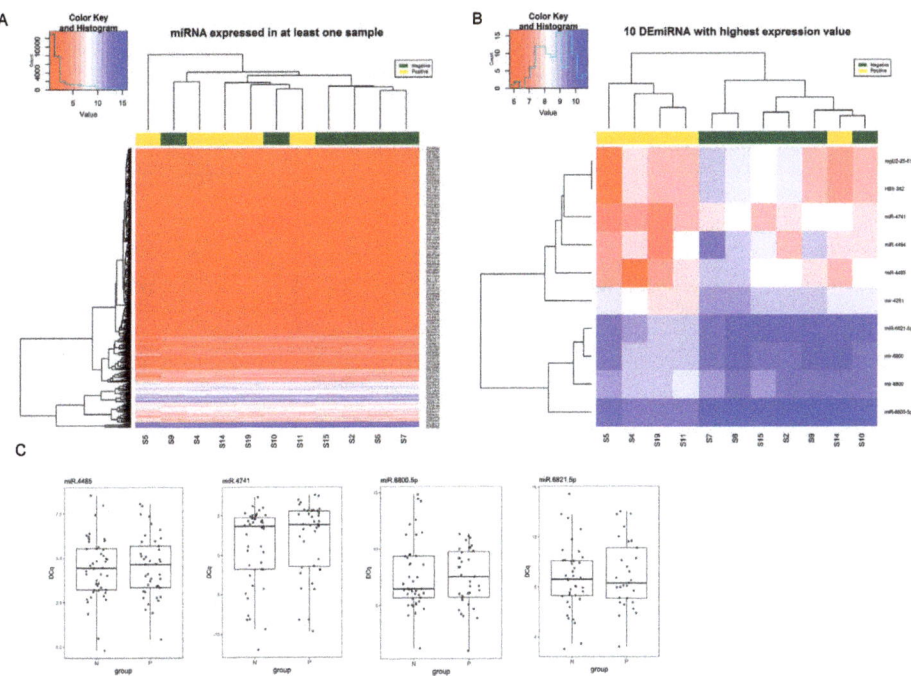

Figure 2. Results of miRNA expression profile by microarrays. (**A**) Heatmap showing the expression (microarray intensity signal) of miRNA that are expressed in at least one sample. (**B**) Heatmap of the expression of the ten DEmiRNAs showing the highest expression. Hierarchical clustering shows that the expression pattern of these ten miRNAs is able to group patients according to their LS-OCMBs status. (**C**) RT-qPCR validation results of selected candidate miRNAs. P—positive LS-OCMB status. N—negative LS-OCMB status. DE—differentially expressed.

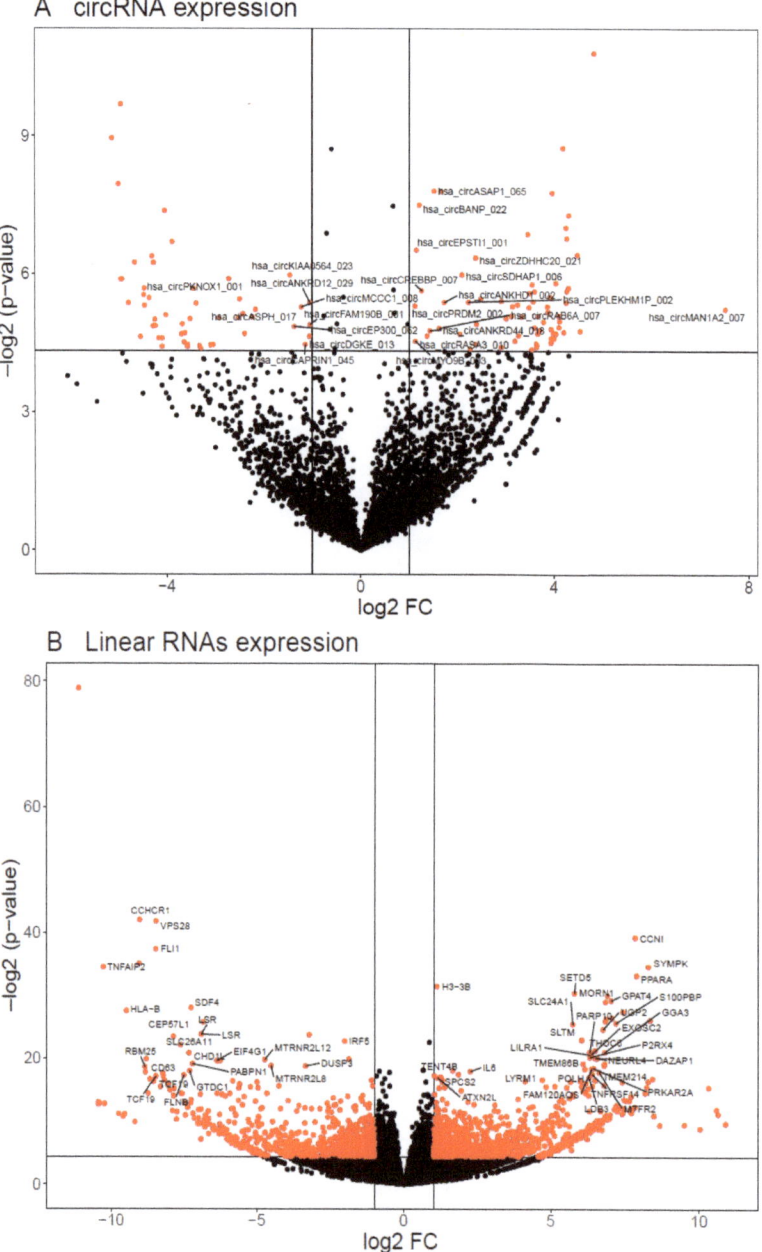

Figure 3. Cont.

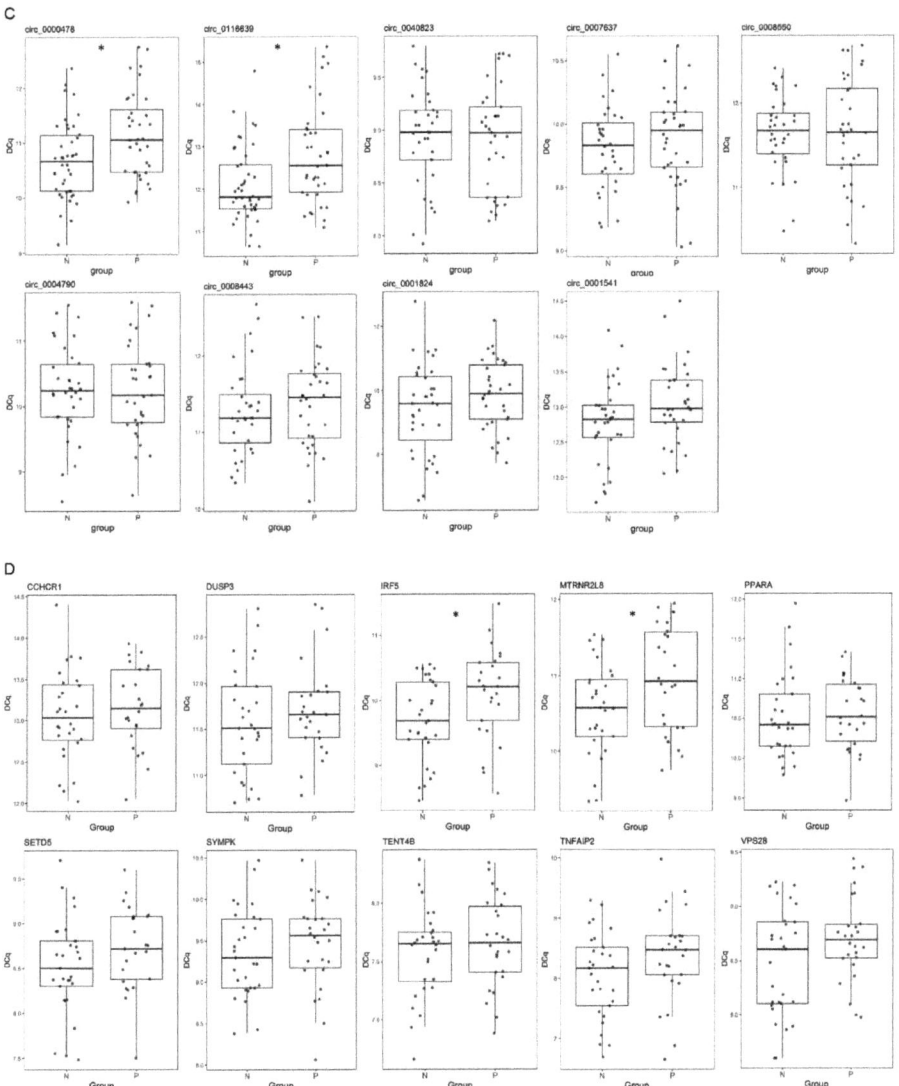

Figure 3. Results of circRNAs and linear RNAs expression profile by RNA-seq. (**A**) Volcano plot showing the expression difference (log2 FC) between positive and negative group of circRNA that show a sum of reads across all samples higher than 10. DEcircRNA are highlighted in red and labels point at those DEcircRNA with a base mean higher than 5. (**B**) Volcano plot showing the expression difference (log2 FC) of linear RNAs between positive and negative groups. Differentially expressed linear RNAs are highlighted in red and labels point at those DE linear RNAs with an adjusted p-value < 0.01. (**C**) RT-qPCR validation results of selected candidate circRNAs. Asterisk indicates a statistically significant difference ($p < 0.01$). circ_0000478 and circ_0116639 validation includes more samples than the rest of the circRNAs because of limitations in sample amount (Table S1). (**D**) RT-qPCR validation results of selected candidate linear RNAs. Asterisk indicates a statistically significant difference ($p < 0.05$). P: positive LS-OCMB status. N: negative LS-OCMB status.

3.3. Linear Transcripts Expression Profile

In the present study, we also analyzed the linear transcriptome by RNA-seq, identifying 115,869 transcripts with ≥10 reads in total. We applied an additional filter using a detection criterion, which permitted to identify 84,863 linear RNAs with a consistent expression pattern, from which 92.8% were detected in both groups. Among them, 2441 transcripts were differentially expressed ($p < 0.05$ and FC >| 2|), from which 1421 were detected in both groups (Figure 3B). The rest of the transcripts are specific to one of the groups, 382 being expressed only in PBMCs from patients with negative LS-OCMBs status while 638 transcripts are only expressed in patients with positive LS-OCMBs.

We selected ten candidate linear RNAs to confirm their differential expression by RT-qPCR in a larger cohort. As it can be observed in Figure 3D, the lower expression of IRF5 and MTRNR2L8 was confirmed in PBMCs from patients with positive LS-OCMBs (FC = −1.33 in both transcripts; $p < 0.05$).

Differentially expressed linear RNAs are enriched in biological processes regarding mainly the immune system. The most significant and enriched terms (FDR < 0.01 and fold-enrichment > 2) are shown in Figure 4. Complement activation, humoral immune response and type I interferon signaling pathway appear among the top enriched terms.

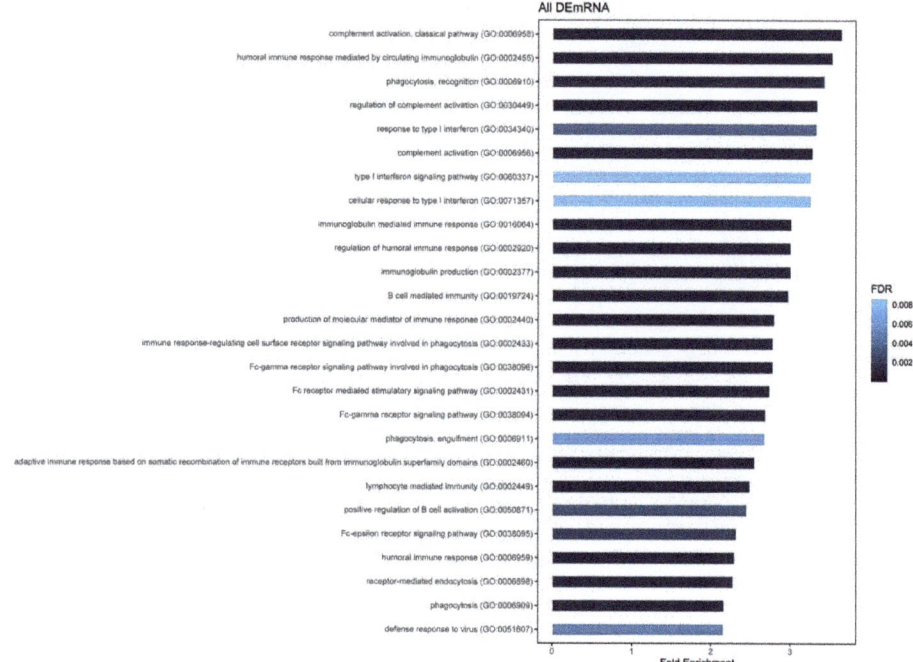

Figure 4. Results from gene overrepresentation test of 2441 DEmRNA. The most significant (fold-enrichment > 2) and enriched (FDR < 0.01) GO biological processes are shown. Bars are colored according to their FDR value. DE—differentially expressed. FDR—false discovery rate.

3.4. Evaluation of circRNA and Linear RNAs as Biomarkers of a Highly Active Disease

In order to assess the potential of the four validated RNAs as blood biomarkers of the LS-OCMB status we performed the ROC curve analysis. As shown in Table 2, different combinations of RNAs were tested to find the best performance in discriminating both groups. We found that different combinations of both circRNAs and linear RNAs improves the performance, reaching AUC values of around 70%.

Table 2. ROC analysis results of the four candidate transcripts and different combinations. ROC—receiver operating characteristic.

Marker/Combination	Transcripts	Sample Size	AUC (%)	CI (%)
circRNA-1	circ_0000478	80 (43 LS-OCMB−; 37 LS-OCMB+)	65.9	53.9–77.9
circRNA-2	circ_0116639		66.4	54.2–78.5
Combi_circ	circ_0000478-circ_0116639		68.9	57.2–80.5
linearRNA-1	IRF5	55 (29 LS-OCMB−; 26 LS-OCMB+)	65.6	50.7–80.6
linearRNA-2	MTRNR2L8		67.0	52.4–81.7
Combi_linear	IRF5-MTRNR2L8		68.6	54.1–83.1
circRNA-1	circ_0000478	51 (26 LS-OCMB−; 25 LS-OCMB+)	65.1	49.8–80.4
circRNA-2	circ_0116639		66.2	50.6–81.7
linearRNA-1	IRF5		67.1	51.8–82.3
linearRNA-2	MTRNR2L8		69.0	54.1–83.9
CombiALL	circ_0000478-circ_0116639-IRF5-MTRNR2L8		69.8	55.3–84.4
combi1	circ_0000478-circ_0116639		66.3	51.1–81.6
combi2	IRF5-MTRNR2L8		70.3	55.6–85.0
combi3	circ_0000478-IRF5		68.3	52.8–83.8
combi4	circ_0000478-MTRNR2L8		68.6	53.7–83.6
combi5	circ_0116639-IRF5		69.8	55.0–84.7
combi6	circ_0116639-MTRNR2L8		67.8	52.8–82.9
combi7	circ_0000478-circ_0116639-IRF5		69.8	55.0–84.6
combi8	circ_0000478-circ_0116639-MTRNR2L8		68.2	53.3–83.0
combi9	circ_0000478-IRF5-MTRNR2L8		68.8	53.7–83.8
combi10	circ_0116639-IRF5-MTRNR2L8		68.8	53.8–83.7

4. Discussion

In this work, we characterized the whole-transcriptome of PBMCs from MS patients with distinct LS-OCMB status. This profiling and the validation experiments revealed that the global transcriptome of PBMCs from patients with positive LS-OCMBs is different from those patients with negative LS-OCMB status.

RNA-seq results reveal that there are 124 circRNAs and 2441 linear RNAs differentially expressed between the two groups. Interestingly, 58% of linear RNAs are detected only in one of the groups, highlighting that there is a specific expression pattern in PBMCs from patients with different LS-OCMB status. It is true; however, that our RNA-seq sample size is limited and these observations should be taken with care.

To the best of our knowledge, none of the circRNAs have been previously related with MS. Circ_0000478 is located in chromosome 13 and its host gene is von Willebrand factor A domain containing 8 (*VWA8*). Interestingly, the linear transcript of this gene is also among the differentially expressed linear RNAs in our dataset, having a fold-change of −3.23 ($p = 0.047$). This transcript has been recently described and codes a mitochondrial protein with still uncertain function [32]. Regarding circ_0116639, it is located in chromosome 22, overlapping the *EP300* gene. EP300 is a histone acetyltransferase, which is detected in our study but is not differentially expressed. These differences in expression patterns of the circRNA with their host genes reveals that the biogenesis of circRNAs is independently regulated from that of their host genes, as it has been previously described [33].

Of note, interferon regulatory factor 5 (*IRF5*) is one of the confirmed downregulated transcripts, and polymorphisms in this gene has been associated to the risk of developing MS in last genome-wide association analysis, performed by the International Multiple Sclerosis Genetics Consortium, as well as in replication studies in Spanish cohorts [34,35]. Additionally, SNPs in this gene have been related to increased levels of CXCL13 in CSF, a chemokine related to highly active disease [36]. On top of that, it has been shown in animal models that IRF5 is related with the microglial polarization towards a pro-inflammatory state (M1) in response to stroke and in Alzheimer's disease [37,38]. This could suggest microglial implication in a more aggressive disease course, as it has been suggested by other authors in a exome sequencing project [39]. Nonetheless, our findings are made in peripheral PBMCs, so the *IRF5* source might be peripheral monocytes or macrophages. In any case, further research is needed to uncover *IRF5* implication in a highly active MS disease course.

On the other hand, MT-RNR2 like 8 transcript (*MTRNR2L8*), the other validated linear transcript showing lower expression in the LS-OCMB+ group, is coded in chromosome 11, and, interestingly, it spans the location of the miR-4485 stem-loop location, one of the four miRNAs selected for validation in the present study. According to microarray data, miR-4485 is downregulated in LS-OCMB+ groups, as it is *MTRNR2L8*. The fact that *MTRNR2L8* is a host gene for mir-4485 may explain that both transcripts appear downregulated in this group of patients, even if the miRNA could not have been validated. These results point at a possible interaction between these two RNAs that might be related to a more active disease, but further research is needed to confirm this hypothesis. According to UniProt, MTRNR2L8 has a role as a neuroprotective and antiapoptotic factor and it has been found to be increased in a specific area of the brain from patients with major depressive disorder [40]. Although the function of this gene is still unclear, the possible role as a neuroprotective factor is very interesting in the case of MS, since we find this gene downregulated in PBMCs. But again, further studies should be conducted to uncover the possible link between *MTRNR2L8* expression in peripheral blood and disease activity, as well as the mechanisms underlying this relationship.

Gene overrepresentation test shows that biological processes related to complement activation, humoral immune response and type I interferon response are among the most enriched term. Of note, intrathecal synthesis of IgM antibodies has previously been correlated with intrathecal complement activation [41], and its role in demyelination and axonal damage has been clearly demonstrated [42]. Interestingly, different components of the complement system have been related to MS and plasma levels of some of the components have been proposed as MS disease state biomarkers [43]. Of note, these processes are enriched among altered genes in PBMC from patients with a marker of a high activity disease. This analysis may reveal that those patients may have an altered immune response that may explain their higher disease activity, but further and other kind of studies will be needed to explore this hypothesis.

The main aim of this study was to identify in blood a biomarker or a group of them that could differentiate between positive and negative LS-OCMB patients, thus could be used as a more accessible marker of highly active disease. ROC curve analysis revealed that these markers in combination have around 70% of accuracy, which is considered, in general, an acceptable performance [44]. Taking into account that these are measured in blood, they may help in the clinics to perform repeated measurements, while taking serial samples of CSF has serious drawbacks. Efforts are being made to define patients with a highly active disease course, given that their effective therapeutic window might be narrower than a more benign or less active disease form [45]. In line with this, several biomarkers have been proposed to identify individuals with aggressive disease course, such as CSF levels of neurofilament light chain, CXCL13 or CHI3L1 [46–48]. Other authors have also reported differences in non-coding transcriptome between patients with different disease activity. Quintana and colleagues studied the expression in CSF of a panel of miRNAs patients with MS with LS-OCMB characterization and patients with other neurological diseases (ONDs) [49]. They found differences in the expression of miR-30a-5p, miR-150, miR-645 and miR-191 between the OND group and the LS-OCMB+ group, but they could not find any difference between patients with positive and negative LS-OCMBs. Due to differences in the profiling platforms between their study and the present one, we are unable to check the expression of our candidate miRNA in data from Quintana and colleagues. Another study reported that serum levels of miR-24-3p correlate with disease progression index, calculated dividing EDSS value by disease duration, but the status of LS-OCMB is not measured [50]. More recently, the expression in blood of long non-coding RNAs has also been described to show the capacity of discriminating highly active MS patients from others with less active disease course, based on a age-related MS severity score [51].

All these studies highlight the need of biomarkers that are able to identify patients with highly active disease and the effort that the scientific community is doing in this direction. In addition, it is also important to have a consensus on the definition of what is an aggressive disease course, given that each study uses different parameters to measure and classify patients in each of the groups, which makes the comparison between them really challenging [52,53]. An early recognition of a patient in this group could benefit from different therapeutic advice and; therefore, the possibility to improve the long-term outcome of the disease.

Our miRNA profiling study discovered some miRNA differentially expressed between the two groups, although they have not been validated by RT-qPCR experiments. In this regard, other techniques such as droplet digital PCR (ddPCR) may help in reducing variability and discover small differences between groups. Although it has been reported that the sensitivity is not increased with ddPCR in gene expression studies, and that the performance is similar provided that the amount of starting material is enough and there are no contaminants in the reaction [54,55]. Nonetheless, it is a technique that could be considered in future validation projects aiming at definitely discarding or including those miRNAs as biomarkers for a more aggressive MS course.

5. Conclusions

In summary, we have identified two circRNAs and two linear RNAs which are downregulated in patients with positive LS-OCMB status. Our findings are important in the field of biomarkers for multiple sclerosis, given that they could contribute to the identification of patients with highly active disease. Additionally, an important advantage compared to other biomarkers is that they are detected in blood, allowing serial tests to monitor their levels, while this task is not so recommended for lumbar puncture. Future studies in larger cohorts will be needed to confirm their utility, but we consider that they may serve as a first screening tool to decide which patients should go into a lumbar puncture to confirm their LS-OCMB status.

Supplementary Materials: Supplementary materials can be found at http://www.mdpi.com/2227-9059/8/12/540/s1. Table S1: A complete list of samples and the experiment in which each of them were included. Table S2: Assays and primers used in RT-qPCR experiments. Figure S1: Agarose gel electrophoresis image of PCR product and Sanger Sequencing results showing the back-spliced junction of circRNAs.

Author Contributions: Conceptualization, D.O. (David Otaegui) and M.M.-C.; methodology, D.O. (David Otaegui), M.M.-C., L.I., T.B., D.O. (Danel Olaverri), and L.M.V.; validation, L.I. and L.S.; formal analysis, L.I., D.O. (Danel Olaverri), T.B., M.M.-C., M.E. and L.C.-F.; investigation, L.I., M.M.-C., M.E., L.C.-F.; resources, A.P., T.C.-T., M.E., L.C.-F., L.M.V. and D.O. (David Otaegui); writing—original draft preparation, L.I., D.O. (David Otaegui) and M.M.-C.; writing—review and editing, D.O. (Danel Olaverri), T.B., Á.P., T.C.-T., L.M.V.; visualization, L.I., D.O. (Danel Olaverri), M.M.-C.; supervision, D.O. (David Otaegui), L.I., M.M.-C. and L.M.V.; project administration, D.O. (David Otaegui) and M.M.-C.; funding acquisition, L.M.V., D.O. (David Otaegui) and M.M.-C. All authors have read and agreed to the published version of the manuscript.

Funding: This research was funded by Instituto de Salud Carlos III (PI17/00189 and PI15/00513), Red Española de Esclerosis Múltiple (REEM) (RD16/0015/0007 and RD16/0015/0001), Diputación Foral de Gipuzkoa (109/18) and the Basque Government (PRE_2019_2_0206) and ELKARTEK program.

Acknowledgments: Authors want to acknowledge the staff of Genomic Platform at Biodonostia Health Research Institute.

Conflicts of Interest: The authors declare no conflict of interest. The funders had no role in the design of the study; in the collection, analyses, or interpretation of data; in the writing of the manuscript, or in the decision to publish the results.

References

1. Filippi, M.; Bar-Or, A.; Piehl, F.; Preziosa, P.; Solari, A.; Vukusic, S.; Rocca, M.A. Multiple sclerosis. *Nat. Rev. Dis. Prim.* **2018**, *4*, 1–27. [CrossRef] [PubMed]

2. Comabella, M.; Montalban, X. Body fluid biomarkers in multiple sclerosis. *Lancet Neurol.* **2014**, *13*, 113–126. [CrossRef]
3. Paul, A.; Comabella, M.; Gandhi, R. Biomarkers in Multiple Sclerosis. *Cold Spring Harb. Perspect. Med.* **2019**, *9*. [CrossRef] [PubMed]
4. Villar, L.M.; Sadaba, M.C.; Roldan, E.; Masjuan, J.; Gonzalez-Porque, P.; Villarrubia, N.; Espino, M.; Garcia-Trujillo, J.A.; Bootello, A.; Alvarez-Cermeno, J.C. Intrathecal synthesis of oligoclonal IgM against myelin lipids predicts an aggressive disease course in MS. *J. Clin. Investig.* **2005**, *115*, 187–194. [CrossRef]
5. Polivka, J.J.P., Jr.; Krakorova, K.; Peterka, M.; Topolcan, O. Current status of biomarker research in neurology. *EPMA J.* **2016**, 1–13. [CrossRef]
6. Kemppinen, A.K.; Kaprio, J.; Palotie, A.; Saarela, J. Systematic review of genome-wide expression studies in multiple sclerosis. *BMJ Open* **2011**, *1*, e000053. [CrossRef]
7. Nickles, D.; Chen, H.P.; Li, M.M.; Khankhanian, P.; Madireddy, L.; Caillier, S.J.; Santaniello, A.; Cree, B.A.; Pelletier, D.; Hauser, S.L.; et al. Blood RNA profiling in a large cohort of multiple sclerosis patients and healthy controls. *Hum. Mol. Genet.* **2013**, *22*, 4194–4205. [CrossRef] [PubMed]
8. Irizar, H.; Muñoz-Culla, M.; Sáenz-Cuesta, M.; Osorio-Querejeta, I.; Sepúlveda, L.; Castillo-Triviño, T.; Prada, A.; Lopez de Munain, A.; Olascoaga, J.; Otaegui, D. Identification of ncRNAs as potential therapeutic targets in multiple sclerosis through differential ncRNA—mRNA network analysis. *BMC Genom.* **2015**, *16*, 250. [CrossRef] [PubMed]
9. Dolati, S.; Marofi, F.; Babaloo, Z.; Aghebati-Maleki, L.; Roshangar, L.; Ahmadi, M.; Rikhtegar, R.; Yousefi, M. Dysregulated Network of miRNAs Involved in the Pathogenesis of Multiple Sclerosis. *Biomed. Pharmacother.* **2018**, *104*, 280–290. [CrossRef]
10. Du, C.; Liu, C.; Kang, J.; Zhao, G.; Ye, Z.; Huang, S.; Li, Z.; Wu, Z.; Pei, G.; Du, C.; et al. MicroRNA miR-326 regulates T H -17 differentiation and is associated with the pathogenesis of multiple sclerosis. *Nat. Immunol.* **2009**, *1259*, 1252–1259. [CrossRef] [PubMed]
11. Muñoz-Culla, M.; Irizar, H.; Sáenz-Cuesta, M.; Castillo-Triviño, T.; Osorio-Querejeta, I.; Sepúlveda, L.; López De Munain, A.; Olascoaga, J.; Otaegui, D. SncRNA (microRNA &snoRNA) opposite expression pattern found in multiple sclerosis relapse and remission is sex dependent. *Sci. Rep.* **2016**, *6*. [CrossRef]
12. De Felice, B.; Mondola, P.; Sasso, A.; Orefice, G.; Bresciamorra, V.; Vacca, G.; Biffali, E.; Borra, M.; Pannone, R. Small non-coding RNA signature in multiple sclerosis patients after treatment with interferon-β. *BMC Med. Genom.* **2014**, *7*, 1–9. [CrossRef] [PubMed]
13. Jonas, S.; Izaurralde, E. Towards a molecular understanding of microRNA-mediated gene silencing. *Nat. Rev. Genet.* **2015**, *16*, 421–433. [CrossRef]
14. Floris, G.; Zhang, L.; Follesa, P.; Sun, T. Regulatory Role of Circular RNAs and Neurological Disorders. *Mol. Neurobiol.* **2017**, *54*, 5156–5165. [CrossRef]
15. Xia, X.; Tang, X.; Wang, S. Roles of CircRNAs in Autoimmune Diseases. *Front. Immunol.* **2019**, *10*, 1–8. [CrossRef] [PubMed]
16. Paraboschi, E.M.; Cardamone, G.; Soldà, G.; Duga, S.; Asselta, R. Interpreting Non-coding Genetic Variation in Multiple Sclerosis Genome-Wide Associated Regions. *Front. Genet.* **2018**, *9*, 1–10. [CrossRef]
17. Cardamone, G.; Paraboschi, E.M.; Rimoldi, V.; Duga, S.; Soldà, G.; Asselta, R. The Characterization of GSDMB Splicing and Backsplicing Profiles Identifies Novel Isoforms and a Circular RNA That Are Dysregulated in Multiple Sclerosis. *Int. J. Mol. Sci.* **2017**, *18*, 576. [CrossRef]
18. Iparraguirre, L.; Muñoz-Culla, M.; Prada-Luengo, I.; Castillo-Triviño, T.; Olascoaga, J.; Otaegui, D. Circular RNA profiling reveals that circular RNAs from ANXA2 can be used as new biomarkers for multiple sclerosis. *Hum. Mol. Genet.* **2017**, *26*. [CrossRef]
19. Kacperska, M.J.; Walenczak, J.; Tomasik, B. Plasmatic microRNA as potential biomarkers of multiple sclerosis: Literature review. *Adv. Clin. Exp. Med.* **2016**, *25*, 775–779. [CrossRef]
20. Stoicea, N.; Du, A.; Lakis, D.C.; Tipton, C.; Arias-Morales, C.E.; Bergese, S.D. The MiRNA Journey from Theory to Practice as a CNS Biomarker. *Front. Genet.* **2016**, *7*, 1–8. [CrossRef]
21. Zhang, Z.; Yang, T.; Xiao, J. Circular RNAs: Promising Biomarkers for Human Diseases. *EBioMedicine* **2018**, *34*, 267–274. [CrossRef] [PubMed]
22. Villar, L.M.; González-Porqué, P.; Masjuán, J.; Álvarez-Cermeño, J.; Bootello, A.; Keir, G. A sensitive and reproducible method for the detection of oligoclonal IgM bands. *J. Immunol. Methods* **2001**, *258*, 151–155. [CrossRef]

23. Kent, W.J.; Sugnet, C.W.; Furey, T.S.; Roskin, K.M.; Pringle, T.H.; Zahler, A.M.; Haussler, A.D. The Human Genome Browser at UCSC. *Genome Res.* **2002**, *12*, 996–1006. [CrossRef] [PubMed]
24. Dobin, A.; Davis, C.A.; Schlesinger, F.; Drenkow, J.; Zaleski, C.; Jha, S.; Batut, P.; Chaisson, M.; Gingeras, T.R. STAR: Ultrafast universal RNA-seq aligner. *Bioinformatics* **2013**, *29*, 15–21. [CrossRef]
25. Li, H.; Durbin, R. Fast and accurate short read alignment with Burrows—Wheeler transform. *Bioinformatics* **2009**, *25*, 1754–1760. [CrossRef]
26. Zhang, X.; Dong, R.; Zhang, Y.; Zhang, J.; Luo, Z.; Zhang, J.; Chen, L.; Yang, L. Diverse alternative back-splicing and alternative splicing landscape of circular RNAs. *Genome Res.* **2016**, *26*, 1277–1287. [CrossRef]
27. Gao, Y.; Zhang, J.; Zhao, F. Circular RNA identification based on multiple seed matching. *Brief. Bioinform.* **2017**, 1–8. [CrossRef]
28. Hansen, T.B. Improved circRNA Identification by Combining Prediction Algorithms. *Front. Cell Dev. Biol.* **2018**, *6*, 1–9. [CrossRef]
29. Love, M.I.; Huber, W.; Anders, S. Moderated estimation of fold change and dispersion for RNA-seq data with DESeq2. *Genome Biol.* **2014**, *15*, 1–21. [CrossRef]
30. Bray, N.L.; Pimentel, H.; Melsted, P.; Pachter, L. Near-optimal probabilistic RNA-seq quantification. *Nat. Biotechnol.* **2016**, *34*, 525–528. [CrossRef]
31. Mi, H.; Thomas, P. PANTHER Pathway: An ontology-based pathway database coupled with data analysis tools. *Nat. Protoc.* **2019**, *14*, 703–721. [CrossRef] [PubMed]
32. Luo, M.; Ma, W.; Sand, Z.; Finlayson, J.; Wang, T.; Diaz, R.; Willis, W.T.; Mandarino, L.J. Von Willebrand factor A domain-containing protein 8 (VWA8) localizes to the matrix side of the inner mitochondrial membrane. *Biochem. Biophys. Res. Commun.* **2020**, *521*, 158–163. [CrossRef]
33. Moldovan, L.I.; Hansen, T.B.; Venø, M.T.; Okholm, T.L.H.; Andersen, T.L.; Hager, H.; Iversen, L.; Kjems, J.; Johansen, C.; Kristensen, L.S. High-throughput RNA sequencing from paired lesional- and non-lesional skin reveals major alterations in the psoriasis circRNAome. *BMC Med. Genom.* **2019**, *12*, 1–17. [CrossRef] [PubMed]
34. International Multiple Sclerosis Genetics Consortium. The Multiple Sclerosis Genomic Map implicates peripheral immune cells and microglia in susceptibility. *Science* **2019**, *365*, 1–10. [CrossRef]
35. Vandenbroeck, K.; Alloza, I.; Swaminathan, B.; Antiguedad, A.; Otaegui, D.; Olascoaga, J.; Barcina, M.G.; de las Heras, V.; Bartolome, M.; Fernandez-Arquero, M.; et al. Validation of IRF5 as multiple sclerosis risk gene: Putative role in interferon beta therapy and human herpes virus-6 infection. *Genes Immun.* **2011**, *12*, 40–45. [CrossRef]
36. Lindén, M.; Khademi, M.; Bomfim, I.L.; Piehl, F.; Jagodic, M.; Kockum, I.; Olsson, T. Multiple sclerosis risk genotypes correlate with an elevated cerebrospinal fluid level of the suggested prognostic marker CXCL13. *Mult. Scler. Jounrla* **2012**, *19*, 863–870. [CrossRef]
37. Al Mamun, A.; Chauhan, A.; Yu, H.; Xu, Y.; Sharmeen, R.; Liu, F. Interferon regulatory factor 4/5 signaling impacts on microglial activation after ischemic stroke in mice. *Eur. J. Neurosci.* **2018**, *47*, 140–149. [CrossRef]
38. Zhu, D.; Yang, N.; Liu, Y.-Y.; Zheng, J.; Ji, C.; Zuo, P.-P. M2 Macrophage Transplantation Ameliorates Cognitive Dysfunction in Amyloid-β-Treated Rats Through Regulation of Microglial Polarization. *J. Alzheimer's Dis.* **2016**, *52*, 483–495. [CrossRef]
39. Gil-Varea, E.; Urcelay, E.; Vilariño-Güell, C.; Costa, C.; Midaglia, L.; Matesanz, F.; Rodríguez-antigüedad, A.; Oksenberg, J.; Espino-paisan, L.; Sadovnick, A.D.; et al. Exome sequencing study in patients with multiple sclerosis reveals variants associated with disease course. *J. Neuroinflamm.* **2018**, *15*, 1–10. [CrossRef]
40. Pantazatos, S.P.; Huang, Y.-Y.; Rosoklija, G.B.; Dwork, A.J.; Arango, V.; Mann, J.J. Whole-transcriptome brain expression and exon-usage profiling in major depression and suicide: Evidence for altered glial, endothelial and ATPase activity. *Mol. Psychiatry* **2017**, *22*, 760–773. [CrossRef]
41. Sellebjerg, F.; Christiansen, M.; Garred, P. MBP, anti-MBP and anti-PLP antibodies, and intrathecal complement activation in multiple sclerosis. *Mult. Scler.* **1998**, *4*, 127–131. [CrossRef] [PubMed]
42. Mead, R.J.; Singhrao, S.K.; Neal, J.W.; Lassmann, H.; Morgan, B.P. The Membrane Attack Complex of Complement Causes Severe Demyelination Associated with Acute Axonal Injury. *J. Immunol.* **2002**, *168*, 458–465. [CrossRef] [PubMed]
43. Ingram, G.; Hakobyan, S.; Hirst, C.L.; Harris, C.L.; Loveless, S.; Mitchell, J.P.; Pickersgill, T.P.; Robertson, N.P.; Morgan, B.P. Systemic complement profiling in multiple sclerosis as a biomarker of disease state. *Mult. Scler. J.* **2012**, *18*, 1401–1411. [CrossRef] [PubMed]

44. Mandrekar, J.N. Receiver Operating Characteristic Curve in Diagnostic Test Assessment. *J. Thorac. Oncol.* **2010**, *5*, 1315–1316. [CrossRef] [PubMed]
45. Iacobaeus, E.; Ryschkewitsch, C.; Gravell, M.; Khademi, M.; Wallstrom, E.; Olsson, T.; Brundin, L.; Major, E. Analysis of cerebrospinal fluid and cerebrospinal fluid cells from patients with multiple sclerosis for detection of JC virus DNA. *Mult. Scler. J.* **2009**, *15*, 28–35. [CrossRef]
46. Håkansson, I.; Tisell, A.; Cassel, P.; Blennow, K.; Zetterberg, H.; Lundberg, P.; Dahle, C.; Vrethem, M.; Ernerudh, J. Neurofilament levels, disease activity and brain volume during follow-up in multiple sclerosis. *J. Neuroinflamm.* **2018**, *15*, 1–10. [CrossRef]
47. Khademi, M.; Kockum, I.; Andersson, M.L.; Iacobaeus, E.; Brundin, L.; Sellebjerg, F.; Hillert, J.; Piehl, F.; Olsson, T. Cerebrospinal fluid CXCL13 in multiple sclerosis: A suggestive prognostic marker for the disease course. *Mult. Scler. J.* **2011**, *17*, 335–343. [CrossRef]
48. Cantó, E.; Tintore, M.; Villar, L.M.; Costa, C.; Nurtdinov, R.; Deisenhammer, F.; Hegen, H.; Khademi, M.; Olsson, T.; Piehl, F.; et al. Chitinase 3-like 1: Prognostic biomarker in clinically isolated syndromes. *Brain* **2015**, *138*, 918–931. [CrossRef]
49. Quintana, E.; Ortega, F.J.; Robles-Cedeño, R.; Villar, M.L.; Buxó, M.; Mercader, J.M.; Alvarez-Cermeño, J.C.; Pueyo, N.; Perkal, H.; Fernández-Real, J.M.; et al. miRNAs in cerebrospinal fluid identify patients with MS and specifically those with lipid-specific oligoclonal IgM bands. *Mult. Scler. J.* **2017**, *23*, 1716–1726. [CrossRef]
50. Vistbakka, J.; Sumelahti, M.; Lehtimäki, T.; Elovaara, I.; Hagman, S. Evaluation of serum miR-191-5p, miR-24-3p, miR-128-3p and miR-376c-3 in multiple sclerosis patients. *Acta Neurol. Scand.* **2018**, 1–7. [CrossRef]
51. Gupta, M.; Martens, K.; Metz, L.M.; Jason, A.P.; Koning, D.; Pfeffer, G. Long noncoding RNAs associated with phenotypic severity in multiple sclerosis. *Mult. Scler. Relat. Disord.* **2019**, *36*, 101407. [CrossRef] [PubMed]
52. Iacobaeus, E.; Arrambide, G.; Amato, M.P.; Derfuss, T.; Vukusic, S.; Hemmer, B.; Tintore, M. Aggressive multiple sclerosis (1): Towards a definition of the phenotype. *Mult. Scler. J.* **2020**, 1031–1044. [CrossRef] [PubMed]
53. Díaz, C.; Zarco, L.A.; Rivera, D.M. Highly active multiple sclerosis: An update. *Mult. Scler. Relat. Disord.* **2019**, *30*, 215–224. [CrossRef]
54. Hindson, C.M.; Chevillet, J.R.; Briggs, H.A.; Gallichotte, E.N.; Ruf, I.K.; Hindson, B.J.; Vessella, R.L.; Tewari, M. Absolute quantification by droplet digital PCR versus analog real-time PCR. *Nat. Methods* **2013**, 1–6. [CrossRef]
55. Taylor, S.C.; Laperriere, G.; Germain, H. Droplet Digital PCR versus qPCR for gene expression analysis with low abundant targets: From variable nonsense to publication quality data. *Sci. Rep.* **2017**, 1–8. [CrossRef] [PubMed]

Publisher's Note: MDPI stays neutral with regard to jurisdictional claims in published maps and institutional affiliations.

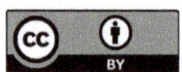

© 2020 by the authors. Licensee MDPI, Basel, Switzerland. This article is an open access article distributed under the terms and conditions of the Creative Commons Attribution (CC BY) license (http://creativecommons.org/licenses/by/4.0/).

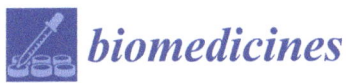

Review

Current Advances in Pediatric Onset Multiple Sclerosis

Kristen S. Fisher [1], Fernando X. Cuascut [2], Victor M. Rivera [2] and George J. Hutton [2],*

1. Baylor College of Medicine, Texas Children's Hospital, Houston, TX 77030, USA; kristen.fisher@bcm.edu
2. Baylor College of Medicine, Maxine Mesinger Multiple Sclerosis Center, Houston, TX 77030, USA; fernando.cuascut@bcm.edu (F.X.C.); vrivera@bcm.edu (V.M.R.)
* Correspondence: ghutton@bcm.edu; Tel.: +1-713-798-2273

Received: 10 March 2020; Accepted: 26 March 2020; Published: 28 March 2020

Abstract: Multiple sclerosis (MS) is an autoimmune inflammatory disease affecting the central nervous system leading to demyelination. MS in the pediatric population is rare, but has been shown to lead to significant disability over the duration of the disease. As we have learned more about pediatric MS, there has been a development of improved diagnostic criteria leading to earlier diagnosis, earlier initiation of disease-modifying therapies (DMT), and an increasing number of DMT used in the treatment of pediatric MS. Over time, treatment with DMT has trended towards the initiation of higher efficacy treatment at time of diagnosis to help prevent further disease progression and accrual of disability over time, and there is evidence in current literature that supports this change in treatment patterns. In this review, we discuss the current knowledge in diagnosis, treatment, and clinical outcomes in pediatric MS.

Keywords: multiple sclerosis; pediatric multiple sclerosis; neuroimmunology; demyelinating disease; pediatric neurology; child neurology

1. Introduction

Multiple sclerosis (MS) is a chronic autoimmune disease of the central nervous system resulting in inflammation and demyelination in the brain and spinal cord. Although it is most commonly seen in adults, between 3–5% of patients have an onset of disease under the age of 18, and less than 2% of patients under 10 years of age [1–4]. Pediatric MS is rare, much less common than adult MS. The incidence of pediatric MS has been reported in ranges of 0.13 to 0.6 cases per 100,000 children per year [5]. Due to this, there have been fewer research, publications, and natural history data on pediatric MS. With the development of the International Pediatric MS Study Group (IPMSSG) in 2005, the knowledge base surrounding pediatric MS has increased. While the pathophysiology of the disease in the pediatric population is in line with that of the adult population, there are different challenges in the diagnosis, treatment, disease course, and clinical outcomes. In this review, we discuss the currently known environmental and genetic risk factors of pediatric MS, varying clinical presentations, diagnostic criteria and differential diagnoses, diagnostic evaluations, current treatment options, cognitive impairments and psychiatric comorbidity, disease course, and outcomes.

2. Epidemiology

In the pediatric MS population diagnosed before puberty, the number of males and females diagnosed is relatively equivalent [6,7]. In adolescents, the ratio of females to males with MS increases to 2 to 3:1, which may suggest that the onset of menarche plays some role in the pathogenesis of MS [6]. Additionally, the prevalence of MS increases after age 10 [8]. A diverse racial and ethnic population are diagnosed with pediatric MS, one study reporting 67% self-identifying as white and 20.6% as African

American [9]. In this cohort, 30.2% identified as Hispanic, while other cohorts have reported up to 52% of pediatric patients with MS or CIS as Hispanic [9,10]. There has been a significant link to the role of obesity in MS and it has been shown that adolescent obesity is a risk factor for pediatric MS [11]. Not only was adolescent obesity a risk to develop MS, but one study found that in pediatric MS, obesity was present in early childhood years [12]. Obesity has been shown to promote an inflammatory state, which could contribute to not only the pathogenesis of MS, but could also play a role in the risk of relapse and long-term management. A retrospective cohort study performed comparing pediatric MS patients who were obese vs. those with normal BMI showed that obese patients had statistically significant higher relapse rates on first-line treatments, and higher relapse rates on second-line treatments [13]. Low levels of vitamin D have been associated with an increased risk of pediatric MS and with increased rates of relapse [14,15]. In the adult population it has been shown that there is an increased risk of MS in those who smoke cigarettes, and coinciding with this, children who are exposed to smoking in the home have been shown to be more likely to develop pediatric MS than a control population [16,17]. Epstein-Barr virus (EBV) may play a role in pathogenesis and risk of MS and pediatric MS, although the mechanism remains unclear at this time [15,18]. Historically, a correlation between EBV and MS was proposed due to the similarities in the epidemiology of the diseases, and studies have shown a strong correlation in support of this [19]. EBV infection can occur at any age, and is generally asymptomatic in young children. The presence of MS-mimics such as Neuromyelitis Optica Spectrum Disorder (NMOSD) and anti-myelin oligodendrocyte antibody syndrome, may contribute to a higher frequency of EBV seronegative- antibody children diagnosed with MS. One of the main genetic risk factors found in pediatric MS is HLA DRB1*1501 [20,21]. HLA DRB1*1501 is additionally seen as a genetic risk factor in adult MS, and postulated to be associated with earlier age of onset in the adult population, although there has been varying evidence in support of this, and thus at this time cannot be attributed to age of onset. The HLA class II proteins play a role in cell-mediated immunity, leading to the suspicion that it could be a genetic marker or predisposition to developing MS [22]. There are 57 previously identified single nucleotide polymorphisms that have been associated with adult-onset MS that have also been identified in a large cohort of children with demyelinating diseases and found to be associated with increased risk of pediatric-onset MS [23]. One recently published cohort identified 32% of patients with at least one relative with MS [22], with a report of incidence in a first-degree relative of 2–5% [24]. In monozygotic twins, a concordance rate of 27% is reported vs. dizygotic twins with a rate of 2.3% [24]. There have been numerous correlated factors in pediatric MS, and likely more that have yet to be determined. Many of these factors also overlap, and more studies are needed in order to determine if there are additional genetic etiologies that may lead to a predisposition to development of pediatric MS in the context of certain environmental factors.

3. Clinical Presentation

In a subset of patients at the initial presentation of a demyelinating event, a diagnosis of pediatric MS can be made. Younger children will often present with multifocal symptoms, but entering adolescence it becomes more common to present with single focal symptoms more similar to that of adults [25,26]. The most commonly reported symptoms in children include sensory (15–30%), motor (30%), and brainstem dysfunction (25–41%) [27]. The clinical course in 95–98% of pediatric MS patients is relapsing remitting, compared to 85–90% in adults [27–29]. Less than 3% of pediatric MS cases are reported as primary progressive, compared to 10–15% in the adult population [28–30]. In children with a progressive course, other diagnoses should be considered. Children have been reported to have a higher relapse rate compared to adult-onset MS, especially within the first few years of diagnosis [31,32]. Studies have reported 2.3–2.8 times higher relapse rate in pediatric MS, and higher rates of relapse early in the disease if without treatment or on lower efficacy treatment [32–34]. These findings suggest that those with pediatric MS have a more significant inflammatory component than those with adult-onset MS [32]. Due to these factors, more recent treatment has trended toward initiation with higher efficacy medications at time of diagnosis to help target this increased inflammatory state, decrease relapse rate, and prevent accrual of disability.

4. Diagnosis

To make the diagnosis of MS, at least one clinical event with symptoms lasting at least 24 h must be present. Dissemination in space is the development of lesions in distinct regions of the CNS, including periventricular, cortical or juxtacortical, infratentorial brain regions, and the spinal cord [35]. Dissemination in time is demonstrated by the presence of enhancing and non-enhancing lesions at any time, or by new T2 hyperintense lesions on follow up MRI [35]. In 2007, the IPMSSG created a consensus definition for pediatric MS, which was updated in 2012 following the publication of the revised 2010 McDonald criteria for the diagnosis of MS [36]. Per the IPMSSG, pediatric MS has been defined by occurrence of any of the following [37]:

1. Two or more clinically isolated syndromes (CIS) separated by greater than 30 days involving multiple areas of the CNS;
2. One CIS associated with MRI findings consistent with dissemination in space and a follow up MRI showing at least one new lesion consistent with dissemination in time;
3. One acute disseminated encephalomyelitis (ADEM) attack followed by 1 CIS more than 3 months after symptom onset with new MRI findings consistent with dissemination in space;
4. CIS with MRI findings consistent with dissemination in time and space if the patient is at least 12 years of age.

In children with acute demyelinating attacks consistent with MS, the 2010 McDonald criteria have been studied and shown to have high sensitivity, specificity, and positive predictive value for children at least 11 years of age [38]. The criteria have only a 55% positive predictive value in children under 11, and should not be applied to those with an ADEM presentation [38]. More recently, the revised 2017 McDonald criteria were compared to the prior 2010 criteria in a pediatric cohort and demonstrated improvement in accuracy (87.2% vs 66.7%) and sensitivity (84.0% vs 46.8%), but the 2017 criteria remain unvalidated in children under 12 years of age [39]. Although there is improved accuracy and sensitivity with these revised criteria, there continues to be misdiagnosis due to overlapping features with numerous mimickers of MS including multiphasic ADEM, NMOSD, vasculitis and other neuroinflammatory diseases, metabolic disorders, and leukodystrophies.

In the pediatric population, there is a wide array of alternative diagnoses to be considered when evaluating a patient for possible pediatric MS. Most commonly reported indications of an alternative etiology include progressive course at disease onset, encephalopathy, fever, negative oligoclonal bands, and significantly elevated CSF white blood cells or protein [40]. Typical lesions are ovoid in shape, and are asymmetric in hemispheric involvement. Typically, lesions are located in periventricular and juxtacortical white matter, corpus callosum, pons, cerebellum and middle cerebellar peduncle, and spinal cord (more commonly the cervical cord). MRI features that could indicate a diagnosis other than pediatric MS include symmetric bilateral lesions, large gray matter involvement at the onset, DWI abnormalities, meningeal enhancement, presence of hemorrhage, prolonged period of contrast enhancement, and presence of edema or mass effect [40]. If the MRI and clinical presentation fall within the criteria for diagnosis, in general, lumbar puncture may not be required to aid in diagnosis; however, lumbar puncture for CSF analysis should be considered in those with atypical presentations. As there are limitations in current diagnostic criteria, evaluation for other mimics of pediatric MS, should be assessed at time of presentation with Aquaporin-4 and anti-MOG antibodies. Anti-MOG antibody can also be present in monophasic and multiphasic ADEM, which differ from MS and NMOSD in prognosis and management. Other studies to be performed at time of presentation may include (if indicated per clinical judgement) the C-reactive protein, erythrocyte sedimentation rate, anti-nuclear antibody, angiotensin-converting enzyme level, folate, vitamin B12, and thyroid-stimulating hormone. Those with a progressive course should be evaluated for mitochondrial, metabolic, and neurodegenerative disorders including leukodystrophies. Other considerations include other autoimmune conditions, including systemic lupus erythematosus, neurosarcoidosis, or Sjogren syndrome.

Clinically Isolated Syndrome (CIS) in pediatrics has been defined by the IPMSSG as a monofocal or polyfocal CNS event of presumed inflammatory/demyelinating cause in a child without encephalopathy and no prior history of CNS demyelination. The MRI should not meet the criteria for MS diagnosis, with both dissemination in time and space absent. Optic neuritis is the most common CIS presentation in pediatrics, followed by transverse myelitis and brainstem syndromes [41]. In a cohort of 770 patients with pediatric CIS who were followed for 10 years to assess the risk of conversion to MS, female gender and multifocal symptoms at onset were risk factors for the occurrence of a second attack [42]. In pediatric optic neuritis, rates of conversion to MS range from 13.8–32% [43,44]. There has been a higher risk of conversion to MS reported in those with abnormal brain MRI at the onset of optic neuritis, bilateral optic neuritis, and those with recurrent optic neuritis [43–45]. Transverse myelitis, similarly, is typically a monophasic disorder. Reported risk factors for relapse of pediatric transverse myelitis include female gender and abnormal brain MRI, which is consistent with that reported in adult studies [46].

Acute disseminated encephalomyelitis (ADEM) is most commonly a monophasic demyelinating disease preceded by viral infection or vaccination. Patients typically present with multifocal symptoms and encephalopathy, and seizures can also be present. MRI findings play a large role in the differentiation of ADEM from MS: diffuse bilateral lesions with ill-defined borders are more commonly seen in ADEM [47]. Susceptibility weighted imaging has been used in the identification of multiple sclerosis, but also has been looked at as a possible tool in helping differentiate ADEM and MS [48]. In patients with multiphasic ADEM, anti-myelin oligodendrocyte glycoprotein (MOG) antibodies can be evaluated to help differentiate from MS. Anti-MOG associated disorders can present as optic neuritis, monophasic ADEM or a neuromyelitis optica spectrum disorder (NMOSD). While some patients with anti-MOG associated disorders will respond to an initial course of steroids, some will require longer-term immunomodulation [49].

Most commonly, patients with NMOSD present with transverse myelitis and optic neuritis. MRI findings are used in differentiating pediatric MS from NMOSD. Patients with NMOSD can have brain MRI abnormalities, most commonly reported in the diencephalic region, dorsal medulla (area postrema), and peri-ependymal circumventricular areas. Typical characteristics of optic nerve lesions in NMOSD include involvement of the optic chiasm and lesions extending greater than half the length of the optic nerve [50]. In NMOSD, spinal cord lesions extend at least three vertebral segments, which is seen in 10% of patients with pediatric MS [47]. Additionally, it has been seen that contrast enhancement in spinal cord lesions in NMO display a rim-enhancement as compared to MS where more uniform enhancement is seen [51]. Due to selective involvement in the area postrema, 38% of pediatric NMO patients present with vomiting [52]. CSF can display significant pleocytosis with neutrophilic or lymphocytic predominance, and oligoclonal bands are less frequently seen than in MS [53,54].

5. Diagnostic Evaluations

MRI is an important tool in pediatric MS and aids in the diagnosis. MRI findings are used for the assessment of dissemination in time and space. Spinal cord imaging typically shows cervical cord lesions, short segment lesions (< 3 vertebral segments in length) that involve only a portion of the diameter of the cord [55]. While MRI brain and spine are the most valuable test in supporting the diagnosis of MS, the MRI spine may be less useful in the diagnosis of pediatric MS, with one study only showing 10% of patients meeting the criteria of dissemination in time and space based on the addition of MRI spine [56]. Based on the initial MRI, pediatric MS patients show a higher number of T2 lesions than adults and more frequently have cerebellar and brainstem involvement [57]. Additionally, pediatric patients have lesions that are larger and more ill-defined [58]. The presence of at least one periventricular white matter lesion and at least one T1 hypointensity on initial MRI can predict progression to MS at the time of presentation [59].

Cerebrospinal fluid (CSF) pleocytosis is present in 53–66% of patients, with cell count reported as high as 61 [60,61]. A lymphocytic predominance is more commonly seen, but in children under 11 years of age, an elevated neutrophil count may be seen [8]. The presence of oligoclonal bands in the CSF is significant for ongoing neuroinflammation and has been reported in numerous CNS inflammatory conditions, including pediatric and adult MS. The presence of oligoclonal IgG bands in the CSF has been reported in 64% to 92% of pediatric MS patients, and is seen to be less frequent in younger children [60]. Oligoclonal bands in the CSF can be used to aid in the diagnosis of pediatric MS. In children aged 12–17 years old with clinical suspicion of MS, the presence of oligoclonal bands strongly supports a diagnosis [62]. In patients with a pediatric radiologically isolated syndrome, the presence of oligoclonal bands increases the specificity of MRI criteria, and can help in predicting conversion to MS [63]. It is important to note that while oligoclonal bands can be used to make the diagnosis of pediatric MS, other conditions that are classified as mimickers of pediatric MS can also have a presence of oligoclonal bands, thus, this presence does not eliminate other diagnoses.

6. Treatment Options

The primary goal of treatment with disease modifying therapy is to achieve a state of no evidence of clinical or radiographic disease activity. No evidence of disease activity (NEDA) is characterized by the absence of clinical relapses, no progression of clinical disability, no new or enlarging T2 lesions on MRI, and no contrast-enhancing lesions on MRI [64]. There are varying approaches to disease modifying therapy, including an escalation or "step-up" vs. an induction or "step-down" approach [6]. The first approach involves starting with what is considered to be first-line therapy, and escalating treatment if the patient were to have evidence of clinical relapse or interval development of new demyelinating lesions on MRI despite patient compliance with the medication and adequate duration of treatment [6]. The second involves using the more efficacious treatments first to induce a state of no evidence of disease activity. At this time, fingolimod is the only FDA approved treatment for pediatric MS, but other treatments, including interferons, glatiramer acetate, dimethyl fumarate, teriflunomide, natalizumab, rituximab, and cyclophosphamide, have been used and reports have shown the benefits of these treatments. Currently, consensus statements suggest first-line therapies as interferons or glatiramer acetate, but more recent studies have led to a discussion of the need for revision of these guidelines in light of studies showing that a large number of patients on injectable therapies require escalation of therapy [65,66]. Additionally, there is no standard definition of treatment failure across treatment centers, and with this, no guidelines for the transition of medications. The IPMSSG has proposed definitions for breakthrough disease, including an increase or no reduction in relapse rate, development of new T2 or contrast-enhancing lesions on MRI, or two or greater clinical or MRI relapses within 12 months [67]. Some children achieve a state of NEDA on first-line medications, but some require a transition of medications due to the breakthrough of disease, while other patients may change medications due to poor tolerance or non-compliance.

Interferons in injectable formulations along with glatiramer acetate are commonly used first-line treatments in pediatric MS as has been displayed with observational studies [68]. Interferons are well tolerated, with 25–35% of children reporting flu-like symptoms [69,70]. To mitigate adverse effects, the dose can be titrated over 4 weeks until reaching full dose, and pretreatment with analgesics is recommended. Regulatory laboratory monitoring is required as interferon beta can result in elevation of liver transaminases, thyroid function abnormalities and decreased peripheral blood cell counts [69–72]. Interferons should be used with caution in children with a known history of depression as there have been reported mood side effects [6]. In 44 pediatric MS patients treated with interferon-beta-1b, no serious adverse events were reported [70]. In a retrospective study named REPLAY, adult doses of interferon beta-1a were tolerated without adverse reactions in pediatric MS [69].

Glatiramer acetate is a synthetic amino acid polymer that resembles myelin basic protein, which is delivered via subcutaneous injection. Retrospective studies have shown reduction of annualized relapse rate (ARR) similar to those of the adult trials ranging from 0.2–0.25 [73,74]. In the pediatric population, full adult dosing is used and generally well-tolerated [75]. The most commonly reported side effect are injection site reactions. Rarely, an immediate post-injection systemic reaction occurs with flushing, chest pain, palpitations, and shortness of breath, but this usually self-resolves. Regular laboratory monitoring is not required. As interferons and glatiramer acetate are generally well tolerated and shown to decrease relapse rates in retrospective studies, they were commonly used as first line treatments until the more recent development and introduction of newer treatment options.

Fingolimod, a once-daily oral medication, was approved by the FDA in 2018 as a first-line treatment in pediatric MS based on the results of the PARADIGMS trial. Fingolimod binds to sphingosine-1-phosphate receptors, sequestering lymphocytes in the lymph node and prevents activated lymphocytes from crossing into the CNS. In pediatric MS, an 82% reduction in annualized relapse rate in comparison to those treated with interferon beta-1a was demonstrated [76]. Additionally, over a two-year interval at all time points, patients treated with fingolimod had lower EDSS scores compared to those treated with interferon beta-1a [77]. While the PARADIGMS trial showed improved efficacy of treatment and improved EDSS at follow up with treatment with fingolimod compared to interferon beta-1a, it additionally has increased risks with treatment. The serious adverse events in the pediatric population included leukopenia and seizures. It is required that patients be monitored for bradycardia for 6 h with the first dose. Patients should be monitored for macular edema with annual ophthalmology exams, although there was only one report of macular edema in the PARADIGMS trial [76]. Routine laboratory monitoring of liver transaminases and lymphocyte counts are recommended. Additionally, there is a risk for progressive multifocal leukoencephalopathy (PML), which has been more commonly reported in patients on fingolimod for longer duration and with positive John Cunningham Virus (JCV) antibodies. PML is an opportunistic infection of the CNS that is potentially fatal and is caused by the reactivation of latent JCV.

Dimethyl fumarate is a twice-daily oral medication that was approved by the FDA in 2013 for the treatment of MS in adults. The specific mechanism of action is unknown, but it is shown to affect cytokines and lower lymphocyte counts. Phase 3 studies in adults have shown dimethyl fumarate significantly reduces relapse rates and the development of new T2 hyperintense lesions on MRI. Common side effects include flushing, which can be abated with pretreatment with aspirin. There have been cases of PML in patients on dimethyl fumarate, all occurring in patients with lymphocyte counts under 800, thus, routine laboratory monitoring is recommended. An open-label study, FOCUS, was performed to evaluate the effect of dimethyl fumarate on MRI activity in the pediatric population, and showed a reduction in the development of new T2 hyperintense lesions [78]. While there are data showing a reduction in the breakthrough disease on MRI, there are yet to be data on the reduction of clinical relapse in the pediatric MS population. CONNECT is an open-label randomized controlled study comparing dimethyl fumarate versus interferon beta-1a in the pediatric population that is currently ongoing [79].

Teriflunomide is a once-daily oral pill that reduces the activation and proliferation of lymphocytes by inhibiting pyrimidine synthesis. In studies in the adult MS population, teriflunomide has been shown to significantly reduce the relapse rate, disability progression, and new activity on MRI in comparison to placebo [80]. Common side effects include hair thinning, nausea, diarrhea, and elevated liver transaminases. There is a significant risk of teratogenicity, and if pregnancy is desired. a period of washout with cholestyramine should be performed. Teriflunomide is not commonly prescribed in the pediatric population. TERIKIDS, a randomized, double-blind, placebo-controlled trial, is currently ongoing, evaluating efficacy and safety of teriflunomide in pediatric MS [79].

Natalizumab is a humanized monoclonal antibody that has been shown to decrease clinical relapse by 68% and decrease the development of new T2 hyperintense lesions by 83% compared to placebo in adults, and small open-label studies in pediatric MS population have shown good efficacy and tolerability [81–84]. In a study of 55 pediatric patients, only three relapses occurred, all within 6 months of initiation of natalizumab [82]. At one year follow up, 83% were free of new T2 lesions on MRI and 74% at two years follow up [82]. No serious adverse effects were reported in this study group. Additionally, a recently published cohort of 20 treatment naïve pediatric MS patients showed that over a treatment period of 24 months with natalizumab, patients had a significant reduction in mean EDSS overall, and NEDA-3 plus status (no evidence of relapse, no disease progression, no new MRI activity, and no cognitive decline) was maintained in 80% of patients, demonstrating natalizumab as a highly effective treatment in pediatric MS [85]. JCV antibodies should be monitored at least every 6 months given the elevated risk of PML in those who are JCV antibody positive, and if seroconversion were to occur, then transitioning to alternative therapy should be considered. Additional risk factors in the setting of positive JCV status include prolonged duration of natalizumab use and prior immunosuppression.

Rituximab is a monoclonal antibody that depletes CD20+ B cells that has been shown in both pediatric and adult MS populations to reduce both clinical relapses and MRI lesions [86,87]. In a case series of 14 pediatric MS patients treated with rituximab, no patients had subsequent relapses [88]. The most common adverse effects include hypogammaglobulinemia and infusion reactions [87,89]. The risk of PML is present with rituximab; however, in pediatric MS a larger population and longer follow up is needed to better understand this risk [89].

Cyclophosphamide, an alkylating agent, has been shown to be effective in reducing the relapse rate in pediatric MS patients with aggressive disease [90]. It is given as a monthly infusion, and affects cytokine expression, in addition to T-cell and B-cell function [80]. While it is effective, there are significant risks of secondary malignancies, infection, and sterility [90]. Additional side effects include nausea, vomiting, alopecia, osteoporosis, and amenorrhea [80].

7. Cognitive Impairment, Fatigue, and Psychiatric Comorbidities

Cognitive function is affected in approximately 30% of pediatric MS patients. Children present with differing deficits than those with adult MS, as children can show greater deficits in vocabulary and language-based cognition [91]. Other commonly reported impairments in those with longer disease duration include attention, processing speed, visual-motor skills, executive functions, and memory [92]. Cohorts of pediatric MS patients who have undergone neuropsychology evaluation have found a strong association between cognitive impairment and EDSS score, number of relapses, and disease duration [93]. Studies have looked at cognitive functioning at the time of diagnosis and in follow up. One recent study compared initial neuropsychological evaluations in 19 patients who were either treatment naïve or on solely interferon beta, all of which had follow up assessments performed. Six patients were escalated to a higher efficacy treatment (three to natalizumab and three fingolimod), and the remainder did not require escalation of treatment (10 on interferon beta-1a, two on glatiramer acetate, and one on dimethyl fumarate). While cognitive impairment was seen early in the disease at initial evaluation, those patients who did not have an escalation of treatment had a higher degree of impairment at time of follow up in comparison to those who had an escalation of therapy [94]. Studies additionally have shown that those with pediatric MS are at a higher risk of cognitive disability than adult MS patients [95,96]. Cognitive impairment is more significant in the pediatric MS population, and findings show that those who have been escalated to a higher efficacy treatment to have a lower degree of cognitive impairment; thus, this argues towards an induction or "step-down" treatment approach to help protect from development or further cognitive decline, although larger studies are warranted to confirm this hypothesis.

There are additional features of pediatric MS that can impact everyday functioning. Fatigue is a common complaint in the MS population and can significantly affect daily functioning and can also be a contributing factor in cognitive functioning. In one study comparing pediatric MS patients with healthy controls, there was no significant difference between the two groups in regard to self-reported fatigue, although an additional study reported that at least half of pediatric MS patients report at least mild fatigue [97,98]. Importantly in this study, self- and parent-reported fatigue were associated with higher scores on the Children's Depression Inventory [97]. Additional studies have shown signs of depression are higher in the pediatric MS population [99,100]. In combination, depression or anxiety disorders are present in approximately half of pediatric MS patients. The most commonly reported psychiatric diagnoses are anxiety disorders, attention deficit hyperactivity disorder, and mood disorders [101]. When looking at overall quality of life, one study reported that approximately half of pediatric MS patients reported difficulties in school and emotional functioning [99]. Additional studies have shown that in addition to fatigue and depression, increased EDSS can contribute to decrease in health-related quality of life [102].

8. Clinical Outcomes

Despite elevated relapse rates, the pediatric population tends to have a complete recovery from relapse within 12 months with little accrual of disability during childhood years [36]. Generally, as children do not accumulate disability, they will not develop secondary progressive MS in childhood years, and it generally will take the pediatric MS population approximately 10 years longer than the adult MS population to convert to secondary progression [28,103]. Despite this, the time of progression from mild to severe disability is the same in adults and children [28]. Given this, those with pediatric MS will reach disability milestones at a younger age than those with adult-onset MS [30,103,104]. An increased risk of disability in pediatric MS was associated with a progressive course at onset and an increased number of relapses in the first five years, while a reduced risk was present in those that had complete remission from the initial event [103]. These findings further support the importance of early recognition and treatment in pediatric MS.

Patients with pediatric MS have a smaller brain volume than expected for their age [105], and this carries into adulthood. In comparing the adult brain volume of pediatric MS patients with age-matched adult MS patients, those with the pediatric-onset disease have reduced brain and deep grey matter volume, particularly thalamic volume [106].

9. Conclusions

Pediatric MS is a rare disorder, but the long-term clinical implications in those who are diagnosed lead to significant cognitive and physical disability in adulthood, even with current first-line treatments. The ultimate aim of the treatment of pediatric MS is to reach a state of NEDA. More recently, the goals have been aimed towards NEDA-4, which is a state of no clinical relapse, no disease progression, no new MRI activity, no cognitive decline, and no evidence of brain atrophy present [107,108]. Given the elevated annualized relapse rate, increased rate of cognitive disability, and younger age at reaching disability milestones in pediatric MS, to achieve NEDA-4, the treatment paradigm may need to shift towards that of treatment with higher efficacy medications.

Author Contributions: K.S.F. designed and wrote the manuscript. F.X.C. reviewed the manuscript. V.M.R. reviewed the manuscript. G.J.H. reviewed the manuscript. All authors have read and agreed to the published version of the manuscript.

Funding: This research received no external funding.

Conflicts of Interest: The authors declare no conflict of interest.

References

1. Boiko, A.; Vorobeychik, G.; Paty, D.; Devonshire, V.; Sadovnick, D.; UBC MS Clinic Neurologists. Early onset multiple sclerosis: A longitudinal study. *Neurology* **2002**, *59*, 1006–1010. [CrossRef] [PubMed]
2. Bigi, S.; Banwell, B. Pediatric multiple sclerosis. *J. Child. Neurol.* **2012**, *27*, 1378–1383. [CrossRef]
3. Tenembaum, S. Multiple sclerosis in childhood and adolescence. *J. Neurol. Sci.* **2011**, *311*, S53–S57. [CrossRef]
4. Gordon-Lipkin, E.; Banwell, B. An update on multiple sclerosis in children: Diagnosis, therapies, and prospects for the future. *Expert Rev. Clin. Immunol.* **2017**, *13*, 975–989. [CrossRef] [PubMed]
5. Waldman, A.; Ghezzi, A.; Bar-Or, A.; Mikaeloff, Y.; Tardieu, M.; Banwell, B. Multiple sclerosis in children: An update on clinical diagnosis, therapeutic strategies, and research. *Lancet Neurol.* **2014**, *13*, 936–948. [CrossRef]
6. Wang, C.X.; Greenberg, B.M. Pediatric Multiple Sclerosis: From Recognition to Practical Clinical Management. *Neurol. Clin.* **2018**, *36*, 135–149. [CrossRef] [PubMed]

7. Huppke, B.; Ellenberger, D.; Rosewich, H.; Friede, T.; Gärtner, J.; Huppke, P. Clinical presentation of pediatric multiple sclerosis before puberty. *Eur. J. Neurol.* **2014**, *21*, 441–446. [CrossRef]
8. Chitnis, T.; Krupp, L.; Yeh, A.; Rubin, J.; Kuntz, N.; Strober, J.B.; Chabas, D.; Weinstock-Guttman, B.; Ness, J.; Rodriguez, M.; et al. Pediatric Multiple Sclerosis. *Neurol. Clin.* **2011**, *29*, 481–505. [CrossRef]
9. Belman, A.L.; Krupp, L.B.; Oslen, C.S.; Rose, J.W.; Aaen, G.; Benson, L.; Chitnis, T.; Gorman, M.; Graves, J.; Harris, Y.; et al. Network of Pediatric MS Centers. Characteristics of children and adolescents with multiple sclerosis. *Pediatrics* **2016**, *138*, 1–8. [CrossRef]
10. Langer-Gould, A.; Brara, S.M.; Beaber, B.E.; Koebnick, C. Childhood obesity and risk of pediatric multiple sclerosis and clinically isolated syndrome. *Neurology* **2013**, *80*, 548–552. [CrossRef]
11. Chitnis, T.; Graves, J.; Weinstock-Guttman, B.; Belman, A.; Olsen, C.; Misra, M.; Aaen, G.; Benson, L.; Candee, M.; Gorman, M.; et al. Network of Pediatric MS Centers. Distinct effects of obesity and puberty on risk and age at onset of pediatric MS. *Ann. Clin. Transl.Neurol.* **2016**, *3*, 897–907. [CrossRef] [PubMed]
12. Brenton, J.N.; Woolbright, E.; Briscoe-Abath, C.; Qureshi, A.; Conaway, M.; Goldman, M.D. Body mass index trajectories in pediatric multiple sclerosis. *Dev. Med. Child. Neurol.* **2019**, *61*, 1289–1294. [CrossRef] [PubMed]
13. Huppke, B.; Ellenberger, D.; Hummel, H.; Stark, W.; Robl, M.; Gartner, J.; Huppke, P. Association of Obesity with Multiple Sclerosis Risk and Response to First-line Disease Modifying Drugs in Children. *JAMA Neurol.* **2019**, *76*, 1157–1165. [CrossRef] [PubMed]
14. Mowry, E.M.; Krupp, L.B.; Milazzo, M.; Chabas, D.; Strober, J.B.; Belman, A.L.; McDonald, J.C.; Oksenberg, J.R.; Bacchetti, P.; Waubant, E. Vitamin D status is associated with relapse rate in pediatric-onset multiple sclerosis. *Ann. Neurol.* **2010**, *67*, 618–624. [CrossRef] [PubMed]
15. Banwell, B.; Bar-Or, A.; Arnold, D.L.; Sadovnick, D.; Narayanan, S.; McGowan, M.; O'Mahony, J.; Magalhaes, S.; Hanwell, H.; Vieth, R.; et al. Clinical, environmental, and genetic determinants of multiple sclerosis in children with acute demyelination: A prospective national cohort study. *Lancet Neurol.* **2011**, *10*, 436–445. [CrossRef]
16. Hedström, A.K.; Olsson, T.; Alfredsson, L. Smoking is a major preventable risk factor for multiple sclerosis. *Mult. Scler.* **2016**, *22*, 1021–1026. [CrossRef]
17. Mikaeloff, Y.; Caridade, G.; Tardieu, M.; Suissa, S. Parental smoking at home and the risk of childhood-onset multiple sclerosis in children. *Brain* **2007**, *130*, 2589–2595. [CrossRef]
18. Ahmed, S.I.; Aziz, K.; Gul, A.; Samar, S.S.; Bareeqa, S.B. Risk of Multiple Sclerosis in Epstein–Barr Virus Infection. *Cureus* **2019**. [CrossRef]
19. Ascherio, A.; Munger, K.L.; Lennette, E.T.; Spiegelman, D.; Hernan, M.A.; Olek, M.J.; Hankinson, S.E.; Hunter, D.J. Epstein-Barr virus antibodies and risk of multiple sclerosis: A prospective study. *J. Am. Med. Assoc.* **2001**, *286*, 3083–3088. [CrossRef]
20. Waubant, W.; Ponsonby, A.L.; Pugliatti, M.; Hanwell, H.; Mowry, E.M.; Hintzen, R.Q. Environmental and genetic factors in pediatric inflammatory demyelinating diseases. *Neurology* **2016**, *87*, S20–S27. [CrossRef]
21. Gianfrancesco, M.A.; Stridh, P.; Shao, X.; Rhead, B.; Graves, J.S.; Chitnis, T.; Waldman, A.; Lotze, T.; Schreiner, T.; Belman, A.; et al. Genetic risk factors for pediatric-onset multiple sclerosis. *Mult. Scler. J.* **2018**, *24*, 1825–1834. [CrossRef] [PubMed]
22. Boiko, A.N.; Gusev, E.I.; Sudomoina, M.A.; Alekseenkov, A.D.; Kulakova, O.G.; Bikova, O.V.; Maslova, O.I.; Guseva, M.R.; Boiko, S.Y.; Guseva, M.E.; et al. Association and linkage of juvenile MS with HLA-DR2(15) in Russians. *Neurology* **2002**, *58*, 658–660. [CrossRef] [PubMed]
23. van Pelt, E.D.; Mescheriakova, J.Y.; Makhani, N.; Ketelslegers, I.A.; Neuteboom, R.F.; Kundu, S.; Broer, L.; Janssens, C.; Catsman-Berrevoets, C.E.; van Duijn, C.M.; et al. Risk genes associated with pediatric-Onset MS but not with monophasic acquired CNS demyelination. *Neurology* **2013**, *81*, 1996–2001. [CrossRef] [PubMed]
24. Vargas-Lowy, D.; Chitnis, T. Pathogenesis of pediatric multiple sclerosis. *J. Child. Neurol.* **2012**, *27*, 1394–1407. [CrossRef] [PubMed]
25. Mikaeloff, Y.; Suissa, S.; Vallee, L.; Lubetzki, C.; Ponsot, G.; Confavreux, C.; Tardieu, M.; KIDMUS Study Group. First episode of acute CNS inflammatory demyelination in childhood: Prognostic factors for multiple sclerosis and disability. *J. Pediatr.* **2004**, *144*, 246–252. [CrossRef] [PubMed]
26. Gadoth, N. Multiple sclerosis in children. *Brain Dev.* **2003**, *25*, 229–232. [CrossRef]
27. Banwell, B.; Ghezzi, A.; Bar-Or, A.; Mikaeloff, Y.; Tardieu, M. Multiple sclerosis in children: Clinical diagnosis, therapeutic strategies, and future directions. *Lancet Neurol.* **2007**, *6*, 887–902. [CrossRef]

28. Renoux, C.; Vukusic, S.; Mikaeloff, Y.; Edan, G.; Clanet, M.; Dubois, B.; Debouverie, M.; Brochet, B.; Lebrun-Frenay, C.; Pelletier, J.; et al. Natural history of multiple sclerosis with childhood onset. *N. Engl. J. Med.* **2007**, *356*, 2603–2613. [CrossRef]
29. Miller, D.H.; Leary, S.M. Primary-progressive multiple sclerosis. *Lancet Neurol.* **2007**, *6*, 903–912. [CrossRef]
30. Harding, K.E.; Liang, K.; Cossburn, M.D.; Ingram, G.; Hirst, C.L.; Pickersgill, T.P.; Te Water Naude, J.; Wardle, M.; Ben-Shlomo, Y.; Robertson, N.P. Long-term outcome of paediatric-onset multiple sclerosis: A population-based study. *J. Neurol. Neurosurg. Psychiatry* **2013**, *84*, 141–147. [CrossRef]
31. Waldman, A.; Ness, J.; Pohl, D.; Simone, I.L.; Anlar, B.; Pia Amato, M.; Ghezzi, A. Pediatric multiple sclerosis Clinical features and outcome. *Neurology* **2016**, *87*, S74–S81. [CrossRef] [PubMed]
32. Gorman, M.P.; Healy, B.C.; Polgar-Turcsanyi, M.; Chitnis, T. Increased relapse rate in pediatric-onset compared with adult-onset multiple sclerosis. *Arch. Neurol.* **2009**, *66*, 54–59. [CrossRef] [PubMed]
33. Yeh, E.A.; Chitnis, T.; Krupp, L.; Ness, J.; Chabas, D.; Kuntz, N.; Waubant, E. Pediatric multiple sclerosis. *Nat. Rev. Neurol.* **2009**, *5*, 621–631. [CrossRef] [PubMed]
34. Benson, L.A.; Healy, B.C.; Gorman, M.P.; Baruch, N.F.; Gholipour, T.; Musallam, A.; Chitnis, T. Elevated relapse rates in pediatric compared to adult MS persist for at least 6 years. *Mult. Scler. Relat. Disord.* **2014**, *3*, 186–193. [CrossRef] [PubMed]
35. Thompson, A.J.; Banwell, B.L.; Barkhof, F.; Carroll, W.M.; Coetzee, T.; Comi, G.; Correale, J.; Fazekas, F.; Filippi, M.; Freedman, M.S.; et al. Diagnosis of multiple sclerosis: 2017 revisions of the McDonald criteria. *Lancet Neurol.* **2018**, *17*, 162–173. [CrossRef]
36. Narula, S. New Perspectives in Pediatric Neurology-Multiple Sclerosis. *Curr. Probl. Pediatr. Adolesc. Health Care* **2016**, *46*, 62–69. [CrossRef]
37. Tardieu, M.; Banwell, B.; Wolinsky, J.S.; Pohl, D.; Krupp, L. Consensus definitions for pediatric MS and other demyelinating disorders in childhood. *Neurology* **2016**, *87*, S8–S11. [CrossRef]
38. Sadaka, Y.; Verhey, L.H.; Shroff, M.M.; Branson, H.M.; Arnold, D.L.; Narayanan, S.; Sled, J.G.; Bar-Or, A.; Sadovnick, A.D.; McGowan, M.; et al. 2010 McDonald criteria for diagnosing pediatric multiple sclerosis. *Ann. Neurol.* **2012**, *72*, 211–223. [CrossRef]
39. Hacohen, Y.; Brownlee, W.; Mankad, K.; Chong, W.K.K.; Thompson, A.; Lim, M.; Wassmer, E.; Hemingway, C.; Barkhof, F.; Ciccarelli, O. Improved performance of the 2017 McDonald criteria for diagnosis of multiple sclerosis in children in a real-life cohort. *Mult. Scler.* **2018**, 1–9. [CrossRef]
40. Padilha, I.G.; Fonseca, A.P.A.; Pettengill, A.L.M.; Fragoso, D.C.; Pacheco, F.T.; Nunes, R.H.; Maia, A.C.M., Jr.; da Rocha, A.J. Pediatric multiple sclerosis: From clinical basis to imaging spectrum and differential diagnosis. *Pediatric Radiology* **2020**. [CrossRef]
41. Trabatti, C.; Foiadelli, T.; Valentina Sparta, M.; Gagliardone, C.; Rinaldi, B.; Delmonte, M.; Lozza, A.; Savasta, S. Paediatric clinically isolated syndromes: Report of seven cases, differential diagnosis and literature review. *Childs Nerv. Syst.* **2016**, *32*, 69–77. [CrossRef] [PubMed]
42. Iaffaldano, P.; Simone, M.; Lucisano, G.; Ghezzi, A.; Coniglio, G.; Brescia Morra, V.; Salemi, G.; Patti, F.; Lugaresi, A.; Izquierdo, G.; et al. Prognostic indicators in pediatric clinically isolated syndrome. *Ann. Neurol.* **2017**, *81*, 729–739. [CrossRef] [PubMed]
43. Lee, J.Y.; Han, J.; Yang, M.; Oh, S.Y. Population-based Incidence of Pediatric and Adult Optic Neuritis and the Risk of Multiple Sclerosis. *Ophthalmology* **2019**, 1–9. [CrossRef] [PubMed]
44. Absoud, M.; Cummins, C.; Desai, N.; Gika, A.; McSweeney, N.; Munot, P.; Hemingway, C.; Lim, M.; Nischal, K.K.; Wassmer, E. Childhood optic neuritis clinical features and outcome. *Arch. Dis. Child.* **2011**, *96*, 860–862. [CrossRef]
45. Lucchinetti, C.F.; Kiers, L.; O'Duffy, A.; Gomez, M.R.; Cross, S.; Leavitt, J.A.; O'Brien, P.; Rodriguez, M. Risk factors for developing multiple sclerosis after childhood optic neuritis. *Neurology* **1997**, *49*, 1413–1418. [CrossRef]
46. Absoud, M.; Greenberg, B.M.; Lim, M.; Lotze, T.; Thomas, T.; Deiva, K. Pediatric transverse myelitis. *Neurology* **2016**, *87*, S46–S52. [CrossRef]
47. Banwell, B.; Arnold, D.L.; Tillema, J.; Rocca, M.A.; Filippi, M.; Weinstock-Guttman, B.; Zivadinov, R.; Pia Sormani, M. MRI in the evaluation of pediatric multiple sclerosis. *Neurology* **2016**, *87*, S88–S96. [CrossRef]
48. Kelly, J.E.; Mar, S.; D'Angelo, G.; Zhou, G.; Rajderkar, D.; Benzinger, T.L.S. Susceptibility-weighted imaging helps to discriminate pediatric multiple sclerosis from acute disseminated encephalomyelitis. *Pediatr. Neurol.* **2015**, *52*, 36–41. [CrossRef]

49. Narayan, R.; Simpson, A.; Fritsche, K.; Salama, S.; Pardo, S.; Mealy, M.; Paul, F.; Levy, M. MOG antibody disease: A review of MOG antibody seropositive neuromyelitis optica spectrum disorder. *Mult. Scler. Relat. Disord.* **2018**, *25*, 66–72. [CrossRef]
50. Wingerchuk, D.M.; Banwell, B.; Bennett, J.L.; Cabre, P.; Carroll, W.; Chitnis, T.; de Seze, J.; Fujihara, K.; Greenberg, B.; Jacob, A.; et al. International consensus diagnostic criteria for neuromyelitis optica spectrum disorders. *Neurology* **2015**, *85*, 177–189. [CrossRef]
51. Lotze, T.E.; Northrop, J.L.; Hutton, G.J.; Ross, B.; Schiffman, J.S.; Hunter, J.V. Spectrum of pediatric neuromyelitis optica. *Pediatrics* **2008**, *122*. [CrossRef] [PubMed]
52. Galardi, M.M.; Gaudioso, C.; Ahmadi, S.; Evans, E.; Gilbert, L.; Mar, S. Differential Diagnosis of Pediatric Multiple Sclerosis. *Children* **2019**, *6*, 75. [CrossRef] [PubMed]
53. Chitnis, T.; Ness, J.; Krupp, L.; Waubant, E.; Hunt, T.; Olsen, C.S.; Rodriguez, M.; Lotze, T.; Gorman, M.; Benson, L.; et al. Clinical features of neuromyelitis optica in children US Network of Pediatric MS Centers report. *Neurology* **2015**, *86*, 245–252. [CrossRef] [PubMed]
54. Bradshaw, M.J.; Vu, N.; Hunley, T.E.; Chitnis, T. Child Neurology: Neuromyelitis optica spectrum disorders. *Neurology* **2017**, *88*, e10–e13. [CrossRef]
55. Verhey, L.H.; Branson, H.M.; Makhija, M.; Shroff, M.; Banwell, B. Magnetic resonance imaging features of the spinal cord in pediatric multiple sclerosis: A preliminary study. *Neuroradiology* **2010**, *52*, 1153–1162. [CrossRef]
56. Hummel, H.M.; Brück, W.; Dreha-Kulaczewski, S.; Gärtner, J.; Wuerfel, J. Pediatric onset multiple sclerosis: McDonald criteria 2010 and the contribution of spinal cord MRI. *Mult. Scler. J.* **2013**, *19*, 1330–1335. [CrossRef]
57. Waubant, E.; Chabas, D.; Okuda, D.; Glenn, O.; Mowry, E.; Henry, R.G.; Strober, J.B.; Soares, B.; Wintermark, M.; Pelletier, D. Difference in disease burden and activity in pediatric patients on brain magnetic resonance imaging at time of multiple sclerosis onset vs adults. *Arch. Neurol.* **2019**, *66*, 967–971. [CrossRef]
58. Langille, M.M.; Rutatangwa, A.; Francisco, C. Pediatric Multiple Sclerosis: A. Review. *Adv. Pediatr.* **2019**, *66*, 209–229. [CrossRef]
59. Verhey, L.H.; Branson, H.M.; Shroff, M.M.; Callen, D.J.A.; Sled, J.G.; Narayanan, S.; Sadovnick, A.D.; Var-Or, A.; Arnold, D.L.; Marrie, R.A.; et al. MRI parameters for prediction of multiple sclerosis diagnosis in children with acute CNS demyelination: A prospective national cohort study. *Lancet Neurol.* **2011**, *10*, 1065–1073. [CrossRef]
60. Pohl, D.; Rostasy, K.; Reiber, H.; Hanefeld, F. CSF characteristics in early-onset multiple sclerosis. *Neurology* **2004**, *63*, 1966–1967. [CrossRef]
61. Krajnc, N.; Oražem, J.; Rener-Primec, Z.; Kržan, M.J. Multiple sclerosis in pediatric patients in Slovenia. *Mult. Scler. Relat. Disord.* **2018**, *20*, 194–198. [CrossRef] [PubMed]
62. Boesen, M.S.; Born, A.P.; Hylgaard Jensen, P.E.; Sellebjerg, F.; Blinkenberg, M.; Lydolph, M.C.; Jorgensen, M.K.; Rosenberg, L.; Thomassen, J.Q.; Borresen, M.L. Diagnostic Value of Oligoclonal Bands in Children: A Nationwide Population-Based Cohort Study. *Pediatr. Neurol.* **2019**, *97*, 56–63. [CrossRef] [PubMed]
63. Makhani, N.; Lebrun, C.; Siva, A.; Narula, S.; Wassmer, E.; Brassat, D.; Brenton, J.N.; Cabre, P.; Dalliere, C.C.; de Seze, J.; et al. Oligoclonal bands increase the specificity of MRI criteria to predict multiple sclerosis in children with radiologically isolated syndrome. *Mult. Scler. J. Exp. Transl. Clin.* **2019**, *5*, 1–9. [CrossRef] [PubMed]
64. Havrdova, E.; Galetta, S.; Stefoski, D.; Comi, G. Freedom from disease activity in multiple sclerosis. *Neurology* **2010**, *74*, 3–7. [CrossRef] [PubMed]
65. Krupp, L.B.; Vieira, M.C.; Toledano, H.; Peneva, D.; Druyts, E.; Wu, P.; Boulos, F.C. A Review of Available Treatments, Clinical Evidence, and Guidelines for Diagnosis and Treatment of Pediatric Multiple Sclerosis in the United States. *J. Child. Neurol.* **2019**, *34*, 612–620. [CrossRef]
66. Baroncini, D.; Zaffaroni, M.; Moiola, L.; Lorefice, L.; Fenu, G.; Iaffaldano, P.; Simone, M.; Fanelli, F.; Patti, F.; D'Amico, E.; et al. Long-term follow-up of pediatric MS patients starting treatment with injectable first-line agents: A multicentre, Italian, retrospective, observational study. *Mult. Scler. J.* **2019**, *25*, 399–407. [CrossRef]
67. Macaron, G.; Feng, J.; Moodley, M.; Rensel, M. Newer Treatment Approaches in Pediatric-Onset Multiple Sclerosis. *Curr. Treat. Options Neurol.* **2019**, *21*. [CrossRef]
68. Krysko, K.M.; Graves, J.; Rensel, M.; Weinstock-Guttman, B.; Aaen, G.; Benson, L.; Chitnis, T.; Gormna, M.; Goyal, M.; Krupp, L.; et al. Use of newer disease-modifying therapies in pediatric multiple sclerosis in the US. *Neurology* **2018**, *91*, E1778–E1787. [CrossRef]

69. Tenembaum, S.N.; Banwell, B.; Pohl, D.; Krupp, L.B.; Boyko, A.; Meinel, M.; Lehr, L.; Rocak, S.; Verdun di Cantogno, E.; Stam Maraga, M. Subcutaneous interferon beta-1a in pediatric multiple sclerosis: A retrospective study. *J. Child. Neurol.* **2013**, *28*, 849–856. [CrossRef]
70. Banwell, B.; Reder, A.T.; Krupp, L.; Tenembaum, S.; Eraksoy, M.; Alexey, B.; Pohl, D.; Freedman, M.; Schelensky, L.; Antonijevic, I. Safety and tolerability of interferon beta-1b in pediatric multiple sclerosis. *Neurology* **2006**, *66*, 472–476. [CrossRef]
71. Francis, G.; Grumser, Y.; Alteri, E.; Micaleff, A.; O'Brien, F.; Alsop, J.; Moraga, M.; Kaplowitz, N. Hepatic reactions during treatment of multiple sclerosis with interferon-β-1a: Incidence and clinical significance. *Drug Saf.* **2003**, *26*, 815–827. [CrossRef] [PubMed]
72. Pohl, D.; Rostasy, K.; Gärtner, J.; Hanefeld, F. Treatment of early onset multiple sclerosis with subcutaneous interferon beta-1a. *Neurology* **2005**, *64*, 888–890. [CrossRef] [PubMed]
73. Ghezzi, A.; Amato, M.P.; Capobianco, M.; Gallo, P.; Marrosu, G.; Martinelli, V.; Milani, N.; Milanese, C.; Moiola, L.; Patti, F.; et al. Disease-modifying drugs in childhood-juvenile multiple sclerosis: Results of an Italian co-operative study. *Mult. Scler.* **2005**, *11*, 420–424. [CrossRef] [PubMed]
74. Ghezzi, A.; Pia Amato, M.; Annovazzi, P.; Capobianco, M.; Gallo, P.; La Mantia, L.; Marrosu, M.G.; Martinelli, V.; Milani, N.; Moiola, L.; et al. Long-term results of immunomodulatory treatment in children and adolescents with multiple sclerosis: The Italian experience. *Neurol. Sci.* **2009**, *30*, 193–199. [CrossRef]
75. Kornek, B.; Bernert, G.; Balassy, C.; Geldner, J.; Prayer, D.; Feucht, M. Glatiramer acetate treatment in patients with childhood and juvenile onset multiple sclerosis. *Neuropediatrics* **2003**, *34*, 120–126. [CrossRef] [PubMed]
76. Chitnis, T.; Arnold, D.L.; Banwell, B.; Bruck, W.; Ghezzi, A.; Giovannoni, G.; Greenberg, B.; Krupp, L.; Rostasy, K.; Tardieu, M.; et al. Trial of fingolimod versus interferon beta-1a in pediatric multiple sclerosis. *N. Engl. J. Med.* **2018**, *379*, 1017–1027. [CrossRef] [PubMed]
77. Deiva, K.; Huppke, P.; Banwell, B.; Chitnis, T.; Gartner, J.; Krupp, L.; Waubant, E.; Stites, T.; Pearce, G.L.; Merschhemke, M. Consistent control of disease activity with fingolimod versus IFN β-1a in paediatric-onset multiple sclerosis: Further insights from PARADIG MS. *J. Neurol. Neurosurg. Psychiatry* **2020**, *91*, 58–66. [CrossRef]
78. Alroughani, R.; Das, R.; Penner, N.; Pultz, J.; Taylor, C.; Eraly, S. Safety and Efficacy of Delayed-Release Dimethyl Fumarate in Pediatric Patients With Relapsing Multiple Sclerosis (FOCUS). *Pediatr. Neurol.* **2018**, *83*, 19–24. [CrossRef]
79. Waubant, E.; Banwell, B.; Wassmer, E.; Sormani, M.P.; Amato, M.P.; Hintzen, R.; Krupp, L.; Rostasy, K.; Tenembaum, S.; Chitnis, T. Clinical trials of disease-modifying agents in pediatric MS: Opportunities, challenges, and recommendations from the IPMSSG. *Neurology* **2019**, *92*, E2538–E2549. [CrossRef]
80. Brenton, J.N.; Banwell, B.L. Therapeutic Approach to the Management of Pediatric Demyelinating Disease: Multiple Sclerosis and Acute Disseminated Encephalomyelitis. *Neurotherapeutics* **2016**, *13*, 84–95. [CrossRef]
81. Polman, C.H.; Paul, M.D.; Havrdova, E.; Hutchinson, M.; Kappos, L.; Miller, D.; Phillips, T.; Lublin, F.D.; Giovannoni, G.; Wajgt, A.; et al. A randomized, placebo-controlled trial of natalizumab for relapsing multiple sclerosis. *N. Engl. J. Med.* **2006**, *354*, 899–910. [CrossRef] [PubMed]
82. Ghezzi, A.; Pozzilli, C.; Grimaldi, L.M.E.; Moiola, L.; Brescia-Morra, V.; Lugaresi, A.; Lus, G.; Rinaldi, F.; Rocca, M.A.; Trojano, M.; et al. Natalizumab in pediatric multiple sclerosis: Results of a cohort of 55 cases. *Mult. Scler. J.* **2013**, *19*, 1106–1112. [CrossRef] [PubMed]
83. Ghezzi, A.; Pozzilli, C.; Grimaldi, L.M.E.; Brescia Morra, V.; Bortolon, F.; Capra, R.; Filippi, M.; Moiola, L.; Rocca, M.A.; Rottoli, M.; et al. Safety and efficacy of natalizumab in children with multiple sclerosis. *Neurology* **2010**, *75*, 912–917. [CrossRef] [PubMed]
84. Ghezzi, A.; Moiola, L.; Pozzilli, C.; Brescia-Morra, V.; Gallo, P.; Grimaldi, L.M.E.; Filippi, M.; Comi, G.G. Natalizumab in the pediatric MS population: Results of the Italian registry. *BMC Neurol.* **2015**, *15*, 1–6. [CrossRef] [PubMed]
85. Margoni, M.; Rinaldi, F.; Riccardi, A.; Franciotta, S.; Perini, P.; Gallo, P. No evidence of disease activity including cognition (NEDA-3 plus) in naïve pediatric multiple sclerosis patients treated with natalizumab. *J. Neurol.* **2020**, *267*, 100–105. [CrossRef] [PubMed]
86. Hauser, S.L.; Waubant, E.; Arnold, D.L.; Vollmer, T.; Antel, J.; Fox, R.J.; Bar-Or, A.; Panzar, M.; Sarkar, N.; Agarwal, S.; et al. B-cell depletion with rituximab in relapsing-remitting multiple sclerosis. *N Engl. J. Med.* **2008**, *358*, 676–688. [CrossRef]

87. Beres, S.J.; Graves, S.; Waubant, E. Rituximab use in pediatric central demyelinating disease. *Pediatr. Neurol.* **2014**, *51*, 114–118. [CrossRef]
88. Salzer, J.; Lycke, J.; Wickström, R.; Naver, H.; Piehl, F.; Svenningsson, A. Rituximab in paediatric onset multiple sclerosis: A case series. *J. Neurol.* **2016**, *263*, 322–326. [CrossRef]
89. Dale, R.D.; Brilot, F.; Duffy, L.V.; Twilt, M.; Waldman, A.T.; Narula, S.; Muscal, E.; Deiva, K.; Andersen, E.; Eyre, M.R.; et al. Utility and safety of rituximab in pediatric autoimmune and inflammatory CNS disease. *Neurology* **2014**, *83*, 142–150. [CrossRef]
90. Makhani, N.; Gorman, M.P.; Branson, H.M.; Stazzone, L.; Banwell, B.L.; Chitnis, T. Cyclophosphamide therapy in pediatric multiple sclerosis. *Neurology* **2009**, *72*, 2076–2082. [CrossRef]
91. Parrish, J.B.; Farooq, O.; Weinstock-Guttman, B. Cognitive deficits in pediatric-onset multiple sclerosis: What does the future hold? *Neurodegener. Dis. Manag* **2014**, *4*, 137–146. [CrossRef] [PubMed]
92. Ekmekci, O. Pediatric Multiple Sclerosis and Cognition: A Review of Clinical, Neuropsychologic, and Neuroradiologic Features. *Behav. Neurol.* **2017**. [CrossRef] [PubMed]
93. MacAllister, W.; Belman, A.; Milazzo, M.; Weisbrot, D.; Christodoulou, C.; Scherl, W.; Preston, T.; Cianciulli, C.; Krupp, L. Cognitive functioning in children and adolescents with multiple sclerosis. *Neurology* **2005**, *64*, 1422–1425. [CrossRef] [PubMed]
94. Johnen, A.; Elpers, C.; Riepl, E.; Landmeyer, N.C.; Kramer, J.; Polzer, P.; Lohmann, H.; Omran, H.; Wiendl, H.; Gobel, K.; et al. Early effective treatment may protect from cognitive decline in paediatric multiple sclerosis. *Eur. J. Paediatr. Neurol.* **2019**, *23*, 783–791. [CrossRef] [PubMed]
95. Ruano, L.; Branco, M.; Portaccio, E.; Goretti, B.; Niccolai, C.; Patti, F.; Chisari, C.; Gallo, P.; Grossi, P.; Ghezzi, A.; et al. Patients with paediatric-onset multiple sclerosis are at higher risk of cognitive impairment in adulthood: An Italian collaborative study. *Mult. Scler. J.* **2018**, *24*, 1234–1242. [CrossRef] [PubMed]
96. McKay, K.A.; Manouchehrinia, A.; Berrigan, L.; Fisk, J.D.; Olsson, T.; Hillert, J. Long-term Cognitive Outcomes in Patients with Pediatric-Onset vs Adult-Onset Multiple Sclerosis. *JAMA Neurol.* **2019**, *76*, 1028–1034. [CrossRef]
97. Goretti, B.; Portaccio, E.; Ghezzi, A.; Lori, S.; Moiola, L.; Falautano, M.; Viterbo, R.; Patti, F.; Vecchio, R.; Pozzilli, C.; et al. Fatigue and its relationships with cognitive functioning and depression in paediatric multiple sclerosis. *Mult. Scler. J.* **2012**, *18*, 329–334. [CrossRef]
98. MacAllister, W.S.; Christodoulou, C.; Troxell, R.; Milazzo, M.; Block, P.; Preston, T.E.; Bender, H.A.; Belman, A.; Krupp, L.B. Fatigue and quality of life in pediatric multiple sclerosis. *Mult Scler* **2009**, *15*, 1502–1508. [CrossRef]
99. Florea, A.; Maurey, H.; Le Sauter, M.; Bellesme, C.; Sevin, C.; Deiva, K. Fatigue, depression, and quality of life in children with multiple sclerosis: A comparative study with other demyelinating diseases. *Dev. Med. Child. Neurol.* **2020**, *62*, 241–244. [CrossRef]
100. Weisbrot, D.M.; Ettinger, A.B.; Gadow, K.D.; Belman, A.L.; MacAllister, W.S.; Milazzo, M.; Reed, M.L.; Serrano, D.; Krupp, L.B. Psychiatric comorbidity in pediatric patients with demyelinating disorders. *J. Child. Neurol.* **2010**, *25*, 192–202. [CrossRef]
101. Weisbrot, D.; Charvet, L.; Serafin, D.; Milazzo, M.; Preston, T.; Cleary, R.; Moadel, T.; Seibert, M.; Belman, A.; Krupp, L. Psychiatric diagnoses and cognitive impairment in pediatric multiple sclerosis. *Mult. Scler. J.* **2014**, *20*, 588–593. [CrossRef] [PubMed]
102. Storm van's Gravesande, K.; Blaschek, A.; Calabrese, P.; Rostasy, K.; Huppke, P.; Kessler, J.; Kalbe, E.; Mall, V. Fatigue and depression predict health-related quality of life in patients with pediatric-onset multiple sclerosis. *Mult. Scler. Relat. Disord.* **2019**, *36*, 101368. [CrossRef] [PubMed]
103. McKay, K.A.; Hillert, J.; Manouchehrinia, A. Long-term disability progression of pediatric-onset multiple sclerosis. *Neurology* **2019**, *92*, E2764–E2773. [CrossRef] [PubMed]
104. Ghezzi, A.; Amato, M.P. Pediatric multiple sclerosis: Conventional first-line treatment and general management. *Neurology* **2016**, *87*, 2068. [CrossRef]
105. Kerbrat, A.; Aubert-Broche, B.; Fonov, V.; Narayanan, S.; Sled, J.G.; Arnold, D.A.; Banwell, B.; Collins, D.L. Reduced head and brain size for age and disproportionately smaller thalami in child-onset MS. *Neurology* **2012**, *78*, 194–201. [CrossRef]
106. Fenu, G.; Lorefice, L.; Loi, L.; Sechi, V.; Contu, F.; Coghe, G.; Frau, J.; Spinicci, G.; Barracciu, M.A.; Marrosu, M.G.; et al. Adult brain volume in multiple sclerosis: The impact of paediatric onset. *Mult. Scler. Relat. Disord.* **2018**, *21*, 103–107. [CrossRef]

107. Pandit, L. No evidence of disease activity (NEDA) in multiple sclerosis-Shifting the goal posts. *Ann. Indian Acad. Neurol.* **2019**, *22*, 261–263. [CrossRef]
108. Kappos, L.; De Stefano, N.; Freedman, M.; Cree, B.; Radue, E.; Sprenger, T.; Sormani, M.; Smith, T.; Haring, D.; Piani Meier, D.; et al. Inclusion of brain volume loss in a revised measure of 'no evidence of disease activity' (NEDA-4) in relapsing-remitting multiple sclerosis. *Mult. Scler.* **2016**, *22*, 1297–1305. [CrossRef]

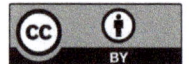

© 2020 by the authors. Licensee MDPI, Basel, Switzerland. This article is an open access article distributed under the terms and conditions of the Creative Commons Attribution (CC BY) license (http://creativecommons.org/licenses/by/4.0/).

MDPI
St. Alban-Anlage 66
4052 Basel
Switzerland
Tel. +41 61 683 77 34
Fax +41 61 302 89 18
www.mdpi.com

Biomedicines Editorial Office
E-mail: biomedicines@mdpi.com
www.mdpi.com/journal/biomedicines

www.ingramcontent.com/pod-product-compliance
Lightning Source LLC
LaVergne TN
LVHW070623100526
838202LV00012B/706